GENERAL OPHTHALMOLOGY

6
Edition

GENERAL
OPHTHALMOLOGY

DANIEL VAUGHAN, MD

*Associate Clinical Professor of
Ophthalmology, University of California
School of Medicine (San Francisco)*

TAYLOR ASBURY, MD

*Professor of Ophthalmology and
Director, Department of Ophthalmology
College of Medicine
University of Cincinnati*

ROBERT COOK, MD

Lange Medical Publications

Los Altos, California

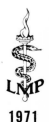

1971

A Concise Medical Library for Practitioner and Student

Current Diagnosis & Treatment 1971 M.A. Krupp, M.J. Chatton, S. Margen, Editors	$11.00
Current Pediatric Diagnosis & Treatment, 1970 C.H. Kempe, H.K. Silver, D. O'Brien, Editors	$11.00
Review of Physiological Chemistry, 13th Edition, 1971 H.A. Harper	$8.00
Review of Medical Physiology, 5th Edition, 1971 W.F. Ganong	$8.50
Review of Medical Microbiology, 9th Edition, 1970 E. Jawetz, J.L. Melnick, E.A. Adelberg	$7.50
Review of Medical Pharmacology, 2nd Edition, 1970 F.H. Meyers, E. Jawetz, A. Goldfien	$8.50
General Urology, 6th Edition, 1969 D.R. Smith	$8.00
General Ophthalmology, 6th Edition, 1971 D. Vaughan, T. Asbury, R. Cook	$8.00
Correlative Neuroanatomy & Functional Neurology, 14th Edition, 1970 J.G. Chusid	$7.50
Principles of Clinical Electrocardiography, 7th Edition, 1970 M.J. Goldman	$7.00
Handbook of Psychiatry, 2nd Edition, 1971 P. Solomon, V.D. Patch, Editors	$7.50
Handbook of Surgery, 4th Edition, 1969 J.L. Wilson, Editor	$6.00
Handbook of Obstetrics & Gynecology, 4th Edition, 1971 R.C. Benson	$6.50
Physician's Handbook, 16th Edition, 1970 M.A. Krupp, N.J. Sweet, E. Jawetz, E.G. Biglieri	$6.00
Handbook of Medical Treatment, 12th Edition, 1970 M.J. Chatton, S. Margen, H. Brainerd, Editors	$6.50
Handbook of Pediatrics, 9th Edition, 1971 H.K. Silver, C.H. Kempe, H.B. Bruyn	$6.50
Handbook of Poisoning: Diagnosis & Treatment, 7th Edition, 1971 R.H. Dreisbach	$6.00

Foreword

In the past 50 years there has been no dearth of English language ophthalmology texts designed for the medical student and general physician. Some have been well received; others have not survived their first editions. The present text, which first appeared in 1958, was an immediate success and has long since won worldwide acceptance. It covers admirably the whole difficult subject of ophthalmology, with its ramifications in the basic sciences, clinical medicine, and surgery. It is recommended by many professors and is the most popular ophthalmology book among medical students.

The format of this useful volume is particularly felicitous since it permits frequent revisions and a reasonable selling price. By virtue of their own wide interests in a variety of ophthalmologic subspecialties, their free use of consultants, and the happy choice of format, the authors have produced an authoritative volume that presents the principles and practices of ophthalmology to the medical profession in a most attractive form.

In view of the increasingly rapid progress being made in the field of ophthalmology and the complexity of the current ophthalmological literature, Drs. Vaughan, Asbury, and Cook are to be congratulated on keeping a useful text so efficiently up to date.

Phillips Thygeson

San Francisco
August, 1971

Preface

This book is an attempt to provide a concise yet reasonably complete, up-to-date review of a difficult specialty for use by medical students, general physicians, pediatricians, internists, and resident physicians in ophthalmology. We hope it will serve these groups as a companion volume to the standard texts as well as a quick reference guide to the management of the more common ocular disorders seen in daily practice.

Very little of what is worthwhile in these pages could have been brought to publication without the generous cooperation and assistance, and in some cases the initiative, of our colleagues. Most especially the authors wish to thank Dr. Phillips Thygeson for his energetic and authoritative participation. Drs. Kenneth Rogers and Hans Thalmann gave invaluable service in their review of the entire manuscript and as consultants on specific problems. Specialized sections were read by Drs. Arthur K. Asbury, Bruce Dahrling II, Chandler Dawson, Hans Gassmann, Michael J. Hogan, Richard S. Kerstine, Heinrich König, Richard O'Connor, Conor O'Malley, Patrick O'Malley, Marvin H. Quickert, Sidney Riegelman, Robert N. Shaffer, William H. Spencer, and Mario Valenton.

Daniel Vaughan
Taylor Asbury
Robert Cook

San Francisco
August, 1971

Table of Contents

1...
Anatomy

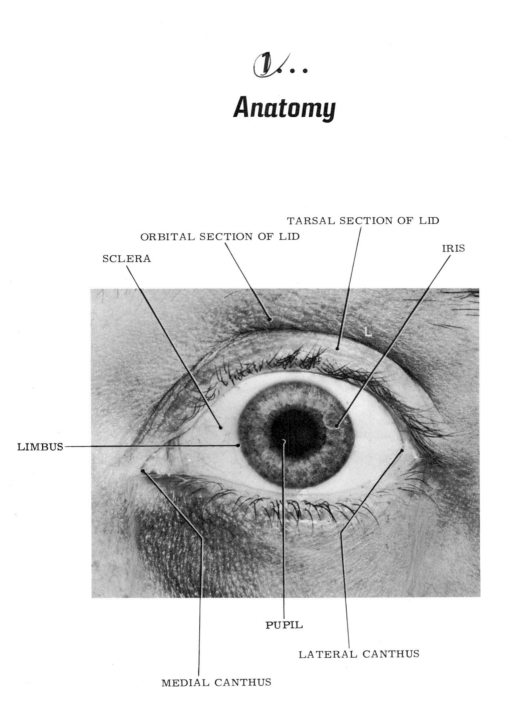

Fig 1-1. **External landmarks of the eye.** (Photo by H. L. Gibson, from Medical Radiography and Photography. Labeling modified slightly.)

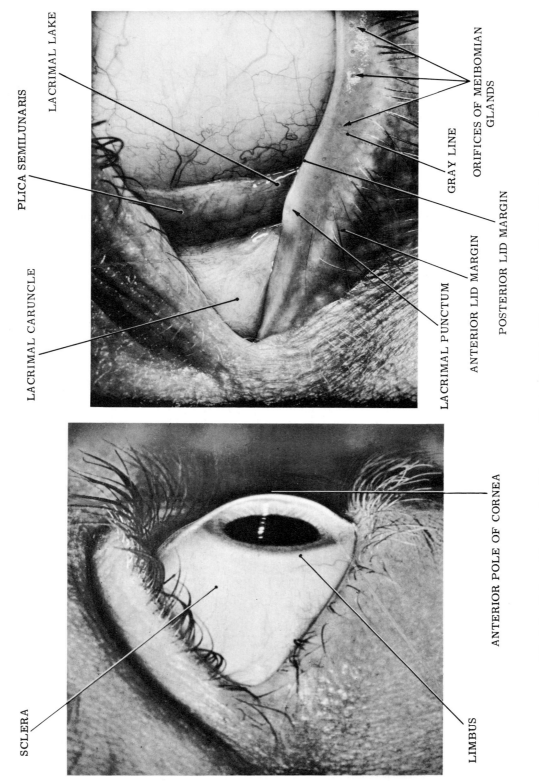

Fig 1-2. External landmarks of the eye. (Photos by H. L. Gibson, from Medical Radiography and Photography. Labeling modified slightly.)

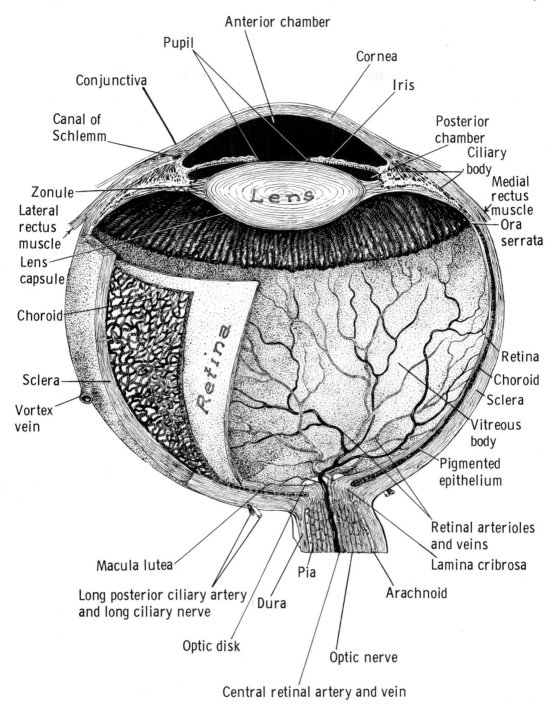

Fig 1-3. Internal structures of the human eye. (Redrawn from an original drawing by Paul Peck and reproduced, with permission, from The Anatomy of the Eye. Courtesy of Lederle Laboratories.)

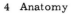

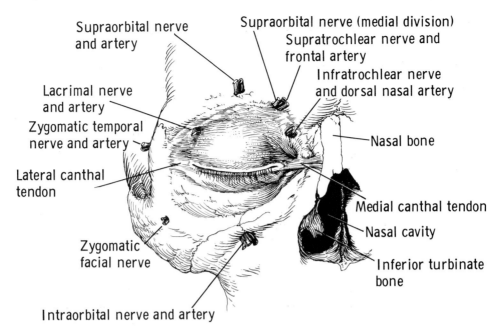

Supraorbital nerve and artery

Supraorbital nerve (medial division)
Supratrochlear nerve and frontal artery

Infratrochlear nerve and dorsal nasal artery

Lacrimal nerve and artery

Zygomatic temporal nerve and artery

Lateral canthal tendon

Nasal bone

Medial canthal tendon

Nasal cavity

Zygomatic facial nerve

Inferior turbinate bone

Intraorbital nerve and artery

Fig 1-4. Vessels and nerves to extraocular structures. (Redrawn and reproduced, with permission, from Wolff: Anatomy of the Eye and Orbit, 4th ed. Blakiston-McGraw, 1954.)

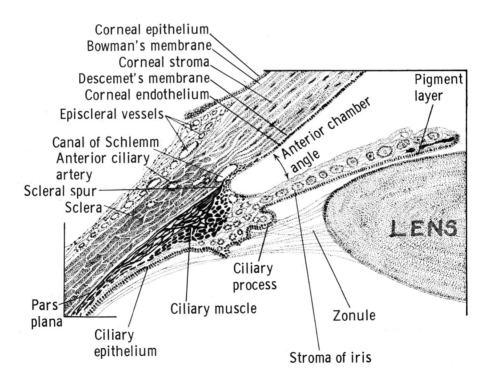

Corneal epithelium
Bowman's membrane
Corneal stroma
Descemet's membrane
Corneal endothelium
Episcleral vessels

Canal of Schlemm
Anterior ciliary artery

Scleral spur
Sclera

Pigment layer

Anterior chamber angle

LENS

Ciliary process

Pars plana

Ciliary muscle

Ciliary epithelium

Zonule

Stroma of iris

Fig 1-5. Anterior chamber angle and surrounding structures. (Redrawn from an original drawing by Paul Peck and reproduced, with permission, from The Anatomy of the Eye. Courtesy of Lederle Laboratories.)

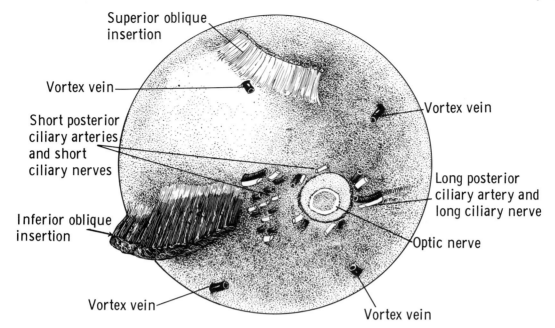

Fig 1-6. **Posterior view of left eye.** (Redrawn and reproduced, with permission, from Wolff: Anatomy of the Eye and Orbit, 4th ed. Blakiston-McGraw, 1954.)

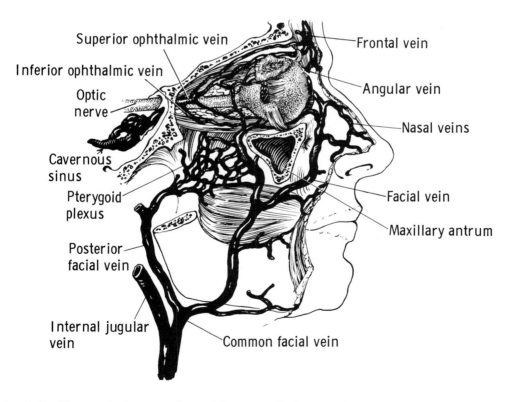

Fig 1-7. **Venous drainage system of the eye.** (Redrawn and reproduced, with permission, from Wolff: Anatomy of the Eye and Orbit, 4th ed. Blakiston-McGraw, 1954.)

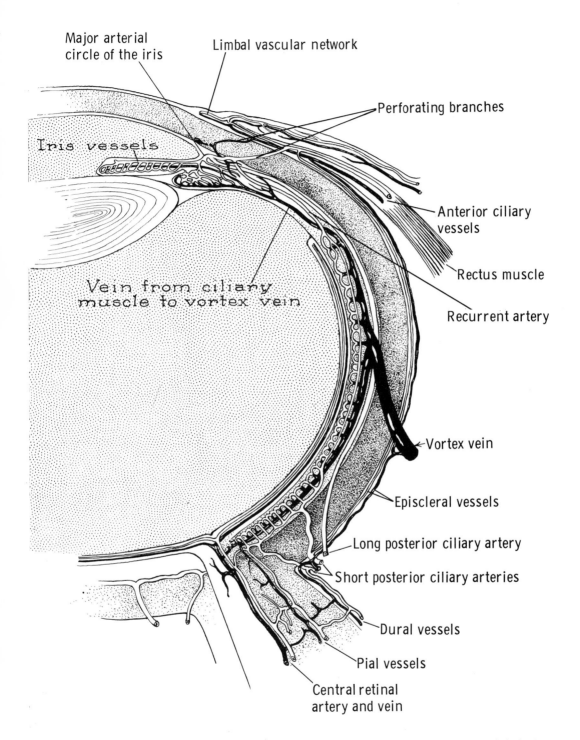

Major arterial
circle of the iris

Limbal vascular network

Perforating branches

Iris vessels

Anterior ciliary
vessels

Rectus muscle

Vein from ciliary
muscle to vortex vein

Recurrent artery

Vortex vein

Episcleral vessels

Long posterior ciliary artery

Short posterior ciliary arteries

Dural vessels

Pial vessels

Central retinal
artery and vein

Fig 1-8. Vascular supply to the eye. All arterial branches originate with the ophthalmic artery. Venous drainage is through the cavernous sinus and the pterygoid plexus. (Redrawn and reproduced, with permission, from Wolff: Anatomy of the Eye and Orbit, 4th ed. Blakiston-McGraw, 1954.)

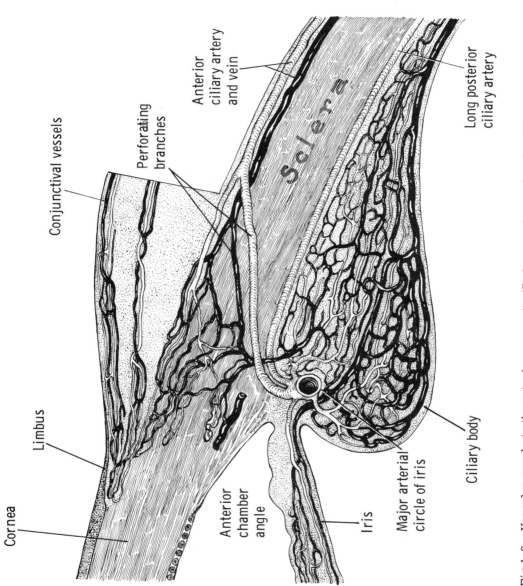

Fig 1-9. Vascular supply to the anterior segment. (Redrawn and reproduced, with permission, from Wolff: Anatomy of the Eye and Orbit, 4th ed. Blakiston-McGraw, 1954.)

2...

Growth, Development, and Senescence

EMBRYOLOGY OF THE EYE
(See Fig 2-1.)

OPTIC VESICLE STAGE

The earliest embryonic stage at which ocular structures can be differentiated from the rest of the fetus is the embryonic plate stage. The site of the eye is indicated by flattened areas on both sides of the anterior end of the neural groove. The neural groove (2.5 mm or 2 week stage) deepens and sinks into the underlying mesoderm, and detaches from the surface ectoderm to form the neural tube from which the CNS develops. Before the anterior end of the neural tube is completely closed, buds of neural ectoderm grow toward the surface ectoderm on either side to form the spherical optic vesicles (4 mm or 3 week stage). These vesicles are connected to the forebrain by the optic stalks. At the 4 mm stage a thickening of the surface ectoderm, the lens plate, begins to form just opposite the ends of the optic vesicles.

OPTIC CUP STAGE

The optic vesicle invaginates to produce the optic cup, so that the original outer wall of the optic vesicle becomes approximated to its inner wall. At the same time the lens plate also invaginates to form first a cup and then a hollow sphere known as the lens vesicle. By the 9 mm (5 week) stage, the lens vesicle separates completely from the surface ectoderm to lie free in the rim of the optic cup.

During the formation of the optic vesicle, the invagination process includes the lower surface of the optic stalk, producing the choroidal fissure. This fissure permits entrance into the optic stalk of the vascular mesoderm which eventually forms the hyaloid system. As invagination becomes complete, the choroidal fissure narrows until it becomes completely closed (13 mm or 6 week stage), leaving one small permanent opening at the anterior end of the optic stalk through which pass the hyaloid artery until the 100 mm (4 month) stage and the central retinal artery and vein thereafter.

At this point the ultimate general structure of the eye has been determined. Further development consists of differentiation into individual structures. In general, differentiation occurs relatively more rapidly in the posterior than in the anterior segment early in gestation and more rapidly in the anterior segment later in gestation.

EMBRYONIC ORIGINS OF
INDIVIDUAL EYE STRUCTURES*

Surface Ectoderm
Lens; corneal epithelium, conjunctiva, lacrimal gland and drainage system; vitreous (mesoderm also contributes to vitreous).

Neural Ectoderm
Vitreous, retina; epithelium of iris, ciliary body, and retina; pupillary muscle sphincter and dilator, optic nerve.

Mesoderm
Sclera; stroma of cornea, conjunctiva, iris, ciliary body, choroid; extraocular muscles, lids (except epithelium and conjunctiva), hyaloid system (gone by birth), sheaths of the optic nerve; connective tissue and blood supply of eye, bony orbit, and vitreous.

---

*Endoderm does not contribute to the formation of the eye.

EMBRYOLOGY OF
SPECIFIC STRUCTURES

Lens

Soon after the lens vesicle lies free in the rim of the optic cup (13 mm or 6 week stage), the cells of its posterior wall elongate, encroach on the empty cavity, and finally fill it in (26 mm or 7 week stage). At about this stage (13 mm or 6 week), a hyaline capsule is secreted by the lens cells. Secondary lens fibers elongate from the equatorial region and grow forward under the subcapsular epithelium, which remains as a single layer of cuboidal epithelial cells, and backward under the lens capsule. These fibers meet to form the lens sutures (upright "Y" anteriorly and inverted "Y" posteriorly), which are complete by the 7th month. (This growth and proliferation of secondary lens fibers continues at a decreasing rate throughout life; the lens therefore continues to enlarge slowly, causing compression and eventually sclerosis of the lens fibers.)

Retina

The outer layer of the optic cup remains as a single layer and becomes the pigmented epithelium of the retina. Pigmentation begins at the 10 mm (5 week) stage. The inner layer undergoes a complicated differentiation into the other 9 layers of the retina. This occurs slowly throughout gestation. By the 7th month the outermost cell layer (consisting of the nuclei of the rods and cones) is present as well as the bipolar, amacrine, and ganglion cells and nerve fibers. The macular region is thicker than the rest of the retina until the 8th month, when macular depression begins to develop. Macular development is not complete until 6 months after birth.

Optic Nerve

The axons of the ganglion cell layer of the retina form the inner nerve fiber layer. The fibers slowly form the optic stalk and then the optic nerve (26 mm or 7 week stage). Mesodermal elements enter from surrounding tissue to form the vascular septa of the nerve. Medullation extends from the brain peripherally down the optic nerve, and at birth has reached the lamina cribrosa. Medullation is completed by the third month of life.

Iris and Ciliary Body

During the third month (50 mm stage) the rim of the optic cup grows forward in front of the lens as a double row of epithelium and lies posterior to mesoderm which becomes the stroma of the iris. These 2 epithelial layers become pigmented in the iris, whereas only the outer layer is pigmented in the ciliary body. Folds appear in the epithelial layers of the ciliary body; mesoderm grows into this fold to form the ciliary processes. By the 5th month (150 mm stage), the sphincter muscle of the pupil is developing from a bud of nonpigmented epithelium derived from the anterior epithelial layer of the iris near the pupillary margin. Soon after the 6th month, the dilator muscle appears in the anterior epithelial layer near the ciliary body.

Choroid

At the 6 mm ($3\frac{1}{2}$ week) stage, a network of capillaries encircles the optic cup and develops into the choroid. By the 13 mm (6 week) stage, the outer neural epithelial layer has secreted Bruch's membrane. By the third month, the intermediate and large venous channels of the choroid are developed, and drain into the vortex veins to exit from the eye.

Vitreous

A. First Stage: (Primary vitreous, 4.5-13 mm or 3-6 week stage.) At about the 4.5 mm stage, fibrils grow in from the inner layer of the optic vesicle to join elements from the lens vesicle which, along with some mesoderm fibrils associated with the hyaloid artery, form the primary vitreous. This stage ends as the lens capsule appears, precluding any further lens participation in vitreous formation. The primary vitreous does not atrophy, and ultimately lies just behind the posterior pole of the lens as the hyaloid canal.

B. Second Stage: (Secondary vitreous, 13-65 mm or 3-10 week stage.) Müller's fibers of the retina become continuous with vitreous fibrils, so that the secondary vitreous is mainly derived from retinal ectoderm. The hyaloid system develops a set of vitreous vessels as well as vessels on the lens capsule surface (tunica vasculosa lentis). The hyaloid system is at its height at 40 mm and then atrophies from posterior to anterior.

C. Third Stage: (Tertiary vitreous, 65 mm or 10 weeks on.) During the third month the marginal bundle of Drualt is forming. This consists of vitreous fibrillar condensations extending from the future ciliary epithelium of the optic cup to the equator of the lens. Condensations then form the suspensory ligament of the lens, which is well developed by the 110 mm or 4 month stage. The hyaloid system atrophies completely during this stage.

Blood Vessels

Long ciliary arteries bud off from the hyaloid at the 16 mm (6 week) stage and anastomose around the optic cup margin with the

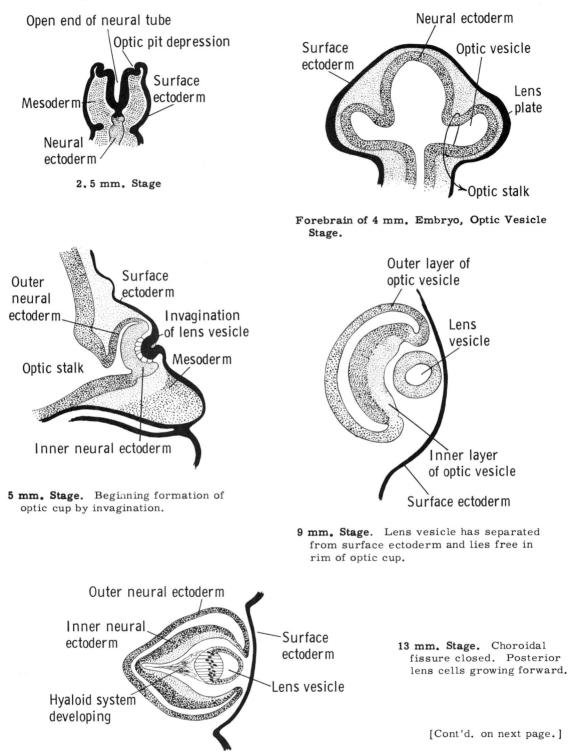

Open end of neural tube
Optic pit depression
Mesoderm
Surface ectoderm
Neural ectoderm

2.5 mm. Stage

Neural ectoderm
Surface ectoderm
Optic vesicle
Lens plate
Optic stalk

Forebrain of 4 mm. Embryo, Optic Vesicle Stage.

Outer neural ectoderm
Surface ectoderm
Invagination of lens vesicle
Optic stalk
Mesoderm
Inner neural ectoderm

5 mm. Stage. Beginning formation of optic cup by invagination.

Outer layer of optic vesicle
Lens vesicle
Inner layer of optic vesicle
Surface ectoderm

9 mm. Stage. Lens vesicle has separated from surface ectoderm and lies free in rim of optic cup.

Outer neural ectoderm
Inner neural ectoderm
Surface ectoderm
Hyaloid system developing
Lens vesicle

13 mm. Stage. Choroidal fissure closed. Posterior lens cells growing forward.

[Cont'd. on next page.]

Fig 2-1. Embryologic development of ocular structures. (Redrawn and reproduced, with permission, from Mann: The Development of the Human Eye, 2nd ed. British Medical Association, 1950.)

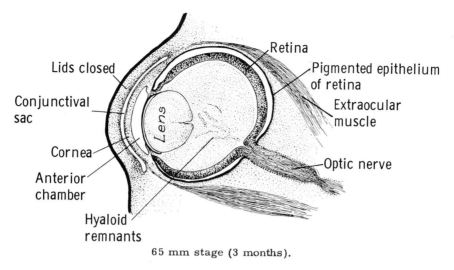

65 mm stage (3 months).

Fig 2-1. Cont'd.

major circle of the iris by the 30 mm (7 week) stage.

The hyaloid system (see Vitreous) atrophies completely by the 8th month. Part of the hyaloid artery within the optic nerve becomes the central retinal artery (100 mm or 4 month stage). Buds begin to grow into the retina and develop the retinal circulation, which reaches the ora serrata at 8 months. The branches of the central retinal vein develop simultaneously.

Cornea

The epithelium is derived from surface ectoderm, whereas the rest of the cornea comes from mesodermal structures. The earliest differentiation is seen about the 12 mm (5 week) stage, when endothelial cells appear. Descemet's membrane is secreted by the flattened endothelial cells by the 75 mm (12 week) stage. The stroma slowly thickens, largely by an increase in the number of elastic fibers, and forms an anterior condensation just under the epithelium which is recognizable at 100 mm (4 months) as Bowman's membrane. A definite corneoscleral junction is present at 4 months.

Anterior Chamber

The anterior chamber of the eye first appears at 20 mm (7 weeks) and remains very shallow until birth. At 65 mm (9-10 weeks), Schlemm's canal appears as a vascular channel at the level of the recess of the angle and gradually assumes a relatively more anterior location as the angle recess develops. The iris, which in the early stages of development is quite anterior, gradually lies relatively more posteriorly as the chamber angle recess develops, most likely because of the difference in rate of growth of the anterior segment structures. The trabecular meshwork develops from the loose vascular mesodermal tissue lying originally at the margin of the optic cup. The aqueous drainage system is ready to function before birth.

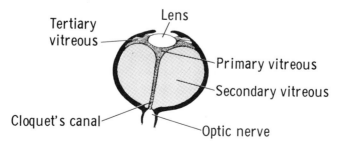

Fig 2-2. **The vitreous.** (Redrawn and reproduced, with permission, from Duke-Elder: Textbook of Ophthalmology, Vol. I. Mosby, 1942.)

Sclera and Extraocular Muscles

The sclera and extraocular muscles form from condensations of mesoderm encircling the optic cup and are first identifiable at the 20 mm (7 week) stage. Development of these structures is well advanced by the 4th month. Tenon's capsule appears about the insertions of the rectus muscles at the 80 mm (12 week) stage and is complete at 5 months.

Lids and Lacrimal Apparatus

The lids develop from mesoderm except for the skin and conjunctiva. The lid buds are first seen at 16 mm (6 weeks) growing in front of the eye, where they meet and fuse at the 37 mm (8 week) stage. During the 5th month, they separate and lashes and meibomian and other lid glands develop. The lacrimal gland (including the accessory glands and the conjunctiva) and drainage system develop from ectoderm. The canaliculi, lacrimal sac, and nasolacrimal duct are developed by burying a solid epithelial cord between the maxillary and nasal processes. This cord canalizes just before birth.

PATHOLOGY OF CONGENITAL OCULAR ABNORMALITIES

Congenital defects of the ocular structures have been described under 2 main headings: (1) developmental anomalies or dysplasias of embryonal origin, and (2) tissue reactions to intrauterine inflammation in the latter months of gestation. Examples of the first type are the colobomas, dermoid tumors, anophthalmos, and microphthalmos. In the second category belong certain lesions of chorioretinitis similar to those seen in postnatal life and some forms of cataract. Heredity plays a major role in many congenital deformities.

In reviewing the embryologic development of the eye, with its complex folds to form the optic vesicles, cornea, lens, and anterior chamber, it is obvious that any failure of regression of primitive vascular tissue at the proper stage, or failure of fusion of embryonic tissue, would lead to a defect of development, eg, of the iris or choroid (coloboma). These developmental defects commonly occur at any point from a segment of the optic nerve itself at the disk, along the choroidal structure and the ciliary body, or in an iris segment. These defects are often seen grossly as a missing wedge of iris tissue, or may be seen with the ophthalmoscope as a large white strip extending radially along the inner surface of the eye toward the periphery.

An eye may be missing (anophthalmos) or smaller than normal (microphthalmos). A small eye is quite often deficient in function.

Congenital lens opacities may occur at any time during the formation of the lens, and the stage at which the opacity began to develop is often measurable by the depth of the opacity. The innermost fetal nucleus of the lens forms early in embryonal life and is surrounded by the embryonal nucleus. Adult addition to the lens is a peripheral subcapsular growth in postnatal life. Certain types of congenital cataracts are familial, whereas others may occur as reactions to intrauterine influences.

Congenital rests, such as dermoids, occur frequently in the ocular structures.

GROWTH AND DEVELOPMENT

Eyeball

At birth the eye is larger in relation to the rest of the body than is the case in children and adults. In relation to its ultimate size (reached at 7-8 years) it is comparatively short, averaging 17.3 mm in anteroposterior length (the only optically significant dimension). This would make the eye quite hyperopic if it were not for the refractive power of the nearly spherical lens.

Cornea

The newborn infant has a relatively large cornea which reaches adult size by the age of 2 years. It is flatter than the adult cornea, and its curvature is greater at the periphery than in the center. (The reverse is true in adults.)

Almost all astigmatic refractive errors are produced by differences in curvature in the various meridians of the cornea. In the infant, the vertical meridian usually has the greatest curvature (producing "physiologic astigmatism"). In adult life the cornea tends to flatten, and the flattening is more marked in the vertical than the horizontal, changing the axis of astigmatism. However, the degree of astigmatism changes very little throughout life.

Lens

At birth the lens is more nearly spherical in shape than later in life, producing a greater refractive power which helps to compensate for the short anteroposterior diameter of the eye. The lens grows throughout life as new fibers are added to the periphery, making it flatter.

The consistency of the lens material changes throughout life. At birth it may be compared with soft plastic; in old age the lens is of a glass-like consistency. This accounts for the greater resistance to change of shape in accommodation as one grows older.

Refractive State

About 80% of children are born hyperopic, 5% myopic, and 15% emmetropic. Hyperopia increases until about 7-8 years of age and then gradually decreases until 19 or 20 years of age. After age 7 or 8, myopia gradually increases until about 25 years. (Hyperopia decreases much less than myopia increases.) There is usually little change in refractive error during the third and fourth decades. Presbyopia occurs in almost all people at age 42-46.

Iris

At birth there is little or no pigment on the anterior surface of the iris; the posterior pigment layer showing through the translucent tissue gives the eyes of most infants a bluish color. As the pigment begins to appear on the anterior surface, the iris assumes its definitive color. If considerable pigment is deposited, the eyes become brown. Less iris stroma pigmentation results in blue, hazel, or green.

Position

During the first 3 months of age, eye movements may be so poorly coordinated (because of the normally slow development of reflexes) that doubt may exist about the straightness of the eyes. Most of the binocular reflexes should be well developed by 6 months of age. A deviating eye after 6 months should be investigated (see Chapter 14).

Nasolacrimal Apparatus

The cord of cells that hollows out to form the nasolacrimal duct between the tear sac and the nose usually becomes patent at about the time of birth. Failure to function may not be noticed for some time because of lack of tear secretion in the first few weeks of life. Failure of tear production by 3 months of age demands attention.

Optic Nerve

The completion of the medullation process around the optic nerve fibers usually occurs within a few weeks after birth.

AGING CHANGES IN THE EYE

Eyelids

Aging of the skin tissues produces gradual loss of elasticity, with wrinkling and drooping folds (dermatochalasia). There may be fatty alteration of the tissues (xanthelasma).

Conjunctivas

Senile plaques and degenerative infiltrates occasionally are found.

Cornea

The cornea may show circular infiltration of degenerative material within the limbus ("arcus senilis"). A flattening of curvature of the vertical meridian tends to produce astigmatism "against the rule."

Lens

The lens continues to grow throughout life, although in senescence the rate of growth decreases. The consistency changes from the soft plastic juvenile lens to an almost "glass-like" character, with increasing difficulty in change of shape with attempted accommodation (presbyopia).

Disturbances of lens metabolism may produce tissue changes with resultant loss of transparency (cataract). Most older people have some degree of cataract.

Vitreous

Increase in "floaters" (muscae volitantes) due to fibrillar condensations, exudates, degenerative deposits (synchysis scintillans, asteroid hyalosis); detachment and liquefaction of vitreous.

Choroid and Retina

Arteriosclerosis of the vessels of the choroid and retina may be followed by degenerative changes in these tissues.

• • •

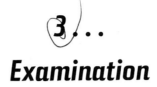

Examination

ROUTINE EYE EXAMINATION

As in other medical examinations, the routine examination of a patient with an eye problem should consist of a careful pertinent history, physical examination, and special examinations as required.

GENERAL INFORMATION

Age

The age of the patient is important not only as an etiologic factor in senile changes but also for the purpose of comparing his abilities with established norms for the age group and in helping to determine what one might expect in the way of performance without discomfort. For example, in cases of amblyopia, occlusive treatment should improve the visual acuity of a child under age 7, whereas the same treatment in a child over 7 would be less effective. In a young child it is not too important to correct the visual acuity to 20/20, as his demands for clear distance visual acuity are much less than is the case with older school children or adults. Age also plays a role in the rate of progression of myopia, which tends to increase during the teens and levels off in the third decade.

Age is also an important factor in visual disability in the prepresbyopic or early presbyopic period, as the symptoms of presbyopia are often quite disconcerting to a person who has had good eyesight all his life. Proper interpretation of these symptoms with explanation to the patient may postpone the need for the first pair of reading glasses or facilitate the adjustment to the first pair.

Occupation

Occupational demands for visual acuity are important in determining the treatment of visual symptoms. Special requirements, such as those involved in working with small objects or at unusual working distances, must be considered in the work-fatigue balance of the visual effort. Even in the same age group, marked differences in symptoms may be noted between 2 individuals with the same refractive error having widely different work demands on their eyes. Small refractive errors producing discomfort in an accountant, for example, may be unnoticed by the housewife.

In presbyopic patients requiring occupational bifocals, special work requirements play an important role in the prescription of bifocal segments.

In industrial injuries a careful record should be made of time and circumstances of injury, previous emergency treatment, and visual acuity.

SYMPTOMS AND SIGNS

Most of the presenting manifestations of eye involvement fall into one of 5 categories: (1) subnormal visual acuity; (2) pain or discomfort; (3) change of appearance of lids, orbit, or eye; (4) diplopia or dizziness; and (5) discharge or increased conjunctival secretion. Some of the important features of each complaint are discussed below.

Subnormal Visual Acuity

A. Duration: Is the patient's visual acuity the same as it has been for most of his life? Was the change in acuity recently noted? Was it found by accidentally covering one eye? Has there been a gradual diminution of acuity over many months or years?

B. Difference in Visual Acuity in the 2 Eyes: Is the patient certain that visual acuity was formerly the same in both eyes? Has he passed an eye examination as part of his driver's test or military physical examination? At that time was the visual acuity the same in both eyes?

C. Disturbances of Vision:

1. Distortion of the normal shapes of objects (metamorphopsia) is most often due to astigmatism or macular lesions.

2. Photophobia is commonly due to corneal inflammation, aphakia, iritis, and ocular albinism. Some drugs may produce increased light discomfort (eg, chloroquine, acetazolamide).

3. Color change (chromatopsia), such as yellow, white, or red vision, may be due to chorioretinal lesions or lenticular changes, or may be associated with systemic disturbances (eg, yellow vision of jaundice) or certain medications (eg, yellow or white vision in digitalis toxicity).

4. Halos, or rings seen when viewing lights or bright objects, are typically thought of as accompanying glaucoma but are also found with other processes causing corneal edema or infiltration as well as with lens changes. Incipient cataract is the most common cause of halos.

5. "Spots" before the eyes, seen as dots or filaments which move with movement of the eye, are almost always due to benign vitreous opacities.

6. Visual field defects may be due to disorders of the cornea, media, retina, optic nerve, or brain.

7. Night blindness, or difficulty seeing in the dark (nyctalopia), may be congenital (retinitis pigmentosa, hereditary optic atrophy) or acquired (vitamin A deficiency, glaucoma, optic atrophy, cataract, retinal degeneration).

8. Momentary loss of vision (amaurosis fugax) may imply impending cerebrovascular accident, spasm of the central retinal artery, or partial occlusion of the internal carotid artery.

Pain or Discomfort

The usual painful symptoms mentioned are headache, "eye-ache," and burning or itching of the eyes or eyelids. Photophobia (sensitivity to light) may cause great discomfort; fatigue symptoms such as "pull," "tired eyes," and "a feeling of pressure" may be described. Acute localized pain intensified by movement of the eye or lid suggests a foreign body or corneal abrasion.

Headache is the most common complaint, aside from poor visual acuity, which causes a patient to present himself to the ophthalmologist for eye examination. If the eye examination discloses no pathologic abnormalities which may account for the symptom, a careful description of the type of headache and a history of its onset, relationship to use of the eyes, duration, and associated symptoms may not only rule out eye disease as a probable cause but may indicate the proper diagnosis.

For example, the headache which occurs upon arising in the morning and disappears soon afterward is seldom caused by eye disorders; a general medical examination is indicated. On the other hand, mild to moderate headaches which occur toward the end of a day of exacting eye work and which are relieved by a few hours of rest or sleep are more probably due to ocular disorders. Any case of severe headache which is becoming worse should suggest an intracranial lesion; visual field tests, ophthalmoscopy and neurologic consultation are indicated.

"Eye-ache" often accompanies extreme fatigue with or without excessive use of the eyes. It is more common in patients with muscle imbalances, but it may be present with inflammatory lesions involving the episclera, iris, or choroid. The eyes may also ache with the increased pressure of glaucoma. In severe acute congestive glaucoma, the pain may be so intense as to radiate throughout the cranium and be accompanied by nausea and vomiting. Ocular pain may also be caused by fever, neuralgia, retrobulbar neuritis, and temporal arteritis. Aching eyes is one of the first symptoms of severe influenza and dengue.

Burning and itching may be a symptom of eyestrain, but the most frequent cause is inflammation of the lids or conjunctivas, eg, chronic blepharitis, conjunctivitis, and allergic reactions of the hay fever type. Itching, in particular, is a symptom of ocular allergy.

A sensation of "pull" is often described in adjusting to a new lens prescription, particularly if the prescription incorporates a change in astigmatic correction. There may also be sensations of pull or actual ache in adjusting to the first pair of bifocals.

Change in Appearance

A. Discoloration: Redness or congestion of the lids, conjunctivas, or scleras may be due to an acute inflammatory reaction to infection, trauma, or allergy or to acute glaucoma. Subconjunctival hemorrhage is sudden in onset and bright red in appearance. (Gross intraocular hemorrhage gives no external ocular sign.) Change of color of the cornea may occur with corneal ulcer or intraocular infection, producing cloudiness of the anterior chamber or an actual level of purulent material in the anterior chamber (hypopyon). Change of color of the "white" of the eye may be noted. Yellow scleras are usually seen with jaundice or antimalarial drug toxicity (eg, quinacrine). Blue scleras are associated with osteogenesis imperfecta. Dark discoloration may follow prolonged local or systemic use of silver compounds (rare), or may be due to scleral thinning and degeneration.

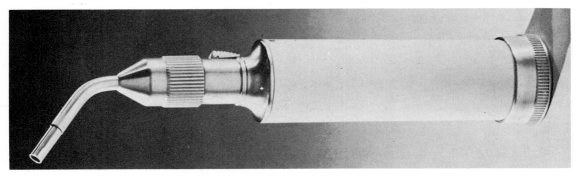

Fig 3-1. Bausch and Lomb metal transilluminator with battery handle.

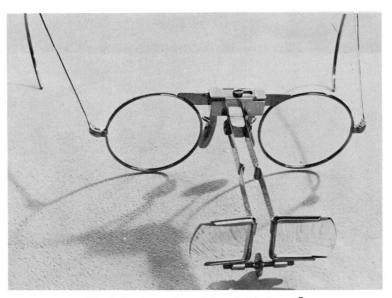

Fig 3-2. Bausch and Lomb Duoloupe®.

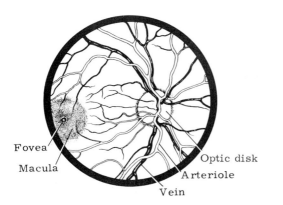

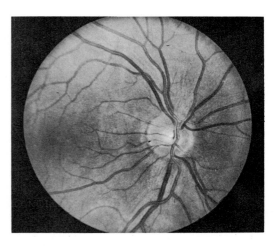

Fig 3-3. The normal fundus. Diagram at left shows landmarks of the photograph at right. (Photo by Diane Beeston.)

B. Swelling: One or both lids may be swollen. Swelling of one lid suggests a local abscess; bilateral swelling indicates a more generalized reaction such as blepharitis, allergy, myxedema, or malignant exophthalmos.

C. Mass: An orbital mass may occur, causing displacement of the globe.

D. Displacement: The eyes may be displaced forward or in other directions. There may be a change of position of the lids, either drooping (ptosis) or retracted (elevated).

Diplopia and Vertigo

It is difficult to differentiate diplopia and vertigo without a careful history. Both may be described by the patient as "dizziness." If double vision is described, it is important to know the time of onset, whether it is constant or intermittent, whether it occurs in certain positions of gaze or at certain distances, and whether the 2 objects seen are horizontal or vertical. Monocular diplopia occurs in lenticular changes, macular lesions, malingering, or hysteria.

Vertigo or light-headedness is often (but seldom justifiably) ascribed to eye disorders, since the patient frequently notes that during this time it is difficult to focus on any object or that "things seem to go around." The attacks are frequently associated with sudden changes in posture, such as arising suddenly from a lying or seated position, or sudden changes in the position of the head or neck muscles.

Discharge (Exudate or Epiphora)

It is important to know the type and amount of discharge, when it occurs, and whether chronic crusting or "granulation" of the lid margins is associated. If the discharge is watery and not associated with redness or pain, it is usually due to epiphora from an excessive formation of tears or a deficiency in the drainage system. The patency of the drainage system may be examined by irrigating the canaliculi and nasolacrimal ducts. If the discharge is watery but accompanied by photophobia or burning, viral conjunctivitis or keratoconjunctivitis may be present. A purulent discharge usually indicates a bacterial infection. A discharge seen with allergic conditions often contains a large number of eosinophils. Samples of the exudate may be stained with methylene blue, Giemsa's, Gram's, or other stains for microscopic identification of cell types and bacteria. If necessary, further identification of bacteria may be done by culture.

Decreased or Increased Lacrimation

Many systemic disorders are characterized by decreased tearing. Dryness of the eyes is a frequent complaint in elderly patients and also occurs in several of the collagen disorders (eg, Sjögren's syndrome), and in patients taking tranquilizers. Excessive tearing may be due to chemical irritation (eg, smog), allergy, acute inflammatory disease of the eye, or obstruction of the lacrimal drainage system.

PHYSICAL EXAMINATION OF THE EYE BY THE GENERAL PHYSICIAN

VISUAL ACUITY

Visual acuity determination should be part of the routine examination of all patients (not only those who present with eye complaints).

Equipment and Materials

The usual method of testing visual acuity is with one of various types of special charts of test letters. (The Snellen chart is most commonly used.) If possible, the well illuminated chart should be so situated that the patient can be placed 20 feet away (eg, at the end of a hall).

Technic

The patient faces the test chart at a distance of 20 feet. If he normally wears glasses, they should be removed. A clean card or occluder is placed in front of his left eye without pressure on the globe, and he is asked to read as far down the chart as possible with the right eye. If he is able to read the line marked "20/20," this is recorded and the same procedure repeated for the left eye. If the patient can read the large letters at the top of the chart but cannot read down to the 20/20 line, the value which corresponds to the smallest line he can read is recorded. If he is unable to read the large letters at the top of the chart, he should be moved progressively closer to the chart until he can read them; this distance is then recorded as the distance from the chart (in feet) over 200 (x/200). If glasses are normally worn, the test should be repeated and the results recorded as "uncorrected" and "corrected." Corrected visual acuity is far more important than uncorrected visual acuity.

Preschool children or illiterates should be instructed in the "E" game, then tested with the illiterate E chart. In this test the patient is taught to point his finger in the direction the bars of the E point. The average 4-year-old child can cooperate satisfactorily in this test. Charts with test pictures have been devised but are not as accurate.

Interpretation of Findings
A corrected visual acuity of less than 20/20 is abnormal.

EXTERNAL OCULAR STRUCTURES

Inspection of external ocular structures (lids, conjunctivas, corneas, scleras, and lacrimal apparatus) should include everting the upper eyelids for inspection of the conjunctival surface with the patient looking down. This can be done easily by grasping the lashes of the upper eyelid with one hand, pulling out and down slightly to put the tissue on a stretch, then pressing on the lid with a thin applicator stick at the superior border of the tarsal plate.

Equipment and Materials
The examination is greatly facilitated by use of a well focused light and a magnifying loupe or slit lamp.

Technic
The exposed surfaces are inspected for defects, foreign bodies, inflammation, discharge, epiphora, dryness, clarity, color, or any other abnormality.

With a history of injury in which the coats of the eye may have been lacerated, great care should be taken in opening the lids to avoid pressure upon the eyeball. In the presence of pain and lid spasm, it may be necessary to instill a few drops of sterile anesthetic solution in order to examine the eye. In small children it may even be necessary to give a short-acting, light general anesthetic.

PUPILS

The pupils should be inspected for size, shape, equality, reaction to the stimulation of light, the effect of accommodation, and for the presence or absence of the consensual light response. (Light directed into the pupil of one eye normally constricts the pupils of both eyes.) Examination for reaction to light is best performed in a darkened room with the examiner to the side of the patient. The pupils may be markedly constricted (miotic) due to the ef-fects of bright illumination, CNS syphilis, or narcotic or parasympathomimetic drugs. They may be dilated as a result of dim illumination, myopia, or sympathomimetic drugs. Unequal pupils (anisocoria) may be a normal finding but suggest neurologic disease if one or both pupils do not react well to light. Argyll Robertson pupil is one in which there is a failure of direct and consensual light response but a normal reaction to accommodation. The tonic pupil of Adie's syndrome, which is a common benign condition, must be differentiated from Argyll Robertson pupil.

POSITION OF THE EYES

The size (microphthalmos or enophthalmos?), prominence (exophthalmos?), and position (orbital tumor, strabismus?) of the eyes should be noted.

The eyes should be observed for alignment as well as for movement of the eyes together in all fields of gaze. Any limitation can be further investigated as described in the section on strabismus evaluation in Chapter 14.

OPHTHALMOSCOPY

Examination of the posterior segment of the eye is done with an ophthalmoscope. This examination is more easily accomplished through a dilated pupil, but with practice a satisfactory examination can be made in most cases through an undilated pupil if the media (aqueous, lens, vitreous) are clear. The illumination in the examining room should be decreased during the examination.

The Use of Mydriatics in the Routine Eye Examination
In examining a patient who has impaired vision of unknown cause it is necessary to dilate the pupil to facilitate ophthalmoscopic and slit lamp examination. (For example, most incipient cataracts and retinal lesions cannot be properly studied through an undilated pupil.) However, for the purposes of routine physical examination it is almost always possible to visualize the ocular media and retina adequately without dilating the pupil if the lighting in the examining room is sufficiently subdued and the light in the ophthalmoscope is strong (fresh batteries).

In young patients, the danger of precipitating an attack of glaucoma by the use of mydriatics is negligible. Before instilling mydriatics into the eyes of older people it is a wise precaution to estimate the depth of the anterior chamber by oblique illumination with a flashlight (Fig 15-7). If the anterior chamber is shallow, mydriatics can precipitate acute angle-closure glaucoma (an ophthalmologic emergency).

Many drugs may be used as mydriatics. Phenylephrine (Neo-Synephrine®), 2.5% or 10%, is a satisfactory drug commonly used for this purpose.

Equipment

There are many types of ophthalmoscopes, but all modern instruments designed for direct ophthalmoscopy (hand ophthalmoscopes) have a source of illumination which is projected by means of a mirror or prism as a beam which nearly coincides with the observer's line of sight through the aperture. With the aperture held as close as possible to the observer's eye and as close as practicable to the subject's eye, the details of the inner eye will be in focus if both eyes (examiner's and patient's) are emmetropic. If either eye is ametropic, the instrument is designed so that a graduated series of convex (plus) or concave (minus) lenses may be rotated into the aperture to bring the details into focus.

Technic

The patient is instructed to fix his gaze on a given object, the direction of gaze depending upon the portion of the eye being examined. The right eye is examined first, with the examiner holding the ophthalmoscope in the right hand and sitting or standing at the right side of the patient. When the left eye is examined, the examiner holds the instrument in the left hand and is in a position to the left side of the patient.

As the examiner rotates a +10 to +12 lens into the aperture, directing the beam toward the patient's eye and bringing the instrument close, the magnified details of the anterior segment of the eye (cornea, iris, and lens) will first be visualized. As he gradually reduces the strength of the plus lenses, the focus of observation gradually extends posteriorly through the vitreous until the retinal details come into view. If the accommodation of the emmetropic observer and of the patient's eye is relaxed ("gaze into the distance"), the strength of lens through which retinal details are first clearly seen may be taken as an indication of the refractive error. (This does not account for small amounts of astigmatism, however. With large astigmatic refractive errors, it will be noted that blood vessels in one meridian may be in focus with one strength of lens, but a different strength of lens will be required to bring the vessels in the opposite meridian into view.)

Aphakic eyes (ie, without lenses) are examined with the +10 to +12 lens in the aperture, or with the patient's own corrective lenses in place.

Details of the structure of the disk are examined. The elevation (choking) may be estimated by comparing the strength of lens through which the central vessels are seen to the strength necessary to focus on the surrounding vessels in the same meridian. The depth of a cupping or depression (eg, glaucomatous cupping of the optic disk) may be measured in a similar manner. The macular area is examined for changes, and the periphery may then be examined by having the patient look in the directions to be examined. When the patient looks down, his upper lid will usually have to be elevated to facilitate examination.

Findings

Opacities in the cornea, lens, and vitreous may be observed in this manner. Localized eye diseases can be seen, as well as ocular changes associated with systemic diseases. An estimation may be made of a refractive error, as described.

CONFRONTATION VISUAL FIELD TESTS

Many conditions are associated with loss of side vision. If special instruments for a careful perimetric field study are not available, the simple confrontation test should be performed as a rough test for gross defects.

Equipment and Materials

A simple wand, such as a pencil with a white eraser, a small white bead or the examiner's finger.

Technic

The observer and patient face each other at arm's length. The patient is then told to hold his hand lightly over his left eye and look with his right eye at the left eye of the examiner, who then holds the target as far to the side as possible midway between himself and the patient. The target is then slowly brought into the line of sight, and the patient is instructed to respond as soon as he is able to identify the target. This is repeated at intervals of 30-45° around the 360° periphery. The fullness of the reported field is compared to that of the observer's. The test is then repeated for the other eye.

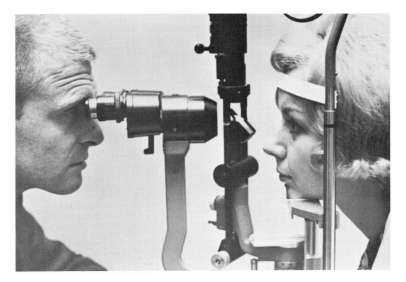

Fig 3-4. Eye examination with Goldmann slit lamp. (Photo by Diane Beeston.)

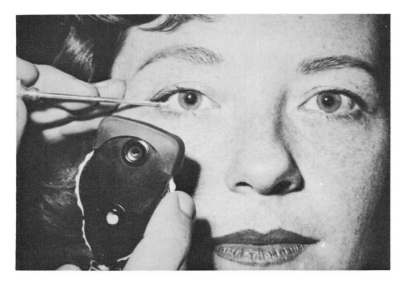

Fig 3-5. Measuring central retinal artery pressure with Bailliart's ophthalmodynamometer. (Photo by Diane Beeston.)

Interpretation of Findings

Gross hemianopsia, bitemporal defects, or large unilateral defects can be detected by confrontation. The test should not be considered a substitute for a careful tangent screen or perimetric visual field test.

SPECIAL EXAMINATIONS BY THE OPHTHALMOLOGIST

SLIT LAMP EXAMINATION
(Biomicroscopy)

The slit lamp consists of a microscope and special light source. It is indicated in any condition of the eyelids or eyeball which can be better diagnosed and treated by having a well illuminated and highly magnified view of the area involved (eg, dendritic keratitis, corneal foreign body, iris tumor, cataract).

Equipment and Materials

A slit lamp is shown in Fig 3-4.

Technic

Both the patient and the examiner are seated. The patient places his chin on a chin rest and his forehead against a frame while the examiner views the eyes through the microscope.

The lids, cornea, anterior chamber, and iris can be easily and quickly studied by moving the focus of both the microscope and the light back and forth. Since the strong light of the slit lamp causes the iris to contract, a mydriatic may be necessary to study lens detail. The Hruby lens (−40 diopters) attachment allows binocular magnified examination of the posterior vitreous and retina. A widely dilated pupil is required.

VISUAL FIELD EXAMINATION

The functions of the retina, optic nerve, and optic pathways are tested by performing peripheral and central visual field tests. Peripheral field examination is most useful in detecting disorders that cause constriction of peripheral vision in one or both eyes (as in retinal detachment, retinitis pigmentosa, or syphilis). Central field examination is useful in detecting disorders causing loss of a portion of the central visual field, particularly in glaucoma, optic neuritis, macular disease, malingering, or hysteria. If intracranial disease is suspected, examination of both the central and peripheral fields is indicated.

Equipment and Materials

Perimeter, tangent screen, light source, and test objects.

Technic

The test must be explained carefully to the patient since it is important to obtain accurate responses.

A. Peripheral Fields: The patient is seated at a perimeter and the left eye covered with a bandage which does not exert pressure on the eyeball. He focuses with his right eye on a spot in the central portion of the perimeter 0.33 meter from his eye. A white test object is brought in from the side at 15° intervals through the 360°, and the patient is asked to signal when he sees the test object. The test object is then passed back along the same meridian from a seeing to a nonseeing area and the patient is asked to signal when it disappears. Both eyes are tested and the visual field plotted on a special chart (see p 294). With the Goldmann perimeter, both the central and peripheral visual fields can be charted in one examination.

B. Central Fields: The central field examination is of greater diagnostic and clinical importance than peripheral field tests. The patient is seated 1-2 meters from a 6 × 8 foot black felt tangent screen, and each eye is covered alternately. The blind spots are outlined, using a 2-3 mm white test object. The entire central visual field is then tested in each eye for visual defects (scotomas). The technic is similar to that employed in the peripheral field examination.

Normal and Abnormal Findings

The peripheral and central visual fields are measured in degrees. Normal values are shown on p 294. The normal blind spot is located at eye level about 13-18° temporal to central fixation and just slightly ($1/3$ disk diameter) inferior to the fixation point. An abnormally large blind spot can be due to papilledema or glaucoma.

Visual field defects must be carefully studied and correlated with other clinical findings to determine the exact site and nature of the lesions causing the defect. These are discussed in Chapter 13.

OPHTHALMODYNAMOMETRY

Ophthalmodynamometry gives an approximate measurement of the relative pressures in the central retinal arteries and is an indirect means of assessing the carotid artery flow on either side. The test consists of exerting pressure on the sclera with a spring plunger while observing with an ophthalmoscope the vessels emerging from the optic disk. The pressure is gradually increased until the central retinal artery begins to pulsate at the point where it or one of its branches leaves the disk. This reading represents the diastolic pressure in the ophthalmic artery on that side, and this pressure is approximately half the brachial blood pressure. The procedure is then repeated in the other eye and the 2 readings recorded directly from the scale in mm Hg.

Examination with Bailliart's ophthalmodynamometer is shown on p 20. The test is performed with the patient in a sitting position with his head supported.

Ophthalmodynamometry is indicated in the neurologic evaluation of patients who complain of "blacking out" (amaurosis fugax) in one eye, spells of weakness on one side of the body, or other symptoms of impending cerebrovascular accident. No significant complications have been reported with its use.

A difference of more than 20% in the diastolic pressures between the 2 eyes suggests, on the side with the lower reading, insufficiency of the carotid arterial system.

SCHIOTZ TONOMETRY

Tonometry is the determination of intraocular pressure by means of an instrument which measures corneal impressibility. It should be part of the general physical examination by internists and general physicians as well as ophthalmologists.

Indications
Tonometer readings should be taken on all patients over the age of 20 having a routine eye examination or general physical examination and on any patient in whom increased intraocular pressure is suspected.

Contraindications and Precautions
Tonometry should not be done on any person with an infected eye, as the infection could be spread to other patients via the tonometer. It is extremely important to clean the tonometer before each use by carefully wiping the footplate with a moist sterile cotton swab and to sterilize the instrument once a day (dry heat).

Corneal abrasions are rare. The only serious infection which can be spread by tonometry is epidemic keratoconjunctivitis, and this can be prevented if the tonometer is cleaned before each use and the physician washes his hands between patients.

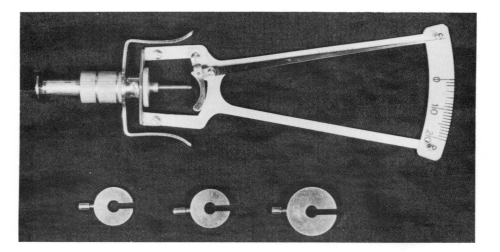

Fig 3-6. Schiotz tonometer and weights. (Photo by Diane Beeston.)

Equipment and Materials

Local anesthetic solution and a tonometer.

Technic

Anesthetic solution is instilled in each eye. The patient lies on his back and is asked to stare at a spot on the ceiling with both eyes or at a finger placed directly in his line of gaze over his head. The tonometer is then placed on the corneal surface of each eye and the scale reading taken from the tonometer. The intraocular tension is determined by referring to a chart that converts the scale reading to mm Hg. If the scale reading is 4 or less, the 7.5 and 10 gm weights are added separately to gain further information concerning the intraocular pressure.

Normal Findings

12 to 20 mm Hg.

Interpretation of Abnormalities

If the tension is 20-25 mm Hg Schiotz or more, further investigation is indicated to determine whether glaucoma is present or not, ie, tonometry is a screening device to select patients for glaucoma testing. Visual field and ophthalmoscopic examinations should be done and the tonometer readings repeated several times at different hours of the day or on different days before the diagnosis of glaucoma can be regarded as established. If the pressure remains high on successive readings and there is a visual field defect or cupping of the optic disks, the diagnosis of glaucoma can be definitely established. In borderline cases, tonography may be helpful in establishing the presence or absence of glaucoma.

Scale readings below 10 are occasionally found without ocular disease but may be pathologic. This can occur following surgery for glaucoma or penetrating injuries and occasionally in severe inflammation.

Accuracy of Method and Sources of Error

Tonometry is accurate for clinical purposes. Sources of error include a poorly calibrated tonometer, improper application of the tonometer to the cornea, or an uncooperative patient who squeezes his lids. (The abnormal pressure of the orbicularis muscles on the eye artificially elevates the tension.)

APPLANATION TONOMETRY

Applanation tonometry measures the force required to flatten rather than indent a small area of the central cornea. It is generally

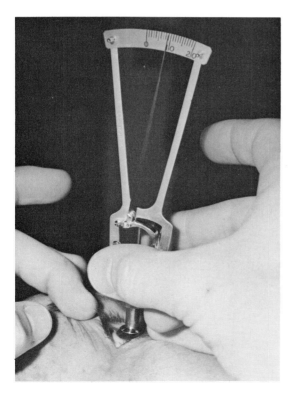

Fig 3-7. Measuring the intraocular pressure with a Schiotz tonometer. (Photo by Diane Beeston.)

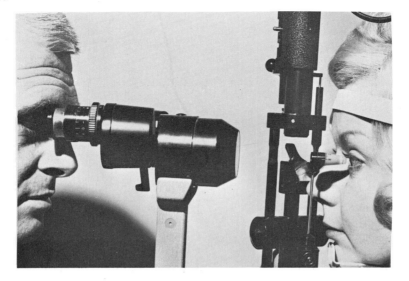

Fig 3-8. Applanation tonometer mounted on a Goldmann slit lamp. (Photo by Diane Beeston.)

more accurate than Schiotz tonometry and is not influenced by scleral rigidity. For example, many myopic eyes have low scleral rigidity which gives deceptively low intraocular pressure readings on the Schiotz tonometer. Borderline cases of glaucoma may be verified by pressure measurement using applanation tonometry. The true nature of some cases of low tension glaucoma (pseudoglaucoma) may also be ascertained.

GONIOSCOPY

Gonioscopy consists of direct visualization of the junction of the iris and cornea (anterior chamber angle). It should be performed in all cases of suspected glaucoma. It is also useful to estimate the extent of involvement of tumors of the iris, to look for suspected foreign bodies in the anterior chamber angle, and to search for aberrant blood vessels, which must be avoided if glaucoma or cataract surgery becomes necessary.

Special Equipment and Materials
Local anesthetic solution, a goniolens, a portable hand microscope, and a Barkan focal illuminator.

Technic
The patient is placed on his back. A local anesthetic is instilled into the eye and the patient's head rotated to the side away from the

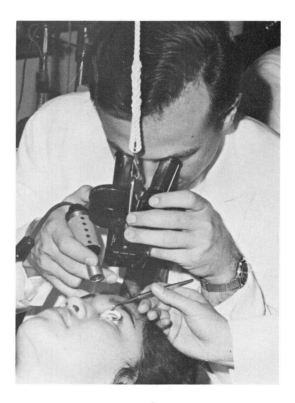

Fig 3-9. Gonioscopy. Examination of the anterior chamber angle with focal illuminator, goniolens, and hand microscope. (Photo by Diane Beeston.)

eye being examined. The goniolens is placed over the cornea and tipped so that sterile saline solution, water, or a contact lens wetting solution can be injected between the cornea and the lens. The patient then looks directly at the ceiling as gentle pressure is exerted upon the goniolens to keep it in place. With the patient fixing his gaze upon a light or spot on the ceiling, the examiner holds the microscope and the illuminating source and views the contents of the anterior chamber, particularly the anterior chamber angle, through a circumference of 360°. Gonioscopy can also be done with the slit lamp utilizing various types of contact lenses.

Normal and Abnormal Findings

Normally (and in most cases of chronic glaucoma) the structures of the anterior chamber angle can be clearly visualized. If the angle is extremely narrow it may be difficult to visualize its inner recesses. In such cases the danger always exists that the angle may close. This would prevent the normal escape of aqueous and cause acute angle-closure glaucoma (an ocular emergency).

AQUEOUS OUTFLOW STUDY
(Tonography)

Tonography permits a rough calculation of the rate of outflow of aqueous from the eye. The test is based upon the change in the intra-ocular pressure which occurs when an electronic tonometer is applied to the eye for 4 minutes.

Equipment and Materials

An electronic tonometer is shown below. This instrument is extremely sensitive and should be used only by qualified experts since precise technic is necessary to avoid inaccurate interpretation.

Techniç

Anesthetic eye drops are instilled and the patient is placed supine and asked to fix his gaze on a spot on the ceiling directly above his head. The tonometer is then allowed to rest on his right cornea for 4 minutes. The intra-ocular pressure is read (in mm Hg) from the electronic scale and recorded every 15 seconds, or an automatic writer can be used to

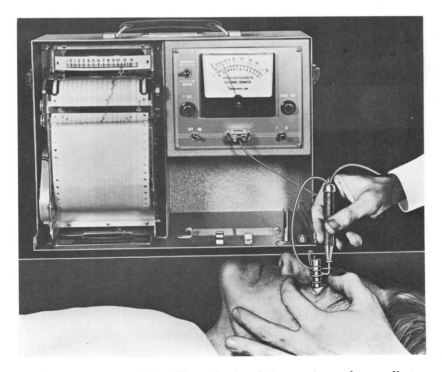

Fig 3-10. Tonography with an electronic tonometer and recording apparatus. (Courtesy of V. Mueller & Co.)

give a continuous record. The procedure is then repeated on the other eye. The difference between the first and the last readings is correlated with the graph to determine the facility of aqueous outflow.

Normal and Abnormal Findings

Normally, the coefficient of outflow factor is above 0.2. If it is below 0.2, the patient is suspected of having glaucoma. If there is no other clinical evidence of glaucoma, the patient should be reexamined periodically in various ways to establish the presence or absence of glaucoma.

SCHIRMER TEST

The Schirmer test is a gross measurement of the quantity of tear fluid in the conjunctival sac. It is indicated in any patient who complains of dry or chronically irritated eyes. These patients are almost always menopausal women with arthritis. The test is performed with standard filter paper cut in strips of about 7 × 50 mm. One end of the filter paper is bent and inserted into the conjunctival sac near the inner angle and left for 5 minutes with the eyes closed. A local anesthetic is not necessary.

The tears from the conjunctival sac should wet at least 10 mm of the filter paper strip in 5 minutes. If less than 10 mm of wetting occurs on repeated examinations, a diagnosis of keratoconjunctivitis sicca (Sjögren's syndrome) should be considered. If the corneal epithelium lacks luster and stains irregularly and the corneal and conjunctival scrapings show desquamated epithelial cells and shreds of mucus, the diagnosis is confirmed.

BACTERIOLOGIC EXAMINATION

Microscopic study is indicated primarily for external ocular infection, and for intraocular infections if a specimen is procurable from the anterior chamber.

Equipment and Materials

Platinum spatula, glass slides; Giemsa's, Gram's, Wright's, and methylene blue stains; binocular microscope and light source, immersion oil. An incubator and culture media are helpful in serious cases but are not necessary for routine conjunctival and lid infections.

Technic

The lid margin, conjunctiva, or cornea is scraped with a platinum spatula and the material smeared on a glass slide and dried. The smear is then stained and examined immediately under the microscope. Most eye organisms can be promptly identified in this manner and the proper treatment instituted without delay. If no organisms are present and there are numerous eosinophils, allergy should be suspected.

CORNEAL STAINING

Corneal staining consists of the instillation of fluorescein or other dyes (merbromin, rose bengal) into the conjunctival sac to outline irregularities of the corneal surface. Staining is indicated in corneal trauma or other corneal disorders (eg, herpes simplex keratitis) when examination with a loupe or slit lamp in the absence of a stain has not been satisfactory.

Precautions

Because the corneal epithelium, the chief barrier to corneal infection, is usually interrupted when corneal staining is indicated, be certain that whatever dye is used (particularly fluorescein) is sterile. Fluorescein is commonly contaminated with Pseudomonas aeruginosa.

Special Equipment and Materials

Fluorescein must be sterile. Fluorescein papers or sterile individual dropper units are safest. Fluorescein solution may be used, but the physician runs the risk of introducing a new organism into the eye.

Technic

The individually wrapped fluorescein paper is wetted with sterile saline or touched to the wet conjunctiva so that a thin film of fluorescein spreads over the corneal surface. Any irregularity in the cornea is stained by the fluorescein and is thus more easily visualized.

Normal and Abnormal Findings

If there is no superficial corneal irregularity, a uniform film of dye covers the cornea. If the corneal surface has been altered, the affected area absorbs more of the dye and will stain a deeper green. It is customary to sketch the staining area on the patient's record for later comparison to show the progress of healing.

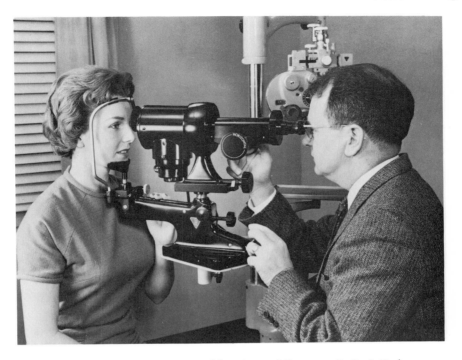

Fig 3-11. Keratometer. (Courtesy of Parsons Optical Co.)

MEASUREMENT OF THE REFRACTIVE POWER OF THE CORNEA

Although originally designed for measuring corneal astigmatism as part of refraction, the keratometer is now used primarily to measure the radii of anterior corneal curvature in millimeters prior to contact lens fitting.

ELECTRORETINOGRAPHY

The electroretinogram (ERG) represents the composite potential generated by the retina from the pigmented epithelium to the bipolar cells. A contact lens electrode is placed on the cornea, and, under conditions of dark and light adaptation, a stroboscopic light is flashed into the eye using various intensities, filters, and time sequences. An initial negative deflection (''a'' wave) is followed by a positive deflection (''b'' wave), a more prolonged wave (''c'' wave), and a final off stimulus (''d'' wave). (Fig 3-12.)

Although of limited clinical value, the electroretinogram depicts the integrity of the

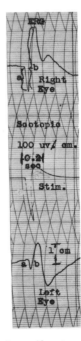

Fig 3-12. Electroretinography. A normal ERG labeled to show a negative a wave, positive b wave, stimulus artifact, and calibration.

neuroepithelium and is, therefore, useful in
determining the presence of various heredo-
degenerative conditions of the retina such as
retinitis pigmentosa, amaurosis congenita
(Leber), and choroideremia. In these conditions, the ERG is either extinguished or is
hardly detectable. This is useful in differentiating secondary degenerative disorders such
as syphilitic retinitis and rubella retinitis,
which give normal or subnormal tracings.
The ERG is also used in primary degeneration
of the macula and color blindness. It has been
of value in establishing the prognosis in central
vein occlusion and as an aid in diagnosis of
late artery occlusion. The composite potential is decreased in certain drug intoxications,
eg, methanol, quinine, chloroquine, and phenothiazines. It is an aid in the differential diagnosis of blindness in infants: In conditions
which involve the neuroepithelium, the potential is absent, whereas in Tay-Sachs disease
it may be normal. Its use has been suggested
in patients with dense cataracts, where observation of the fundus is impossible, and it has
been of diagnostic importance in temporal
arteritis, where a supranormal ERG is obtained in seeing eyes as well as blind eyes.
Other conditions which produce supranormal
ERG's include pheochromocytoma, hypertension, and hyperthyroidism. In multiple sclerosis, abnormal ERG findings often parallel
the optic nerve damage.

THE KLEIN KERATOSCOPE

The Klein keratoscope is used to study the
regularity of the corneal light reflection in the
examination of suspected keratoconus. It is a
round disk with alternating black and white
concentric rings and a hole in the center. The
cornea is examined through the Klein keratoscope much as one would use an ophthalmoscope.

The reflections of the rings are not distorted in a normally curved cornea. Typical
distortions in keratoconus are shown below.

IRRIGATION OF THE LACRIMAL
DRAINAGE SYSTEM

Irrigation of the lacrimal drainage system
is a diagnostic or therapeutic procedure which
consists of injecting fluid through the upper or
lower punctum into the upper or lower canaliculus, whence it will normally flow into the tear
sac and down through the nasolacrimal duct into the nasopharynx. Irrigation is done in patients of all ages who complain of tearing. In
infants who are not cured of dacryocystitis by
the age of 6 months by daily massage of the
tear sac and by antibacterial drops, forceful

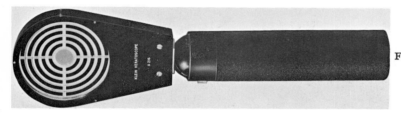

Fig 3-13. Klein keratoscope.

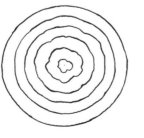

Keratoconus

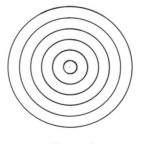

Normal

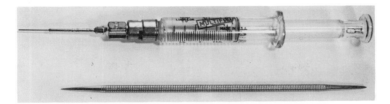

Fig 3-14. Syringe with gold cannula and punctum dilator.

irrigation under general anesthesia should be undertaken in an attempt to open whatever obstruction is present. If this is not successful, as is usually the case, probing of the nasolacrimal duct is indicated while the patient is still anesthetized.

Equipment and Materials

Local anesthetic solution, a punctum dilator, a 2 ml syringe with a lacrimal irrigation cannula, and sterile water or physiologic saline solution. One must be certain that the cannula has a dull tip so that the wall of the canaliculus will not be punctured.

Technic

Adults require one instillation of anesthetic solution in the conjunctival sac. A general anesthetic such as vinyl ether (Vinethene®) is advisable in infants.

The upper and lower puncta in the affected eye are first dilated and the lacrimal needle then passed into the canaliculus. Sterile water or saline solution injected into the canaliculus and tear sac normally passes down the nasolacrimal duct into the nose.

Normal and Abnormal Findings

If the lacrimal drainage system is patent and the patient sits with his head back, he will immediately feel the fluid in his throat; if he sits with his head forward, the fluid will run out of his nose. If the fluid is injected into the lower punctum and comes out of the upper punctum and does not go into the nose or throat, the site of obstruction is in the nasolacrimal duct or the common canaliculus at the entrance to the tear sac. If the fluid will not enter the canaliculus under pressure and does not come out of the opposite punctum or in the throat, the site of obstruction is in the canaliculus.

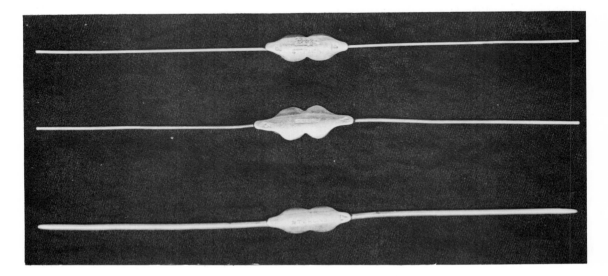

Fig 3-15. Lacrimal probes of various diameters. (Photo by Diane Beeston.)

PROBING OF THE LACRIMAL DRAINAGE SYSTEM

Probing the lacrimal drainage system consists of passing a metal (preferably silver) probe of uniform caliber through the upper or lower punctum and the upper or lower canaliculus into the tear sac and down the nasolacrimal duct into the nose. It is indicated in obstruction of the upper or lower canaliculus or the nasolacrimal duct (particularly in infants) which is not relieved by irrigation.

Probing of the lacrimal drainage system should not be done in patients with acute dacryocystitis. It should always be done gently in order to avoid making a false passage through the canaliculus.

Equipment and Materials

Local anesthetic solution, a punctum dilator, and a flexible silver probe about 15 cm long. The probes vary in diameter and are numbered accordingly from No. 1 (smallest) upward to No. 8.

Technic

In adults, anesthetic drops are instilled into the conjunctival sac and the area of the tear sac is infiltrated with anesthetic. In infants, a general anesthetic such as divinyl ether (Vinethene®) is required.

The upper and lower puncta are dilated and the probe is passed into the tear sac. Lateral pressure on the lid is maintained until the probe is obstructed by the bony nasal wall; the probe is then withdrawn slightly, turned approximately 90°, and passed through the nasolacrimal duct.

Normal and Abnormal Findings

The probe should pass freely and easily through all of the lacrimal passages and should be easily visualized with a nasal speculum in the inferior meatus of the nose. The point of obstruction may be noted when the probe cannot be passed farther without undue force. The most common site of obstruction in patients of all ages is the nasolacrimal duct.

Probing is almost always successful in relieving the obstruction in infants but is seldom successful in adults, for whom dacryocystorhinostomy is usually required.

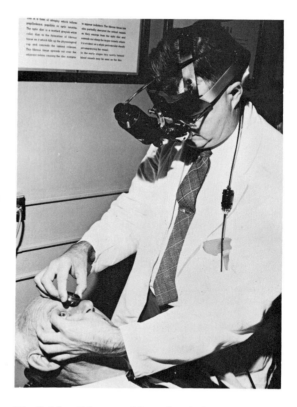

Fig 3-16. **Schepens binocular indirect ophthalmoscope.** Must be used in a darkened room. (Photo by Diane Beeston.)

and a convex lens held before the patient's eye. The observer views an inverted image of the retina which is formed between the lens and the observer's eye.

Binocular indirect ophthalmoscopy can be used to advantage whenever ophthalmoscopic examination is indicated. The advantages of this technic over direct ophthalmoscopy are that the field is larger, the view is stereoscopic, there is more illumination, and the peripheral retina can be more easily visualized. The disadvantages are the inverted image, decreased magnification, more cumbersome equipment, and the fact that the pupil must be dilated with a mydriatic strong enough to overcome the pupillary constrictive effect of the bright light.

BINOCULAR INDIRECT OPHTHALMOSCOPY

Binocular indirect ophthalmoscopy is a means of observing the posterior segment of the eye with a strong source of illumination

LIGHT AND COLOR PERCEPTION

Gross tests of retinal function may be performed by stimulating the macula with light or by merely testing light and color perception.

Retinal function testing is indicated principally in patients with corneal or lens opacities which preclude a view of the retina and for whom surgery is contemplated.

Technic

A. Test of Macular Function: The patient sits with his eyes closed as the examiner massages the eyeball gently with the lighted end of a small flashlight. The patient is then asked to describe what he sees. If the macula is functioning properly, the patient will see a red central area surrounded by the retinal blood vessels. If macular function is impaired, the central area will be dark rather than red and no blood vessels will be seen. One disadvantage of the test is that it is highly subjective and is difficult for some elderly patients to comprehend.

B. Color Perception and Light Projection: A bandage is placed over one eye and the patient's hand placed over the bandage to exclude all light. He is then asked to look straight ahead with the other eye. A light is held in 4 different quadrants and the patient asked to identify the direction from which the light is approaching the eye. A red lens is then held in front of the light, and the patient is asked to differentiate the red from the white light. If he answers all questions correctly, it is reasonably certain that the retina is functioning normally.

Accuracy of Method and Sources of Error

The methods are reasonably accurate as gross tests of retinal function. However, if the opacities of the media are unusually dense, the tests must be cautiously interpreted as it may be that not enough light is reaching the retina to give it proper stimulation.

EXOPHTHALMOMETER

The exophthalmometer is an instrument for determining the degree of anterior projection of the eyes. This is an accurate method of diagnosing and, more particularly, following the course of a patient with exophthalmos.

Equipment and Materials

An exophthalmometer is shown in Fig 3-17.

Technic

The patient stands with his back against the wall and looks into the examiner's eyes. The 2 small concave parts of the exophthalmometer are placed against the lateral orbital margins and the bar reading is noted. This reading represents the distance between the lateral orbital walls. It must be constant for successive examinations on any given patient if the course is to be judged accurately.

The examiner than views the cornea of the patient's right eye in the mirror with the patient fixing his right eye on the examiner's left eye. The cornea is simultaneously lined up in the mirror with a scale that reads directly in millimeters. The left eye is then observed in the same way with the patient fixing his left eye on the examiner's right eye. Both the bar reading and the degree of exophthalmos are recorded in millimeters. (A typical reading: with a bar reading of 96 mm, RE = 17 mm, LE = 17 mm.)

Normal and Abnormal Findings

The normal range of bar readings is 12-20 mm. The reading is usually the same in each eye and indicates the anterior distances from the corneas to the lateral orbital margins. When exophthalmos is diagnosed (bar readings

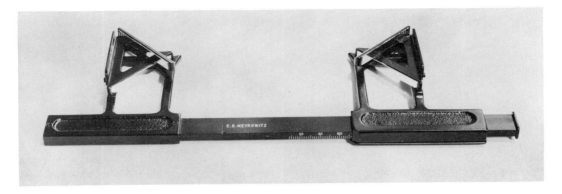

Fig 3-17. Hertel exophthalmometer. (Courtesy of Jenkel-Davidson Optical Co.)

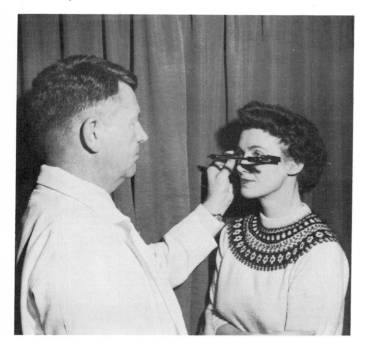

Fig 3-18. Measuring ocular protrusion with the Hertel exophthalmometer.

over 20 mm), one must look for some underlying cause, eg, thyroid disease or orbital
tumor. Periodic exophthalmometer readings
aid greatly thereafter in observing the course
of the disease.

X-RAY EXAMINATION

X-ray examination of the eye and orbit
should be done in unilateral exophthalmos,
optic nerve disease of unknown cause, intraocular or orbital foreign body, or suspected
orbital fractures or tumors.

By utilizing radiopaque markers on the
cornea and taking x-rays at different angles,
intraocular foreign bodies can be accurately
localized. It is often important to determine
if a foreign body is intraocular or intraorbital;
if it is not visible ophthalmoscopically, x-ray
is the best means of localizing the object. Interpretation of x-rays taken about the eye and
orbit in other conditions is beyond the scope of
this book.

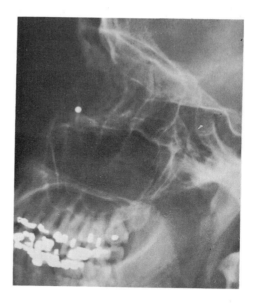

Fig 3-19. Intraocular metallic foreign body as seen by x-ray. (Left lateral view.)

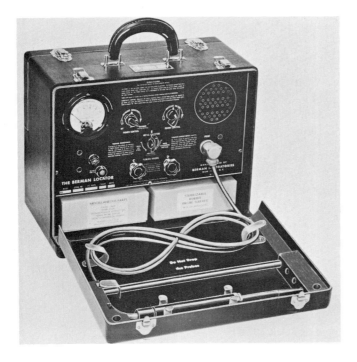

Fig 3-20. The Berman metal locator.

THE BERMAN METAL LOCATOR

The Berman metal locator is an electromagnetic detecting device for localization of metallic foreign bodies. It is used to determine the position of a magnetic metallic foreign body in the eye or orbit which cannot be well localized by x-ray or by ophthalmoscopy. It has a sterilizable tip and is particularly useful during surgical removal of a metallic intraocular foreign body.

COLOR VISION TESTS

Determination of a person's ability to perceive the primary colors and shades thereof is performed as part of the physical examination of military recruits, transportation workers, and others whose occupations require color perception.

Equipment and Materials
The most commonly used polychromatic plates are those of Ishihara, Stilling, and Hardy-Rand-Rittler. The plates are made up of dots of the primary colors printed on a background of similar dots in a confusion of colors.

The dots are set in patterns (eg, numbers) which are confusing to persons with color perception defects.

Technic
Under an illumination of about 30-50 foot candles, the various polychromatic plates are presented to the patient and he is asked to identify them.

Normal and Abnormal Findings
All of the patterns are recognizable to the person with normal color vision. A color-blind person is unable to identify the various figures and forms on the polychromatic plates. The type of color blindness is diagnosed according to the plates used. Red-green blindness is diagnosed in about 8% of the male population and 0.4% of the female population. Blue-yellow or violet blindness is extremely rare.

Accuracy of Method and Sources of Error
An experienced color-defective person may have memorized the plates. If this is suspected, some other test, such as examination with the Eldridge-Green lamp, should be used. Abnormalities of the ocular media, the retina, or the optic nerve can affect the test and should be ruled out if color blindness is discovered.

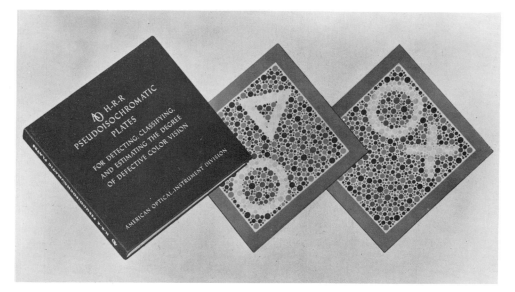

Fig 3-21. H-R-R (Hardy-Rand-Rittler) pseudoisochromatic plates.

TESTS FOR MALINGERING

Utilizing the refractor, place a strong convex lens in front of the good eye and a weak convex lens in front of the "blind" eye. If the patient reads small letters on the test chart, the eye under consideration is not blind. This test can be more subtly done with the refractor than with the trial frame since the strong convex lens is not visible to the patient when the refractor is used.

Place a 10 diopter base-out prism in front of the "blind" eye. If there is sight in the eye, diplopia will result and the eye will be seen to move inward to correct the diplopia.

Place a pair of red-green glasses on the patient, with the red lens in front of the right eye and the green lens in front of the left eye. If the left eye is the suspected eye and the patient can read green letters with this eye, the eye is not blind; the green letters will not be transmitted through the red lens in front of the right eye.

OPHTHALMOSCOPY AFTER INTRAVENOUS FLUORESCEIN INJECTION
(Fluorescein Angiography)

Ophthalmoscopy after fluorescein injection may serve to elucidate some of the subtler vascular aspects of obscure macular lesions, particularly serous macular detachment and lesions simulating it.

Equipment and Materials

Sterile fluorescein solution, 5%; 10 ml syringe with 19 gauge needle; indirect ophthalmoscope with cobalt filter; and, if permanent photographic records are to be made, a Zeiss fundus camera with No. 47A and 15G Kodak Wratten Filters.

Technic

Rapidly inject 10 ml of 5% sterile fluorescein solution in the antecubital vein with the patient in a sitting position and look at the retina with the indirect ophthalmoscope. If

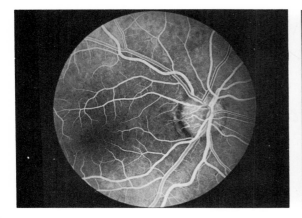

Fig 3-22. Normal retinal vessels filled with fluorescein in arteriovenous phase.
(Courtesy of T. Pettit.)

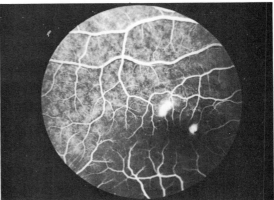

Fig 3-23. Fluorescein leaking into the retina from abnormal vessels in the choroid in a case of serous detachment of the macula.
(Courtesy of T. Pettit.)

permanent records are desired, take a fundus photograph every second for 8 seconds after the fluorescein appears in the retinal vessels, and then every minute for 3 minutes. In some cases, photographs may be desired 30 and 60 minutes later. The photographs may pinpoint the phase of circulation in which abnormal vascular leakage occurs.

Normal and Abnormal Findings

A normal retinal vasculature following fluorescein injection is shown in Fig 3-22. Abnormal leakage of the dye from the choroid into or under the affected retina is a feature of

central serous and hemorrhagic macular degeneration, some diabetic aneurysms, diabetic neovascularization, and aphakic macular edema. If central serous macular detachment (Fig 3-23) persists longer than 6 months, it may be improved by photocoagulating the leakage point very lightly with either laser beam or white (Zeiss zenon-arc) light.

Fluorescein angiography is gradually assuming a more important place as a diagnostic tool. The technic is also useful in demonstrating the vascularity of choroidal and retinal tumors.

•   •   •

Bibliography

Braley, A. E., & others: Stereoscopic Atlas of Slit-lamp Biomicroscopy. Two volumes. Mosby, 1970.

Casellato, L.: Testing visual acuity. Brit J Ophth **55**:44-9, 1971.

Dubois-Poulsen, A.: Critical study of the techniques of peripheral visual tests. Canad J Ophth **1**:24-35, 1966.

Ferrer, O. M.: Serial fluorescein fundus photography of retinal circulation. Am J Ophth **60**:587-91, 1965.

Harrington, D. O.: The Visual Fields. A Textbook and Atlas of Clinical Perimetry, 3rd ed. Mosby, 1971.

Keeney, A. H.: Ocular Examination, Basis and Technique. Mosby, 1970.

Krimsky, E.: Simple eye tests. Postgrad Med **40**:697-703, 1966.

Moses, R. A.: Repeated applanation tonometry. Am J Ophth **66**:89-91, 1968.

Nelson, W. R., & E. Ng: Radiographic interpretation in ophthalmology. Tr Pacific Coast Oto-Ophth Soc **36**:159-73, 1955.

Perkins, E. S.: Tonometry. Proc Roy Soc Med **60**:63-5, 1967.

Pinschmidt, N. W.: Evaluation of the Schirmer tear test. Southern Med J **63**:1256, 1970.

Quickert, M. H.: A fluorescein-anesthetic solution for applanation tonometry. Arch Ophth **77**:734-9, 1967.

Roberts, J.: Visual acuity of children. US Vital Health Statistics **11**:1-35, 1970.

Wallis, N. E.: The electroretinogram (ERG): A review. Brit J Physiol Optics **23**:168-77, 1966.

Zuckerman, J.: Diagnostic Examination of the Eye, 2nd ed. Lippincott, 1964.

4...

Principles of Management of Common Ocular Disorders

It is not necessary to refer every patient with an eye disease to an ophthalmologist for treatment. In general, sties, bacterial conjunctivitis, superficial trauma to the lids, cornea, and conjunctiva, and superficial corneal foreign bodies can be treated just as effectively by the internist or general physician as by the ophthalmologist. On the other hand, more serious eye diseases or symptoms such as the following should be referred as soon as possible for specialized care: iritis, glaucoma, retinal detachment, strabismus, eye pain or blurred vision of undetermined origin, double vision, and corneal trauma or infection.

In the management of acute ocular disorders it is most important to establish a definitive diagnosis before prescribing treatment. The maxim, ''All red eyes are not pink-eye,'' is a useful one; and the physician must be alert for the more serious iritis, keratitis, or glaucoma (see chart on inside front cover). The common practice of prescribing ''shotgun'' topical antibiotic combinations containing corticosteroids is to be discouraged, principally because of the inherent danger of indiscreet steroid treatment.

This chapter is an attempt to summarize for the nonspecialist the basic principles and technics of diagnosis and management of common ocular problems. All of the disorders discussed here are dealt with in greater detail elsewhere in this book.

OFFICE EQUIPMENT AND SUPPLIES

Basic Equipment

A great many specialized instruments have been devised for the investigation of eye disorders. However, most diseases of the eye can be diagnosed with the aid of a few relatively simple instruments:

(1) Hand flashlight.
(2) Binocular loupe.
(3) Ophthalmoscope.
(4) Visual acuity chart (Snellen).

(5) Tonometer. (Tonometry should be done on all patients over 20 years of age having a physical examination.)

Basic Medications

A. Local Anesthetics:
1. Proparacaine (Ophthaine®, Ophthetic®), 0.5%.
2. Benoxinate (Dorsacaine®), 0.4%.

B. Dyes: Sterile fluorescein papers.

C. Mydriatics: Phenylephrine (Neo-Synephrine®), 2.5%, is a satisfactory mydriatic when the examiner wishes to obtain a clearer view of the lens, vitreous, or ocular fundus.

D. Miotics: Pilocarpine, 1%, should be instilled at the end of the examination in all eyes which have been dilated with phenylephrine. This is to prevent possible crowding of the iris into the anterior chamber angle, which can produce an acute angle-closure glaucoma if the anterior chamber angle is narrow.

E. Antibacterial Agents: Sulfisoxazole (Gantrisin®), 4% ophthalmic solution or ointment; or sulfacetamide (Sulamyd®), 10% ophthalmic solution or ointment.

HISTORY AND PHYSICAL EXAMINATION

History

When obtaining a history from a patient who presents with an eye problem, a useful initial question is, ''How do your eyes bother you?'' After he has described his present ocular difficulty, inquire specifically about glasses, blurred vision, pain, red eyes, double vision, trauma to the eyes or head, headaches, and ''eyestrain.'' Information concerning the patient's general health is also relevant, particularly with regard to diabetes mellitus and hypertension. Since many eye diseases have a genetic pattern, the family history should be obtained. The patient's age and occupation are important factors in many ocular difficulties. Patients with glasses should be asked how long it has been since their prescription was changed.

Physical Examination

An adequate gross physical examination of the eye can be performed easily and quickly with a minimum of equipment (see above). By far the most important single examination is visual acuity testing in each eye. This should be done on all patients and the results noted in the clinical record. Visual acuity is tested at a distance of 20 feet using the Snellen chart. It is usually noted with and without glasses. However, corrected visual acuity has greater significance as it is presumably the best possible visual acuity.

Inspection is facilitated by adequate illumination, and should include a mental note of the patient's age, body build, and the structure of his head, face, and eyelids (eg, a patient with Marfan's syndrome is tall and thin and has long fingers). Bell's palsy and acromegaly may also be noted. Observe the eyes grossly for evidence of exophthalmos or enophthalmos.

Using a hand flashlight, examine the lids, conjunctivas, and corneas to rule out inflammation. Observe for icteric scleras (eg, hepatitis), pale conjunctivas (anemia), tumors, and scars. The pupillary light response should also be noted at this time. Gross disorders of the ocular movements can be observed by having the patient hold his head in a fixed position and follow the light of a moving flashlight with his eyes to the right, left, up, down, and inward.

Pressure over the tear sac will produce a mucoid or purulent discharge if significant infection is present.

With the ophthalmoscope one can judge the clarity of the aqueous, lens, and vitreous as well as the appearance of the optic nerve, macula, retina, retinal blood vessels, and choroid. The ophthalmoscopic examination is facilitated by dim illumination in the examining room and a strong, well focused light in the ophthalmoscope. If the ocular fundi cannot be easily visualized through the normal pupil, the pupil should be dilated. **Caution:** Before instilling the mydriatic, examine the anterior chamber by oblique illumination with a hand light (see p 201). If the anterior chamber is shallow (iris and lens quite close to the cornea), dilatation of the pupils should be performed only by an ophthalmologist since in these cases it may precipitate an attack of acute glaucoma.

In any patient over 20 years of age, tonometry should be performed as a screening test for glaucoma. Determining the intraocular tension by finger palpation (tactile tension) of the eyes is not a reliable procedure.

BACTERIOLOGIC AND MICROSCOPIC EXAMINATION

In the management of all serious external eye infections, the first step is to obtain a stained smear of the exudate. In conjunctivitis, for example, the scraping is taken directly from the conjunctival surface, and in corneal ulcer the scraping is taken directly from the advancing border of the lesion. The equipment necessary for the study of stained smears is as follows: platinum spatula, alcohol lamp or Bunsen burner, glass slides, stains (methylene blue, Wright's, Gram's, and Giemsa's), and microscope, light, and imersion oil. Heat the tip of the spatula until it is red-hot, and let it cool. Pull down on the patient's lower lid to expose the conjunctiva, make 3-4 horizontal scrapings, and smear on a clean glass slide. Fix with heat, stain, and dry in air. Prior instillation of local anesthetic drops minimizes discomfort from the scraping.

Cultures and antibiotic sensitivity studies should be done in all cases of corneal ulcer but are necessary in conjunctivitis only in cases which do not respond to treatment within a short time.

Study of the stained smear is far more important than culturing in the average ocular infection, since by this means one can immediately determine whether the causative agent is bacterial, viral, fungal, or allergic, and because in some instances the exact cause can be determined on the spot. This information serves as a guide to treatment. For example, if pneumococci are found, almost any type of antibiotic will be effective, whereas staphylococcal infection will require more specific measures. If there is considerable inflammation of the conjunctiva, if no bacteria are found, and if monocytes are present in increased numbers in the smear, a diagnosis of viral conjunctivitis can be made and the physician knows that the condition will probably last 10-14 days with or without treatment. If many eosinophils are noted in the stained conjunctival smear, the conjunctivitis is probably due to allergy.

TREATMENT OF SPECIFIC
EYE CONDITIONS

LIDS

Marginal Blepharitis

Marginal blepharitis is the most common disorder of the lids. The most important factor in its treatment is cleanliness, which is best maintained by rubbing the scales from the eyelid margins daily with a wet cotton applicator or clean washcloth. Since this disorder is frequently associated with dandruff, a vigorous attempt should be made to keep the scalp clean. An anti-infective ointment should be applied to the lid margins once daily at bedtime until the blepharitis subsides.

Internal Hordeolum

This common condition is essentially a meibomian gland abscess caused by infection with Staphylococcus aureus. The treatment is similar to that of a boil elsewhere on the body. Warm compresses should be applied for 15 minutes 3-4 times daily, followed by the instillation of sulfonamide or antibiotic drops. Incision is required when the hordeolum is pointing. If the hordeolum points toward the conjunctival surface, the incision should be a vertical one on the conjunctival side to avoid cutting across the meibomian glands. If the hordeolum is pointing on the lid side, a horizontal incision is made through the skin as most of the lines of the skin in this region are horizontal.

External Hordeolum (Sty)

Infection of Zeis's or Moll's glands (sty) is smaller and more superficial than internal hordeolum (meibomian gland abscess). Pain and redness are the principal symptoms. Treatment is similar to that outlined for internal hordeolum.

Chalazion

A chalazion is a nontender granulomatous inflammation of a meibomian gland. It should be excised by an ophthalmologist.

Dacryocystitis

A. In Adults: Acute dacryocystitis in adults usually implies that the nasolacrimal duct is completely blocked. The most common secondary invader is Staphylococcus aureus. Systemic administration of penicillin is effective treatment. Local treatment is generally ineffective. Surgical intervention is indicated if the infection does not respond to medical treatment.

B. In Infants: In infantile dacrycystitis the tear sac should be massaged 3-4 times daily. Following the massage, instill sulfonamide or antibiotic drops into the conjunctival sac. If this is not effective in 3-5 weeks, probing of the nasolacrimal duct by an ophthalmologist is indicated.

Tumors

Verrucae and papillomas are common and can usually be easily excised as well by the general physician as by the ophthalmologist as long as they are not near the lid margin. All lid tumors should be examined microscopically to rule out malignancy.

CONJUNCTIVA

Common Types of Conjunctivitis

In any bacterial or viral conjunctivitis, apply warm compresses to the eye for about 15 minutes 3-4 times daily and then instill sulfonamide or antibiotic ointment. Ointments form a film over the cornea, causing blurred vision for 20-30 minutes after instillation, but they are more effective than solutions. Eye drops are prescribed if it is necessary for the patient to use his eyes constantly during the day. The patient is cautioned to wash his hands frequently and not to touch his eyes; this is to prevent spread of the infection to the other eye as well as to his associates and family. Individual washcloths and towels should be used.

In allergic conjunctivitis, use cold compresses for 10-15 minutes 3 times a day, followed by local steroid drops 4 times daily for 2-3 days.

Most cases of bacterial conjunctivitis are self-limited and will disappear in 7-10 days without treatment. Adequate treatment reduces the duration to 1-3 days. If the conjunctivitis does not respond to treatment, the patient should be referred to an ophthalmologist for further care.

CORNEA*

Corneal Foreign Bodies

Note the time and place of the accident and what the patient was doing when it occurred. Visual acuity testing—if possible, before treat-

*All corneal conditions except superficial foreign bodies should be treated by an ophthalmologist.

ment is instituted—is important for legal as well as medical reasons in all cases.

If the patient complains of a foreign body sensation and gives a consistent history, he usually has one even though it may not be readily visible on the initial examination. However, if oblique illumination is used with the hand flashlight, almost all foreign bodies—no matter how small—can be detected. If no corneal foreign bodies are seen and the patient continues to have a foreign body sensation, instill a local anesthetic and turn the upper lid to exclude the possibility of an upper tarsal conjunctival foreign body. If there is no conjunctival foreign body, stain the cornea with fluorescein paper. When the corneal foreign body is found, remove it with a wet cotton applicator or spud under good illumination, using an ocular loupe if one is available. Instill polymyxin-bacitracin (Polysporin®) ointment to prevent contamination with a gram-negative or gram-positive organism. It is not necessary to patch the eye, but it is essential that the patient be observed on the following day to exclude the possibility of secondary infection of the crater. If no infection occurs, the corneal wound will heal by epithelial regeneration in 24-48 hours. If infection occurs the wound area may be weeks or months in healing.

Untreated infection may cause severe corneal ulceration with consequent marked visual loss. Early infection is manifested by a white necrotic area around the foreign body crater and a slight gray exudate. **These patients should be referred immediately to an ophthalmologist**.

Corneal Abrasions

The history should be taken and visual acuity tested before treatment. A patient with a corneal abrasion complains of severe pain, especially with movement of the lid over the cornea. The surface of the cornea may be examined with a light and loupe. If an abrasion is suspected but cannot be seen, stain the cornea with sterile fluorescein. The area of corneal abrasion will have a deeper green stain than the surrounding cornea.

Instill polymyxin-bacitracin (Polysporin®) ophthalmic ointment. Apply a tight pressure bandage to prevent movement of the lid and resultant irritation of the abraded corneal area. Bed rest may be necessary. The patient should be observed on the following day to be certain that the cornea is healing. Corneal abrasions heal in 24-72 hours if a pressure bandage is properly applied. In contrast to corneal foreign body wounds, there is little chance of infection. The main dangers are delayed healing and recurrent corneal erosion due to imperfect healing.

UVEAL TRACT

Any uveal tract disorder may lead to permanent visual impairment. Therefore, the treatment should be supervised by an ophthalmologist.

Acute Anterior Uveitis (Iritis)

This is the most common disorder of the uveal tract and can easily be confused with both conjunctivitis and acute glaucoma. Treatment with local cycloplegics and steroids is usually effective within 10 days. However, recurrences are common.

Posterior Uveitis

This disorder offers more difficulty in diagnosis than anterior uveitis, and the treatment is much less effective.

Neoplasms of the Uveal Tract

Melanoma is a primary tumor of the uveal tract. Its usual location is in the posterior choroid, where it can be seen with the ophthalmoscope. The treatment is enucleation. If a melanoma is situated in the iris, iridectomy is usually successful in removing the entire growth.

VITREOUS

One of the most common of eye complaints is "spots before the eyes." These are usually due to vitreous opacities (visible upon ophthalmoscopic examination). If the spots move about in the field of vision, as is usually the case, the patient may be reassured that they are not serious, only "little spots floating in the jelly-like fluid [vitreous] inside the eye." There is no treatment. With time, the opacities tend to fall inferiorly in the vitreous and thus out of the patient's line of sight. The examiner must bear in mind that vitreous floaters are occasionally the forerunner of retinal detachment.

RETINA

Retinal Detachment

This is an extremely important condition to keep in mind as the diagnosis is fairly simple and surgery is often effective if undertaken soon after the onset. If the patient complains of sudden loss of vision, a shower of floaters, "soot," "lightning flashes," or "a curtain coming up [or down] in front of my eye," he should be examined with the ophthalmoscope through a dilated pupil for the presence of a retinal detachment. This is particularly true if the patient is myopic or has undergone cataract surgery or recent trauma.

A patient with retinal detachment should be hospitalized without delay and prepared for surgery. In transporting a patient with retinal detachment it is preferable for the patient to keep both eyes closed to avoid undue ocular movement. The area of the detachment should be in the dependent position. For example, if the patient has a superior temporal retinal detachment of the right eye he should be supine with the head turned to the right; if the right inferior nasal retina is detached, he should be sitting up with his head turned to the left.

LENS

Cataract
There is no medical treatment for cataract. The only treatment is lens extraction, which is indicated when the opacity decreases visual acuity to the point where the patient can no longer lead a normal life.

Dislocated Lens
This condition may be genetically determined (eg, as one component of Marfan's syndrome) or may be caused by trauma. Visual impairment and secondary glaucoma are the principal indications for lens removal.

OPTIC NERVE

Optic Neuritis
Optic neuritis occurs uncommonly as a unilateral disease in young adults. It may be the first sign of multiple sclerosis. The presenting complaint is sudden loss of central vision. On ophthalmoscopic examination the optic disk may appear normal or may be slightly elevated, with increased vascularity. Systemic steroid treatment has not been effective.

The vision ordinarily returns to normal in a matter of weeks.

Papilledema
Papilledema is most commonly caused by increased intracranial pressure, malignant hypertension, or thrombosis of the central retinal vein. It is manifested as an elevation of the optic disk and dilatation of the veins in the optic disk area. Parapapillary hemorrhages may occur. Papilledema can be visualized easily with the ophthalmoscope through an undilated pupil. Intracranial tumors in the posterior fossa characteristically produce papilledema because of their blocking effect on the CSF. Conversely, frontal lobe tumors usually do not produce papilledema. The rate of onset of papilledema after increased intracranial pressure produced by trauma (eg, subdural hematoma) is extremely variable and is of course related to the magnitude of the process. Moderate degrees of papilledema will not affect visual acuity, but the blind spots will be enlarged as shown by central visual field testing.

Optic Atrophy
In this condition the disk is pale or white. Optic atrophy is usually an end stage process for which no treatment is available. (See fuller discussion on p 142.)

Visual Field Loss in Intracranial Diseases
Some tumors of the CNS which produce gross visual defects in moderately advanced but still treatable stages can be suspected by the general physician by using confrontation field tests. These include pituitary tumors, meningiomas, and posterior fossa tumors. These patients should be referred to a neurosurgeon for treatment.

STRABISMUS

There are 3 prime objectives in the treatment of strabismus: (1) to develop good visual acuity in each eye; (2) to straighten the eyes, for cosmetic purposes; and (3) to develop coordinate function of the 2 eyes (fusion). The best time to initiate nonsurgical treatment of a strabismus patient is by the age of 6 months. If treatment is delayed beyond this time the child will favor the straight eye and suppress the image in the other eye; this results in failure of visual development (amblyopia ex anopsia) in the deviating eye. In such a case patching of the good eye should be instituted without delay.

If the child is under 7 years of age and has an amblyopic eye, the amblyopia can be cured by patching the good eye. At 1 year of age, patching may be successful within 1 week; at 6 years it may take a year to achieve the same result, ie, to equalize the visual acuity in the 2 eyes.

There is no firm rule about the proper time for surgery. Some surgeons operate as early as age 6 months; in some cases there may be valid reasons for deferring strabismus surgery until age 4-5 years. If the visual acuity is equal and the eyes are made reasonably straight with surgery (or with glasses, as in the case of accommodative esotropia), eye exercises (orthoptics) may assist the patient in learning to use his eyes together. This is the seldom achieved ideal result in strabismus therapy. The prognosis is more favorable for strabismus which has its onset at age 2 or 3 than for strabismus which is present at birth; better for divergent than for convergent strabismus; and better for intermittent than for constant strabismus.

GLAUCOMA

Ninety to 95% of glaucoma cases are of the chronic open-angle type. There are no symptoms in the early stages of chronic glaucoma. The best means of detection is by routine tonometry in all persons over the age of 20. Chronic glaucoma comes on insidiously and causes slowly progressive loss of peripheral vision by constant pressure on the optic nerve. The response to miotics is usually good, and surgery is seldom necessary.

Acetazolamide (Diamox®) and other carbonic anhydrase inhibitors, eg, dichlorphenamide (Daranide®, Oratrol®), have been shown to be extremely effective in inhibiting the production of aqueous by the ciliary body. Consequently they are valuable as preoperative adjuncts in the treatment of acute glaucoma and in the management of secondary glaucoma. Because of their side effects (particularly renal calculi), long-term therapy of open-angle glaucoma is not always feasible.

Epinephrine, 0.5-2%, when instilled as drops into the conjunctival sac, also inhibits aqueous production. Epinephrine has been used for many years in the treatment of glaucoma, but has gained much greater popularity in recent years.

It is highly desirable to diagnose glaucoma before significant visual loss has occurred, since visual field loss is not reversible. Next to tonometry, ophthalmoscopy and visual field tests are the most important diagnostic procedures in glaucoma. Gonioscopy and tonography are also helpful in the total evaluation of any glaucoma case.

Approximately 5% of cases are angle-closure glaucoma, which produces pain, injection, and blurred vision. The patient seeks treatment immediately because of the pain. Acute glaucoma is treated surgically. The surgery is preceded by intensive miotic ther-

apy and acetazolamide over a period of hours to lower the pressure in order to minimize complications during surgery. If miotics and carbonic anhydrase inhibitors do not lower the intraocular pressure sufficiently before surgery, glycerine or isosorbide by mouth or intravenous mannitol or urea will nearly always do so within 2 hours.

TRAUMA

Chemical Conjunctivitis and Keratitis

This is best treated with irrigation of the eyes with saline or water immediately after exposure. It is wise not to try to neutralize an acid or alkali by using its chemical counterpart, as the heat generated by the reaction may cause further damage. If the chemical irritant is an alkali, the irrigation should be continued for at least one hour; this is because alkalies are not precipitated by the proteins of the eye, as acids are, but tend to linger in the tissues, producing further damage for hours after exposure. A local anesthetic solution is instilled before the irrigation to relieve pain. The pupil should be dilated with 5% homatropine or 0.2% scopolamine solution. Corticosteroid ointment is placed in the affected eye 2-6 times daily, depending upon the severity of the condition. The patient must be watched carefully for such complications as symblepharon, corneal scarring, closure of the puncta, and secondary infection.

Lids

Lacerations of the lids not involving the lid margins, no matter how deep, can be sutured just as any other skin laceration. If the lid margin is involved, whether the canaliculi are also involved or not, the patient should be referred for specialized care; permanent notching of the lid margin may occur if the edges are not properly sutured.

Conjunctiva

In minor lacerations of the conjunctiva, sutures are not necessary. In order to prevent infection, instill an antibiotic 2-3 times a day until the laceration is healed.

Cornea, Sclera; Intraocular Foreign Bodies

The best emergency treatment for a laceration of the cornea or sclera or an intraocular foreign body is to bandage the eye lightly and cover the bandage with a metal shield which rests on the orbital bones superiorly and inferiorly and is held in place with tape passing over the shield from the forehead to the cheek.

Examination, manipulation, and eye movement should be kept at an absolute minimum, since any undue pressure on the eye may result in extrusion of the intraocular contents.

OCULAR EMERGENCIES

Ocular emergencies may be classified as true emergencies and urgent cases. A true emergency is defined as one in which a few hours' delay in treatment can lead to permanent ocular damage or extreme discomfort to the patient. An urgent case is one in which treatment should be started as soon as possible but in which a delay of a few days can be tolerated.

TRUE EMERGENCIES

Trauma
Corneal foreign bodies and corneal abrasions must be treated early in order to relieve the progressively more severe pain and irritation. Lacerations of the eyeball should be sutured as soon as possible in order to avoid extrusion of the internal contents of the eye. Intraocular foreign bodies should be removed without delay. It is sometimes possible to remove them through the point of entry with a magnet. Because the ocular media become cloudy if the foreign body is not removed, a foreign body which is visible with the ophthalmoscope shortly after the injury might not be visible several hours or a day later. These procedures are best undertaken by an ophthalmologist.

Foreign body beneath the upper lid is suggested by blepharospasm and a history of foreign body but no visible foreign body. Evert the lid by grasping the lashes gently and exerting pressure in the midportion of the outer surface of the upper lid with a cotton applicator. If a foreign body is present on the tarsal conjunctiva, it can be easily visualized when the lid is everted and then removed with a wet cotton applicator.

Corneal Ulcer
Corneal tissue is a good culture medium for bacteria, particularly Pseudomonas aeruginosa. Specific treatment of any corneal wound or infection by an ophthalmologist should be instituted as soon as possible to avoid corneal perforation and possible loss of the eye.

Severe Conjunctivitis
Most cases of conjunctivitis are not urgent. One exception to this rule is gonococcal conjunctivitis, which has the serious complication of corneal ulceration; a delay in treatment of 1-2 days may result in corneal ulceration or perforation.

Orbital Cellulitis
Orbital cellulitis may be complicated by brain abscess. Immediate treatment with systemic antibiotics is indicated. The bacteriology of orbital cellulitis is similar to that of sinusitis. For example, pneumococci and staphylococci are common invaders and require intensive systemic antibiotic therapy.

Chemical Burns
Chemical burns of the external ocular tissues must be treated immediately by copious irrigation with sterile water or saline, if available, or tap water, for at least 5 minutes. Do not use chemical antidotes, since the heat generated by the reaction may increase the degree of injury. After irrigation, instill local anesthetics as necessary to relieve pain, and dilate the pupil to prevent iritis. Local corticosteroid therapy may limit the degree of corneal damage. These patients should be referred to an ophthalmologist as soon as possible after injury.

Acute Iritis
Severe acute iritis causes extreme pain and photophobia. The pupil should be dilated as soon as possible to prevent the formation of posterior synechias, which further increase the possibility of secondary cataract and glaucoma. Slit lamp examination is necessary to confirm the diagnosis.

Acute Glaucoma
If the intraocular pressure is unusually high (60-100 mm Hg Schiotz), permanent optic nerve damage can occur within a period of 24-48 hours. Therefore, these patients should be referred immediately for definitive care.

Occlusion of the Central Retinal Artery
This is a true emergency as the retina is completely without blood as long as the artery is occluded, and the visual receptors in the retina will degenerate within 30-60 minutes if the flow of blood is not restored. The diagnosis is based upon a history of sudden, complete, painless loss of vision in one eye in an older person and the following ophthalmoscopic findings: pallor of the optic disk, edema of the macula, cherry-red fovea, bloodless arterioles which may be difficult to detect, and "boxcar" segmentation of the blood in the veins.

The best treatment (of value only when the patient is seen within 30-60 minutes of onset) is to pass a sharp instrument such as a No. 11 Bard-Parker blade or No. 25 needle with syringe (see p 110) into the anterior chamber. The knife is inserted at the limbus and passed into the anterior chamber on a plane with the iris. The objective is to permit the extrusion of some of the anterior chamber fluid (aqueous) without striking the lens with the knife. This sudden decrease in the intraocular pressure may restore the flow of blood in the central retinal artery. No treatment is required for the wound. There are some favorable reports on the use of anticoagulants in cases of partial occlusion of the central retinal artery or its branches.

Retinal Detachment

Retinal detachment is a true emergency if the macula is threatened. If the macula is detached, permanent loss of central vision usually occurs even though the retina is eventually successfully reattached by surgery.

URGENT CASES

Strabismus or Anisometropia in a Preschool Child With Amblyopia

The sense of sight develops from birth to about 7 years of age. If a child tends to favor one eye as a result of strabismus or anisometropia, vision may fail to develop in the other eye. These children should be treated without delay with glasses, patching the good eye, or both. Surgery is performed if indicated after visual acuity has been equalized in the 2 eyes.

Chronic Glaucoma

Antiglaucoma therapy should be instituted without delay in order to decrease the intraocular pressure and preserve the remaining visual field.

Vitreous Hemorrhage

A patient with hemorrhage into the vitreous body should be referred, as the hemorrhage may later clear to reveal a retinal detachment.

Unilateral Exophthalmos of Recent Origin

The most common cause of bilateral exophthalmos is hyperthyroidism, although it may also appear after thyroidectomy. Unilateral exophthalmos may also be due to an orbital tumor, cavernous sinus thrombosis, or atrioventricular shunt from the internal carotid artery to the cavernous sinus. These disorders are treatable.

Acute Dacryocystitis

Early treatment is indicated to relieve the pain.

Ocular Tumors

Many tumors of the ocular adnexa can be completely excised if they are diagnosed in an early stage. Malignant intraocular tumors (except of the iris) nearly always require enucleation.

Optic Nerve Pathology

Optic nerve disorders are quite serious and may indicate accompanying intracranial or systemic disease. The patient should be examined from a neurologic as well as an ophthalmologic standpoint.

Sympathetic Ophthalmia

With the availability of effective steroid treatment, sympathetic ophthalmia is now a condition which should be referred for immediate local and systemic corticosteroid therapy. Sympathetic ophthalmia should be suspected if the patient has inflammation in both eyes and a history of penetrating injury to one eye.

•   •   •

PRINCIPLES OF ANTIBIOTIC AND CHEMOTHERAPEUTIC TREATMENT OF OCULAR INFECTIONS

In the treatment of infectious eye disease, eg, conjunctivitis, one should always use the drug which is the most effective, the least likely to cause complications, the least likely to be used systemically at a later date, and the least expensive. Of the available antibacterial agents, the sulfonamides come closest to meeting these specifications. Two reliable sulfonamides are sulfisoxazole and sodium sulfacetamide. The sulfonamides have the added advantages of low allergenicity and effectiveness against trachoma. They are available in ointment or solution form.

If sulfonamides are not effective, the antibiotics can be used. Two of the most effective broad-spectrum antibiotics for ophthalmic use are chloramphenicol and neomycin. Both of these drugs have some effect against gram-negative as well as gram-positive organisms. Other antibiotics frequently used are erythromycin, tetracycline, bacitracin, and polymyxin. Combined bacitracin-polymyxin (Polysporin®) ointment is often used prophylactically for the protection it affords against both gram-positive (bacitracin) and gram-negative (polymyxin) organisms.

The great majority of antibiotic and chemotherapeutic medications for eye infections are administered locally. Systemic administration is required for all intraocular infections, corneal ulcer, orbital cellulitis, dacryocystitis, and any serious external infection that does not respond to local treatment.

Ointments have greater therapeutic effectiveness than solutions since in this way contact can be maintained for up to 30-60 minutes. However, they do have the disadvantage of causing blurred vision; where this must be avoided, solutions should be used.

Before one can determine the drug of choice, the causative organisms must be known. For example, a pneumococcal corneal ulcer will respond to treatment with a sulfonamide or any broad-spectrum antibiotic, but this is not true in the case of corneal ulcer due to Pseudomonas aeruginosa, which responds only to vigorous treatment with polymyxin or colistin. Another example is staphylococcal dacryocystitis; staphylococci not sensitive to penicillin are most likely to be susceptible to erythromycin or methicillin.

It is well to keep in mind that **the antibiotics, like the steroids, when used over a prolonged period of time in bacterial corneal ulcers, favor the development of secondary fungal infection of the cornea.** This is another reason for using the sulfonamides whenever they are adequate for the purpose.

COMMON TECHNICS USED IN THE TREATMENT OF OCULAR DISORDERS

Liquid Medications

Place the patient in a sitting position with both eyes open and looking up. Pull down slightly on the lower lid and instill 2 drops in the lower cul-de-sac. The patient is then asked to look down while finger contact on the lower lid is maintained. Do not let the patient squeeze his eye shut.

Ointments

Ointments are instilled in the same way as liquids. While the patient is looking down, lift out the lower lid to trap the medication in the conjunctival sac. The lids should be kept closed for at least one minute to allow the heat of the eyes to melt the ointment.

Eye Bandage

Eye bandages should be applied firmly enough to hold the lid fairly securely against the cornea. A single patch consisting of gauze-covered cotton is usually sufficient. A wrap-around head bandage is seldom necessary. Tape is passed from the cheek to the forehead. If more pressure is desired, use 2 or 3 patches.

Warm Compresses

Use a clean towel or washcloth soaked in hot tap water well below the temperature which will burn the thin skin covering the eyelids. Warm compresses are usually applied for 15 minutes 4 times a day. Their therapeutic value is to increase the amount of blood flow to the affected area and to decrease pain and inflammation.

Removal of Superficial Corneal Foreign Body

The main considerations are good illumination, magnification, anesthesia, position of the patient, and sterile technic. If possible, the patient's visual acuity is always recorded first.

The patient may be in the sitting or supine position. The examiner should use a loupe unless a slit lamp is available. An assistant should direct a strong flashlight into the eye with the rays of light striking the cornea at an oblique angle. The examiner may then see the corneal foreign body and remove it with a wet cotton applicator. If this is not successful, the foreign body may be removed with a metal spud, holding the lids apart with the other hand to prevent blinking. An antibacterial ointment (eg, Polysporin®) is instilled after the foreign body has been removed.

Most patients are more comfortable without a patch on the eye after removal of a foreign body. **It is essential to see the patient the next day to be certain that no infection has occurred and that healing is under way.**

Home Medication

At home the same technics should be used as described above except that drops should be instilled with the patient in the supine position. Experienced patients (eg, those with glaucoma) are usually quite skillful in self-administration of eye drops.

COMMON PITFALLS TO BE AVOIDED IN THE MANAGEMENT OF OCULAR DISORDERS

Dangers in the Use of Local Anesthetics

Unsupervised self-administration of local anesthetics is dangerous because the patient may further injure an anesthetized eye without knowing it. Furthermore, most anesthetics delay healing. This is particularly true of butacaine (Butyn®). Butacaine also elicits a high incidence of allergic responses. **Do not** give patients local anesthetics to take home with them. Eye pain should be controlled by systemic analgesics.

Errors in Diagnosis

Of these the most common is a diagnosis of conjunctivitis when the correct diagnosis is iritis (anterior uveitis), glaucoma, or corneal ulcer (especially herpes simplex). The differentiation between iritis and acute glaucoma may be difficult also.

Misuse of Atropine

Atropine must never be used in routine diagnosis or treatment. It causes cycloplegia of about 14 days' duration and can precipitate an attack of glaucoma if the patient has a narrow anterior chamber angle.

Dangers of Local Corticosteroid Therapy

Local ophthalmologic corticosteroid preparations, eg, prednisolone, have become increasingly popular during recent years because of their anti-inflammatory effect on the conjunctiva, cornea, and iris. In general, it is true that any patient with conjunctivitis, corneal inflammation, or iritis can be made more comfortable by the local use of corticosteroids. However, it must be stressed that the corticosteroids have 4 very serious complications when used in the eye indiscreetly over a long period of time: (1) herpes simplex keratitis, (2) open-angle glaucoma, (3) cataract formation, and (4) fungal infection. The most frequent complications are herpes simplex keratitis and glaucoma. Corticosteroids enhance the activity of the herpes simplex virus, apparently by increasing the destructive effect of collagenase on the collagen of the cornea. This is evidenced by the fact that perforation of the cornea occasionally occurs when the corticosteroids are used during the more active stage of a herpes simplex corneal infection. Corneal perforation was a very rare complication of dendritic keratitis before the corticosteroids came into general use. In the treatment of any corneal inflammation, particularly if the corneal epithelium is not intact, the prolonged use of corticosteroids is sometimes complicated by fungal infection (eg, Candida albicans), and this may lead to loss of the eye. Topical corticosteroids can cause or aggravate open-angle glaucoma and, less commonly, can produce cataracts.

For these reasons, although the corticosteroids are valuable in the treatment of ocular disease, any patient on whom they are being used should be watched carefully for the development of complications. The corticosteroids should not be used unless specifically indicated, eg, in iritis, certain types of keratitis, and acute allergic disorders.

Use of Contaminated Eye Medications

The external coats of the eye, including the sclera and the corneal epithelium, are resistant to infection. However, once the corneal epithelium or sclera is broken by trauma, the tissues become markedly susceptible to bacterial infection. For this reason, ophthalmic solutions which may be used in injured eyes must be prepared with the same degree of caution as fluids intended for intravenous administration.

Sterile, single use disposable units of the common ophthalmic solutions should be used whenever liquid medication is instilled into an injured eye. For routine use in intact eyes, nearly all eye medications are now available in small plastic containers. It is perfectly safe to use these provided they are not kept a long time after opening and are not contaminated accidentally.

•   •   •

Bibliography

Allen, H.: Aseptic technique in ophthalmology. Tr Am Ophth Soc **57**:377-472, 1959.

Becker, V., & D. W. Mills: Elevation of intraocular pressure following corticosteroid eye drops. JAMA **185**:884, 1963.

Girard, L. J., & others: Severe alkali burns. Tr Am Acad Ophth **74**:787-803, 1970.

Hales, R. H.: Ocular injuries sustained in the dental office. Am J Ophth **70**:221-3, 1970.

Havener, W. H.: Ocular Pharmacology, 2nd ed. Mosby, 1970.

Kimura, S. J.: Fluorescein paper: a simple means of insuring the use of sterile fluorescein. Am J Ophth **34**:446-7, 1951.

Leopold, I. H. (editor): Symposium on Ocular Therapy. Mosby, 1966, 1967, 1968, 1969.

Thygeson, P.: Steroid therapy in ophthalmology. Am J Ophth **56**:668, 1963.

Vaughan, D. G., Jr.: Corneal ulcers. Survey Ophth **3**:203-15, 1958.

5...
Lids and Lacrimal Apparatus

I. THE LIDS

Anatomy

The eyelids are moveable folds of tissue which serve to protect the eye. The skin of the lids is loose and elastic, permitting extreme swelling and subsequent return to normal shape and size. The **tarsal plates** consist of dense fibrous tissue with some elastic tissue. They are lined posteriorly by conjunctiva and fuse medially and laterally to form the **medial and lateral palpebral tendons (ligaments)**, which attach to the orbital bones. The **orbital septum** is the fascia lying posterior to the orbicularis oculi muscle and is the barrier between the lid and the orbit.

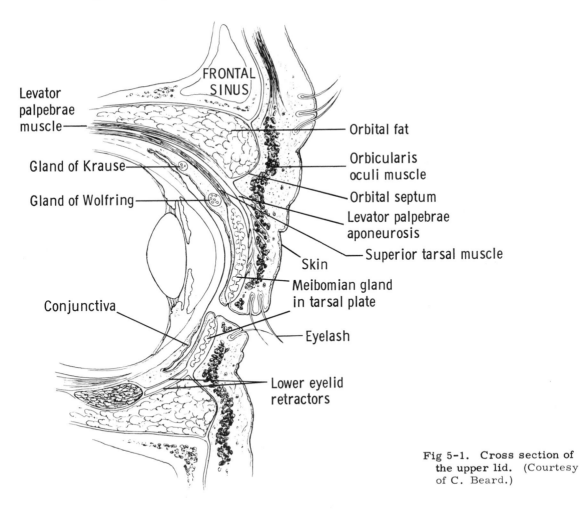

Levator palpebrae muscle

Gland of Krause

Gland of Wolfring

Conjunctiva

FRONTAL SINUS

Orbital fat

Orbicularis oculi muscle

Orbital septum

Levator palpebrae aponeurosis

Superior tarsal muscle

Skin

Meibomian gland in tarsal plate

Eyelash

Lower eyelid retractors

Fig 5-1. Cross section of the upper lid. (Courtesy of C. Beard.)

The **orbicularis oculi** muscle, which is supplied by the 7th cranial nerve, is roughly circular. Its function is to close the lids. The **levator palpebrae** muscle, supplied by the third nerve, inserts into the tarsal plate and the skin and serves to elevate the lid. The superior tarsal muscle (of Müller), supplied by sympathetic nerves, originates in the levator muscle and inserts at the superior edge of the tarsus, coursing deep to the levator aponeurosis.

The 3 types of glands in the lid are the meibomian glands and the glands of Moll and Zeis. The meibomian glands are long sebaceous glands in the tarsal plate. They do not communicate with the hair follicles. There are about 25 in the upper lid and 20 in the lower lid, appearing as yellow vertical streaks deep to the conjunctiva. The meibomian glands produce a sebaceous substance which creates an oil layer on the surface of the tear film. This helps to prevent rapid evaporation of the normal tear layer. The glands of Zeis are smaller, modified sebaceous glands which are connected with the follicles of the eyelashes. The sweat glands of Moll are unbranched sinuous tubules which begin in a simple spiral and not in a glomerulus as do ordinary sweat glands.

There is a **gray line** (mucocutaneous border) on the margins of both the upper and the lower eyelids. If an incision is made along this line, the lid can be cleanly split into a posterior portion, containing the tarsal plate and conjunctiva, and an anterior portion, containing the orbicularis oculi muscle, skin, and hair follicles.

The blood supply to the lids is derived mainly from the ophthalmic and lacrimal arteries. The lymphatics drain into the preauricular, parotid, and submaxillary lymph glands.

Physiology of Symptoms

Lid disorders are among the most common of all ocular problems. The patient with disorders of the eyelids will have varied complaints. There are many pain fibers in the tissues near the lid margins. Consequently, if there is inflammation with stretching of tissues, as in hordeolum, the patient complains of moderately severe pain. In marginal blepharitis there is no pain but the patient complains of red-rimmed eyes; because of the proximity of the lid margins to the conjunctiva, frequent attacks of conjunctivitis are a common complaint.

If the patient has a foreign body sensation, entropion, with eyelashes rubbing on the cornea, should be ruled out. If the lid falls away from the eyeball, as in ectropion, tearing will be the chief complaint, since the tears do not have access to the lower punctum. Exposure keratitis may also occur with ectropion.

Technic of Upper Lid Eversion

Have the patient look down. Grasp the lashes gently and exert pressure posteriorly and medially on the upper lid at the upper tarsal border with a cotton applicator.

INFECTIONS AND INFLAMMATIONS OF THE LIDS

HORDEOLUM

Hordeolum is a common staphylococcal infection of the lid glands which is characterized by a localized red, swollen, and acutely tender area. It is essentially an abscess, as there is pus formation within the lumen of the affected gland. When it affects the meibomian glands it is relatively large and is known as an **internal hordeolum**. The smaller and more superficial **external hordeolum** (sty) is an infection of Zeis's or Moll's glands. Pain is the primary symptom, and the intensity of the pain is in direct proportion to the amount of lid swelling. An internal hordeolum may point to the skin or to the conjunctival side of the lid; external hordeolum always points to the skin side of the lid margin.

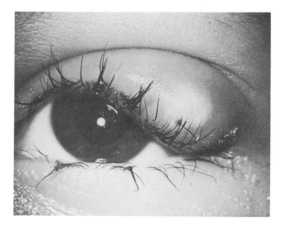

Fig 5-2. Internal hordeolum, left upper eyelid, pointing on skin side. This should be opened by a horizontal skin incision. (Courtesy of A. Rosenberg.)

Treatment of both internal and external hordeolum is with warm compresses for 10-15 minutes 3 times a day, and incision and drainage of the purulent material if the process does not begin to resolve within 48 hours. An ophthalmic antibacterial instilled into the conjunctival sac every 3 hours is beneficial. A large internal hordeolum can be complicated by cellulitis of the entire lid.

CHALAZION

Chalazion is a sterile granulomatous inflammation of a meibomian gland, of unknown cause, characterized by localized swelling in the upper or lower eyelid. It may begin with inflammation and tenderness similar to a hordeolum and develop over a period of weeks. The majority point toward the conjunctival side of the lid. When the lid is everted, the conjunctiva over the chalazion is seen to be reddened and elevated.

If sufficiently large, a chalazion may press upon the eyeball and cause astigmatism.

In general, a fully developed chalazion is differentiated from hordeolum by the absence of acute inflammatory signs.

Chalazion seldom subsides spontaneously; if it is large enough to distort vision or to be a cosmetic blemish, excision is indicated. Pathologically, there is proliferation of the endothelium of the acinus and a granulomatous inflammatory response, including some Langhans type giant cells.

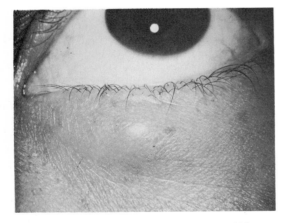

Fig 5-3. **Chalazion, left lower eyelid.** (Courtesy of A. Rosenberg.)

MARGINAL BLEPHARITIS
(Granulated Eyelids)

Blepharitis is a common chronic bilateral inflammation of the lid margins. There are 2 main types: staphylococcal and seborrheic. Staphylococcal blepharitis is usually ulcerative. Seborrheic blepharitis (nonulcerative) is usually associated with the presence of Pityrosporum ovale, although this organism has not been shown to be the etiologic factor. As a rule, both types are present (mixed infection). Seborrhea of the scalp, brows, and ears is frequently associated with seborrheic blepharitis.

The chief symptoms are irritation, burning, and itching of the lid margins. The eyes are "red-rimmed." Many scales or "granulations" can be seen clinging to the lashes of both the upper and the lower lids. In the staphylococcal type, the scales are dry, the lids are red, tiny ulcerated areas are found along the lid margins, and the lashes tend to fall out. In the seborrheic type the scales are greasy, ulceration does not occur, and the lid margins are less red. In the more common mixed type, both dry and greasy scales are present and the lid margins are red and may be ulcerated. Staphylococcus aureus and Pityrosporum ovale can be seen together or singly in stained material scraped from the lid margins.

Conjunctivitis, superficial keratitis of the lower third of the cornea, and chronic meibomianitis are common complications of staphylococcal blepharitis. Seborrheic blepharitis is occasionally complicated by a mild keratitis. Persons with staphylococcal blepharitis are prone to develop chalazions and hordeola.

The scalp, eyebrows, and lid margins must be kept clean, particularly in the seborrheic type, by means of soap and water shampoo. Scales must be removed from the lid margins daily with a damp cotton applicator.

Staphylococcal blepharitis is treated with antistaphylococcal antibiotic or sulfonamide eye ointment applied on a cotton applicator once daily to the lid margins.

Meibomianitis cannot be cured permanently, although expression of the material from the glands may give temporary relief. Staphylococcal conjunctivitis or keratitis usually disappears promptly following local antistaphylococcal medication.

The seborrheic and staphylococcal types usually become mixed, and may run a chronic course over a period of months or years if not treated adequately.

MEIBOMIANITIS

Bilateral, chronic inflammation of the meibomian glands is an uncommon disease of unknown etiology which occurs during or after the middle years of life. It is generally preceded by or associated with blepharitis.

The patient complains of chronically red and irritated eyes and a slight but continuous discharge. The meibomian glands are prominent, the lid margins are red, and there is a frothy conjunctival discharge. A soft, cheesy yellow material which contains no organisms can be expressed from the glands. An irritative conjunctivitis due to contact with the meibomian secretion is a frequent complication.

The only treatment is repeated expression of the meibomian glands. However, because this treatment never produces dramatic results, the patient usually neglects to do it or have it done, and the disease process continues indefinitely with a slight tendency to become worse.

POSITIONAL DEFECTS OF THE LIDS

ENTROPION

Entropion (turning inward of the lid) usually affects the lower lid but may affect the upper lid. It seldom occurs in persons under 40 years of age. The 2 common types are senile (spastic) and cicatricial. Senile entropion is due to a degeneration of fascial attachments between layers in the lower eyelid, allowing preseptal orbicularis to override pretarsal orbicularis and rotate the lid margin inward. Cicatricial entropion is due to scarring of the tarsus palpebrarum and is therefore common in trachoma. Trichiasis (turning in of the lashes so that they rub on the cornea) is a serious complication of entropion. It causes corneal irritation and may encourage corneal ulceration.

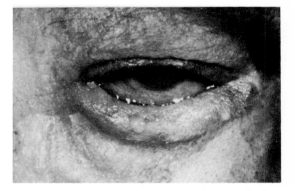

Fig 5-4. **Entropion.** (Courtesy of M. Quickert.)

Surgery to evert the lid is effective in the treatment of both types of entropion. A useful temporary measure is to tape the lower lid to the cheek with tension temporally and inferiorly.

ECTROPION

Ectropion (sagging and eversion of the lower lid), usually bilateral, is a frequent finding in older persons. Ectropion may be caused by relaxation of the orbicularis oculi muscle, either as part of the aging process or following Bell's palsy. The symptoms are tearing and irritation. Exposure keratitis may occur.

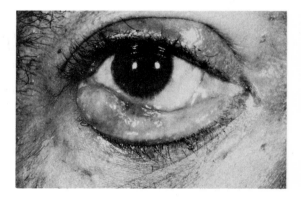

Fig 5-5. **Ectropion.** (Courtesy of M. Quickert.)

Marked ectropion is treated by surgical shortening of the lower lid in a horizontal direction. Minor degrees of ectropion can be treated by several fairly deep electrocautery penetrations through the conjunctiva 4-5 mm from the lid margins at the inferior aspect of the tarsal plate. The fibrotic reaction which follows will frequently draw the lid up to its normal position.

ANATOMIC DEFORMITIES
OF THE LIDS

BLEPHAROCHALASIS
AND DERMATOCHALASIS

Blepharochalasis is redundancy of the skin of the upper or lower lids associated with lymphedema and a defect in the orbital septum. It often occurs in young adults, and a familial tendency is often present. Treatment is surgical, but the condition may recur.

Dermatochalasis is redundancy of upper or lower lid tissues due to aging processes. It may also occur following repeated bouts of angioneurotic edema with consequent stretching of the skin. Excision of a portion of the skin of the lids is required if vision is affected or for cosmetic reasons. Prolapsing orbital fat may be removed at the same time.

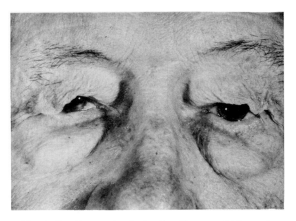

Fig 5-7. Dermatochalasis of upper lids and herniation of orbital fat of lower lids without blepharochalasis. (Courtesy of M. Quickert.)

EPICANTHUS

Epicanthus is characterized by vertical folds of skin over the medial canthi. It is present to some degree in most children. The skin fold is often large enough to cover part of the nasal sclera and cause "pseudoesotropia," as the eyes appear to be crossed when a normal amount of medial sclera is not visible. Prominent epicanthal folds in children gradually decrease as the child grows older and are seldom apparent by school age.

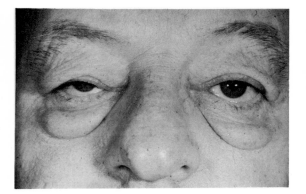

Fig 5-6. Blepharochalasis.
(Courtesy of M. Quickert.)

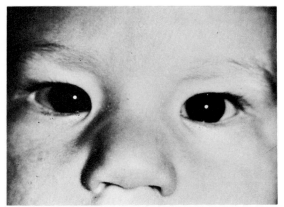

Fig 5-8. Epicanthus.

BLEPHAROSPASM
(Tic)

Blepharospasm is persistent or repetitive involuntary contraction of the orbicularis oculi muscle. It is usually bilateral and is more common in older persons. The cause is not known. It may be due to irritative lesions of the cornea and conjunctiva or of the 7th cranial nerve. Emotional stress and fatigue make it worse. The eyes should be examined carefully to rule out irritative lesions such as corneal foreign body, meibomianitis, and trichiasis.

Treatment consists of removal of the causative factor if possible. If the specific etiology is not known, explanation and reassurance are in order. Intractable cases may require alcohol injection of the orbicularis oculi muscle to produce temporary paralysis. Seventh nerve block with a long-acting local anesthetic should be tried before alcohol injection is resorted to. Plastic surgery designed to weaken orbicularis function and selective removal of 7th nerve branches have been successful in some cases.

If the condition has been present for only a short time, the prognosis for cessation of the blepharospasm is good. Long-standing cases tend to persist regardless of treatment.

PTOSIS

Drooping of the lids when the eyes are open may be unilateral or bilateral and constant or intermittent.

Etiology
A. Congenital ptosis is usually the result of developmental failure of the levator muscle of the lid, alone or in association with anomalies of the superior rectus muscle (most frequent) or complete external ophthalmoplegia (rare). It may be transmitted as a dominant characteristic.

B. Acquired ptosis can be considered in 3 main categories:
1. Mechanical factors - Abnormal weight of the lids may make it difficult for a normal levator muscle to elevate fully. This may be due to acute or chronic inflammatory edema or swelling, tumor, or an extra fold of fatty material, as in xanthelasma.

2. Myogenic factors (eg, muscular dystrophy and myasthenia gravis) - Ptosis of one or both lids is often the first sign of myasthenia gravis and occurs eventually in over 95% of cases. The essential defect in myasthenia gravis seems to be in the humoral transmission at the myoneural junction.

3. Neurogenic (paralytic) factors - Interference with the pathways of the portion of the third cranial nerve supplying the levator muscle at any level from the oculomotor nucleus (midbrain) to the myoneural junction (discussed in greater detail in Chapter 13).

Clinical Findings
Congenital ptosis is evident at birth and is often observed to be associated with weakness of other extraocular muscles. The affected lid has a smooth, flat appearance, and the tarsal fold caused by the pull of a normal levator muscle is absent. This is more noticeable on upward gaze, when the lid fails to retract as the eye moves upward.

If the lid droops enough to partially occlude the pupil, the child usually attempts to compensate by elevating the brow with the frontalis muscle. This produces a marked wrinkling of the forehead, most evident when the condition is unilateral.

If the pupil is completely occluded, amblyopia ex anopsia may occur.

The ptosis of muscular dystrophy progresses very slowly and insidiously but finally becomes complete.

Ptosis in myasthenia gravis is gradual in onset, characteristically appearing in the evening, with fatigue, and improving overnight. Later it becomes permanent. In over 80% of cases, some degree of transient or permanent ophthalmoplegia follows and produces diplopia. A diagnostic test of injection of neostigmine (Prostigmin®) or edrophonium (Tensilon®) IM or IV usually gives a dramatic response by temporarily abolishing the ptosis.

Neurogenic ptosis presents different clinical pictures according to the level of the pathway affected. The findings of other portions of a neurologic syndrome usually help establish the diagnosis.

Treatment
If the condition is so slight that no cosmetic deformity is present and there is no interference with visual acuity, it is best left alone.

Myasthenia gravis should be treated as indicated (with neostigmine or a similar drug).

Some relief may be obtained by wearing special spectacle frames which have a posteriorly attached wire crutch that suspends or ele-

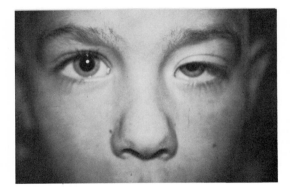 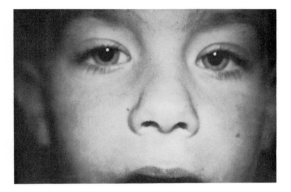

Fig 5-9. **Surgical correction of ptosis.** **Left:** Before operation, ptosis of the left upper lid was present. **Right:** After the operation (levator resection), the ptosis was well corrected and a natural-appearing upper lid fold produced. (Courtesy of C. Beard.)

vates the lid by traction. This may be indicated in temporary paresis or in those who are not good candidates for surgery.

Surgery is the treatment of choice for cosmetic reasons, and should be performed early if vision is occluded. The type of surgery varies with the cause:

(1) If the levator muscle is not completely paralyzed, resection or shortening of the muscle is the procedure of choice.

(2) If the levator muscle has no action, the elevating effect of the frontalis muscle may be utilized by passing some type of traction device (wire, fascia, or suture) subcutaneously from the frontalis to the tissue of the eyelid (tarsus), so that when the brow is raised the lid will be elevated. The advantage of this procedure is that no tissue is destroyed and the traction material may be withdrawn and reinserted if desired. The risk of infection is great unless the patient's own fascia lata is used.

PSEUDOPTOSIS

Pseudoptosis may occur when the upper lid lacks its normal support, as with a shrunken or absent eye or an inadequate prosthesis.

II. THE LACRIMAL APPARATUS

Anatomy

The lacrimal apparatus consists of the lacrimal gland, accessory glands, canaliculi, tear sac, and nasolacrimal duct. The lacrimal gland is a tear-secreting gland located in the anterior superior temporal portion of the orbit. Several secretory ducts connect the gland to the superior conjunctival fornix. The tears pass down over the cornea and bulbar and palpebral conjunctiva, moistening the surfaces of these structures. They drain into the lacrimal canaliculi through the lacrimal puncta, round apertures about 0.5 mm in diameter on the medial aspect of both the upper and lower lid margins. The canaliculi are about 1 mm in diameter and 8 mm long, and join to form a common canaliculus just before opening into the lacrimal sac. Diverticuli may be a part of the normal structure, and are susceptible to fungal infection.

The lacrimal sac is the dilated portion of the lacrimal drainage system which lies in the bony lacrimal fossa.

The nasolacrimal duct is the downward continuation of the lacrimal sac. It opens into the inferior meatus beneath the inferior turbinate bone.

All of the passages of the lacrimal drainage system are lined with epithelium. The tears pass into the puncta by capillary attraction. The combined forces of the capillary attraction in the canaliculi, gravity, and the pumping action of the orbicularis oculi muscle on the lacrimal sac tend to continue the flow of tears down the nasolacrimal duct into the nose and nasopharynx.

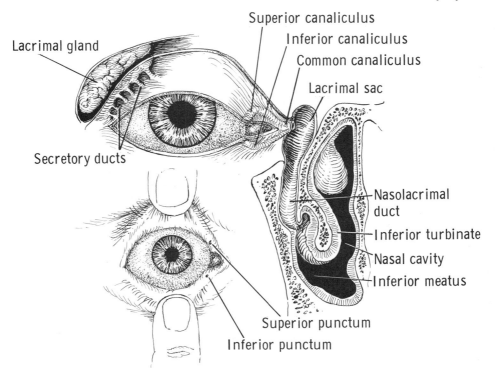

Superior canaliculus

Inferior canaliculus

Common canaliculus

Lacrimal sac

Lacrimal gland

Nasolacrimal duct

Inferior turbinate

Nasal cavity

Inferior meatus

Secretory ducts

Superior punctum

Inferior punctum

Fig 5-10. The lacrimal drainage system. (Redrawn with modifications and reproduced, with permission, from Thompson: Radiography of the Nasolacrimal Passageways. Medical Radiography and Photography 25:66, 1949.)

Physiology of Symptoms

Patients with disorders of the lacrimal apparatus complain of tearing or "dry eyes." In the event of "tearing" without associated symptoms, the pathology is in the lacrimal drainage system or the result of hypersecretion. Paradoxic lacrimation (an occasional late complication of 7th nerve palsy) is a condition in which salivary gland fibers innervate the lacrimal gland. If the eyes are dry, there is faulty production of tears. The physician investigates the symptoms by irrigation to test the patency of the canaliculi and the nasolacrimal ducts and by palpation of the lacrimal gland. If the complaint is of "dry eyes," he also approximates the quantity of tear production (Schirmer test).

There are many causes of tearing, eg, conjunctivitis, keratitis, iritis, and foreign bodies. However, if tearing is the only symptom, the cause in the great majority of cases will be found in the lacrimal drainage apparatus.

INFECTIONS OF THE LACRIMAL APPARATUS

DACRYOCYSTITIS

Infection of the lacrimal sac is a common acute or chronic disease which usually occurs in infants or in persons over 40 (about 9 out of 10 chronic adult cases occur in menopausal women); it is uncommon in the intermediate age groups. It is most often unilateral, and is always secondary to obstruction of the nasolacrimal duct. In many adult cases the etiology of the obstruction remains unknown, but there may be a history of severe trauma to the nose. Acute cases are often preceded by chronic dacryocystitis; some cases are preceded by chronic conjunctivitis (eg, trachoma). In acute dacryocystitis the usual infectious agent is one of the staphylococci; in chronic dacryocystitis, Diplococcus pneumoniae or occasionally Hemophilus influenzae. Candida albicans can cause chronic dacryocystitis and may form a complete cast of the nasolacrimal duct. (Mixed infections do not occur.)

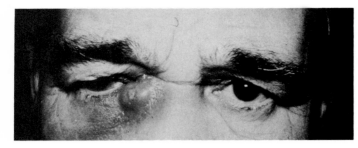

Fig 5-11. Acute dacryocystitis.

It is curious that dacryocystitis is seldom complicated by conjunctivitis even though the conjunctival sac is constantly being bathed with pus exuding through the lacrimal puncta.

Clinical Findings

The chief symptoms are tearing and discharge. In the acute form inflammation, pain, swelling, and tenderness are present in the tear sac area; purulent material can be expressed from the tear sac. In the chronic form tearing is usually the only sign; mucoid material can usually be expressed from the tear sac.

The infectious agent can be identified microscopically by staining a conjunctival smear taken after expression of the tear sac.

Corneal ulcer occasionally occurs following minor corneal trauma in the presence of pneumococcal dacryocystitis. Perforation of the skin and fistula formation may also occur. If a corneal ulcer occurs, vigorous local and systemic treatment is indicated and a dacryocystectomy or dacryocystorhinostomy should be done without delay.

Treatment

A. Adult: Warm compresses to the affected eye at frequent intervals during the acute stage.

1. Acute - Specific treatment for acute staphylococcal or pneumococcal dacryocystitis consists of penicillin, 1 million units daily IM, until the inflammation subsides.

2. Chronic - Since an obstruction of the nasolacrimal duct is the basic cause of dacryocystitis, the disease is usually persistent until the obstruction is relieved. However, probing is notably unsuccessful in adults, and dacryocystorhinostomy is usually necessary if symptoms are severe. If chronic tearing is the only symptom, many patients prefer the tearing to surgery.

B. Infantile: Delayed canalization of the nasolacrimal ducts is very common in infants. The ducts usually open spontaneously in the first month of life, and most of the remainder can be cured by massage of the tear sac by the mother or physician. In a small percentage of patients, the ducts fail to open (usually on one side only) for many weeks or months, long enough for a secondary bacterial (almost always pneumococcal) dacryocystitis to occur. When this happens, frequent (3-4 times a day) and forceful massage of the tear sac is indicated, and antibiotic or sulfonamide drops should be instilled in the conjunctival sac 4-5 times a day. If this is not successful after 3 weeks, probing of the nasolacrimal duct is indicated regardless of the infant's age. First probing of the nasolacrimal duct is effective in about 75% of cases; the remaining 25% can be cured by subsequent probings. Rarely, dacryocystorhinostomy is necessary to establish lacrimal flow.

Course and Prognosis

Acute adult dacryocystitis responds well to systemic antibiotic therapy. Recurrences are common if the nasolacrimal duct obstruction is not removed. The chronic form can be kept latent by using antibiotic eye drops, but relief of the obstruction is the only cure.

CANALICULITIS

Canaliculitis is an uncommon chronic unilateral condition caused by infection with Actinomyces israelii, Candida albicans, or Aspergillus species. It affects the lower canaliculus more often than the upper, occurs exclusively in adults, and causes a secondary purulent conjunctivitis which frequently escapes etiologic diagnosis.

The patient complains of a mildly red and irritated eye with a slight discharge. The organism can be seen microscopically on a direct smear taken from the canaliculus.

Curettage of the necrotic material in the involved canaliculus, followed by irrigation, is

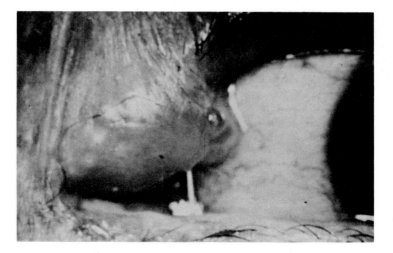

Fig 5-12. Actinomyces israelii (Streptothrix) canaliculitis, left eye.
(Courtesy of P. Thygeson.)

usually effective. Canaliculotomy is sometimes necessary. Tincture of iodine should be applied to the lining of the canaliculus after canaliculotomy.

DACRYOADENITIS

Acute inflammation of a lacrimal gland is a rare unilateral condition which may be seen in children as a complication of mumps, measles, or influenza, and in adults in association with gonorrhea. It may also develop following a perforating injury to the lacrimal gland.

In the acute type there is considerable swelling, pain, and injection over the upper temporal aspect of the eye. This is treated by warm compresses.

If bacterial infection is present, antibiotics are given systemically. Incision may be necessary if pus collects in the gland under tension.

Chronic dacryoadenitis is occasionally seen bilaterally as one manifestation of sarcoidosis. This condition (which, with lacrimal gland swelling, is called Mikulicz's syndrome) usually occurs in Negroes, and is self-limited. The prognosis is good. Chronic dacryoadenitis may also occur in tuberculosis, lymphatic leukemia, and lymphosarcoma.

•   •   •

Bibliography

Aurora, A. L., & F. C. Blodi: Lesions of the eyelids: A clinicopathological study. Survey Ophth 15:94-104, 1970.

Beard, C.: Ptosis. Mosby, 1969.

Berke, R. N.: Results of resection of the levator muscle through a skin incision in congenital ptosis. Arch Ophth 61:177-201, 1959.

Boniuk, M., & L. E. Zimmerman: Eyelid tumors with reference to lesions confused with squamous cell carcinoma. III. Keratoacanthoma. Arch Ophth 77: 29-40, 1967.

Callahan, A.: Reconstructive Surgery of the Eyelids and Ocular Adnexa. Aesculapius Publishing Co., 1966.

Fox, S. A.: Essential (idiopathic) blepharospasm. Arch Ophth 76:318-21, 1966.

Jones, L. T.: The lacrimal secretory system and its treatment. Am J Ophth 62: 47-59, 1966.

Jones, L. T., & M. L. Linn: Diagnosis of the causes of epiphora. Am J Ophth 67: 751, 1969.

Jones, L. T., Reeh, M. J., & J. K. Tsujimura: Senile entropion. Am J Ophth 60:709-10, 1965.

Reese, A. B.: Precancerous and cancerous melanosis. Am J Ophth 61:1272-7, 1966.

Scheie, H. G., & D. M. Albert: Distichiasis and trichiasis: Origin and management. Am J Ophth 61:718-20, 1966.

Sexton, R. R.: Eyelids, lacrima apparatus, and conjunctiva. Annual review. Arch Ophth 83:379-96, 1971.

Thygeson, P.: Complications of staphylococcic blepharitis. Am J Ophth 68:446-9, 1969.

6...

Conjunctiva

Anatomy and Physiology

The conjunctiva is a thin, transparent mucous membrane which lines the anterior sclera up to the limbus and the posterior surface of the lids (Fig 6-1). There are 2 divisions of the conjunctiva: palpebral and bulbar. The palpebral portion lines the lids and the bulbar portion lines the eyeball. At the fornices the conjunctiva is reflected from the lids over the eye. Anteriorly the conjunctiva is continuous with the corneal epithelium. Immediately beneath the bulbar conjunctiva is the anterior portion of Tenon's capsule. Tenon's capsule and the conjunctiva are fused around the limbus in a zone about 3 mm wide. In the region of the inner canthus the conjunctiva is slightly thickened to form the plica semilunaris. The caruncle, a small flesh-like epidermoid structure (see p 2), is attached superficially to the inner portion of the plica. Several small accessory lacrimal glands are present in the superior fornix as well as the openings of the ducts from the lacrimal gland.

Histologically, the conjunctiva consists of 2 layers: the epithelium, composed of cylindrical cells, and the substantia propria, which is divided into adenoidal and fibrous layers. The substantia propria contains goblet cells. These are essentially unicellular mucous glands; the mucinous substance produced assists the tears in keeping the conjunctiva and cornea moist.

The conjunctival blood vessels are derived from the anterior ciliary and palpebral arteries. The nerves are from the ophthalmic division of the 5th cranial nerve. The conjunctiva is rich in lymphatics.

CONJUNCTIVITIS

Conjunctivitis is the most common of all eye diseases in the Western hemisphere. The causes are listed on p 57. The majority are exogenous, but conjunctivitis may rarely be endogenous. Bacterial conjunctivitis, the most frequent type, is self-limited, lasting about 10-14 days untreated. Treatment with one of the many available antibacterial agents usually clears the condition in 1-3 days. Trachoma **and inclusion blennorrhea can be treated successfully with antibiotics.**

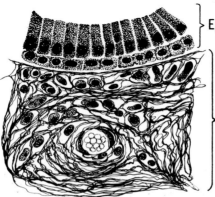

Epithelium

Substantia propria

Fig 6-1. Cross section of conjunctiva. (Redrawn and reproduced, with permission, from Duke-Elder: Textbook of Ophthalmology, Vol. I. Mosby, 1942.)

Viral conjunctivitis is also relatively common. The discharge is usually watery rather than purulent. Viral conjunctivitis is self-limited, lasting 1-3 weeks regardless of treatment. Topical antibiotics are generally used to prevent secondary infection.

Allergic conjunctivitis causes tearing, itching, and injection with a slight stringy discharge. It is usually chronic and bilateral. Corticosteroids instilled locally are effective.

Fungal and parasitic conjunctivitides are usually unilateral and often present as a localized inflammatory granuloma in the conjunctiva. An example of this is the granuloma seen in Leptotrichia conjunctivitis. Fungal and parasitic conjunctivitis are rare in most parts of the world and are given only brief discussions in the following pages.

Physiology of Symptoms

Because of its exposed position, the conjunctiva comes in contact with more microorganisms than any mucous membrane. Organisms commonly found in the urethra seem to thrive on conjunctival tissue, whereas those that grow abundantly on the nasal mucosa do less well in the conjunctival sac. For example, the conjunctiva is relatively immune to the virus of the common cold, whereas the gonococcus and the agent of inclusion blennorrhea, neither of which will grow in the nose, multiply rapidly in the urethra and in the conjunctival sac despite the fact that the tears are constantly washing organisms down the nasolacrimal duct into the nose. In general, organisms pathogenic for the genitourinary tract are also pathogenic for the conjunctiva.

The reaction of the conjunctiva to invading microorganisms is also similar to that of the synovial membranes, as evidenced by the conjunctivitis present as part of Reiter's disease and the purulent conjunctivitis which may develop in association with gonorrheal infection of a bony joint.

The conjunctiva contains many blood vessels and mucus-producing cells but few pain fibers; this accounts for the marked inflammatory response without pain which is characteristic of conjunctivitis. When the lids are closed, as in sleeping, the temperature of the conjunctival sac is elevated. The incubating effect of this increase in temperature promotes the growth of invading bacteria, and this in turn promotes the production of pus cells. This explains the "sticking together of the lids in the morning" in bacterial conjunctivitis.

Conjunctivitis causes an increase in tear production. The antibacterial function of the tears is primarily mechanical, washing conjunctival debris and bacteria into the nasal passages for excretion. The tears also contain lysozyme, which inhibits the growth of many bacteria, including staphylococci. Tear production, the polymorphonuclear response, and the absence of a closed space (when the lids are open) in which to grow all have their role in the self-limiting nature of conjunctivitis, particularly bacterial conjunctivitis.

When the eyes become inflamed, the patient usually seeks treatment early. A diagnosis of conjunctivitis is suggested by a history of red eye of short duration, without pain or photophobia, and by the inflamed appearance of the conjunctiva and the presence of a conjunctival exudate or sticky lids in the morning. The diagnosis can be confirmed and pathogens identified by microscopic examination of stained material from the conjunctival surface. Cultures and antibiotic sensitivity tests should be done in cases that do not respond well to treatment. Keratitis, iritis, and acute glaucoma must be ruled out.

ETIOLOGIC CLASSIFICATION

A. Bacterial: (In approximate order of frequency.)
   1. Pyogenic -
      Diplococcus pneumoniae*
      Staphylococcus aureus*
      Neisseria meningitidis
      Neisseria gonorrhoeae*
      Hemophilus aegyptius (Koch-Weeks bacillus)
      Hemophilus influenzae
      Streptoccus viridans
      Proteus vulgaris
   2. Nonpyogenic -
      Corynebacterium diphtheriae
      Mycobacterium tuberculosis
      Pasteurella tularensis
      Morax-Axenfeld bacillus (Moraxella lacunata)

B. Viral: (In approximate order of frequency.) Viruses of -
      *Pharyngoconjunctival fever (adenoviruses 3 and 7)
      * Epidemic keratoconjunctivitis (adenovirus 8)
      Variola
      Herpes simplex
      Newcastle disease
      Molluscum contagiosum
      Varicella
      Vaccinia

*Causes ophthalmia neonatorum.

C. Chlamydial:
    Chlamydia trachomatis
    Chlamydia oculogenitalis
    Chlamydia lymphogranulomatis

D. Allergic:
    Hay fever
    Vernal
    Phlyctenular keratoconjunctivitis

E. Physical:
    Foreign bodies
    Chemicals
    Other irritants

F. Fungal:
    Candida albicans (ocular candidiasis,
      thrush of eye)
    Sporotrichum schenkii
    Leptotrichia (Sphaerotilus)
    Actinomyces israelii

G. Parasitic:
    Onchocerca caecutiens
    Loa loa
    Wuchereria bancrofti
    Thelazia californiensis
    Thelazia callipaeda
    Nematodes (roundworms)
    Trematodes (flukes) (Schistosoma
      haematobium)
    Cestodes (tapeworms)
    Arthropods (Phthirus pubis, ocular
      myiasis)

H. Spirochetal: Treponema pallidum

I. Unknown Etiology:
    Chronic follicular conjunctivitis
    Conjunctival folliculosis
    Ocular rosacea
    Keratoconjunctivitis sicca (Sjögren's
      syndrome)
    Ocular pemphigus
    Erythema multiforme
    Dermatitis herpetiformis
    Epidermolysis bullosa
    Erythema nodosum
    Psoriasis
    Reiter's disease
    Superior limbic keratoconjunctivitis

BACTERIAL CONJUNCTIVITIS

Bacterial conjunctivitis is an extremely common disorder. It is usually acute but may become chronic. Pathologically it is characterized by conjunctival hyperemia and a subepithelial reaction consisting of fibrin and edema plus polymorphonuclear leukocytes, lymphocytes, and plasma cells. The number and type of cells depend upon the stage of the inflammation. Certain organisms tend to provoke specific tissue responses, such as follicle and papilla formation, membranes, ulcers, and granulomas. Histologically, follicles are nests of lymphocytes surrounded by a vascular network and having a germinal center containing

Table 6-1. Differential diagnosis of conjunctivitis.

| | Viral | Bacterial | | Fungal and Parasitic | Allergic |
		Purulent	Nonpurulent		
Discharge	Minimal	Profuse	Minimal	Minimal	Minimal
Tearing	Profuse	Moderate	Moderate	Minimal	Moderate
Itching	Minimal	Minimal	None	None	Marked
Injection	Generalized	Generalized	Localized	Localized	Generalized
Localized conjunctival lesions	None	None	Frequent	Frequent	None
Preauricular node	Common	Uncommon	Common	Common	None
Stained smear	Monocytes	Bacteria, PMN's	Bacteria, PMN's	Usually negative	Eosinophils
Associated sore throat and fever	Occasionally	Seldom	None*	None	None

*Diphtheritic conjunctivitis occurs only as a complication of diphtheria, and so the other manifestations of the disease are present also. It may be purulent or membranous.

lymphoblasts. Papillae are nodular elevations at the limbus or tarsus, where the conjunctiva is adherent to the underlying tissue; they are caused by subconjunctival exudation, forcing the epithelium into elevations. A conjunctival membrane consists of a superficial fibrinous layer connected to subconjunctival granulation tissue; when this membrane is removed, a raw bleeding surface is exposed.

Clinical Findings

A. Symptoms and Signs:

1. Pyogenic organisms - The pyogenic organisms listed on p 57 account for most cases of conjunctivitis in the USA. They produce bilateral irritation and injection, a purulent discharge with consequent sticking together of the lids upon awakening, and lid edema. The infection usually starts in one eye and is spread to the other eye by the hands. It may be spread from one person to another through towels, doorknobs, and other commonly used articles. Pus production in gonococcal conjunctivitis is unusually profuse. Pneumococcal conjunctivitis is often associated with subconjunctival hemorrhages. Conjunctival membranes may form in the lower palpebral area in streptococcal conjunctivitis.

"Pink eye" is pneumococcal conjunctivitis in temperate climates, Hemophilus aegyptius (Koch-Weeks bacillus) conjunctivitis in warm climates.

2. Nonpurulent types - The Morax-Axenfeld bacillus (Moraxella lacunata) causes a localized angular conjunctivitis associated with fissuring and dermatitis of the external canthi (fairly common) and a scanty conjunctival discharge.

Corynebacterium diphtheriae infection of the eye is very rare. It is characterized by a heavy, gray, bilateral palpebral conjunctival membrane inferiorly and superiorly; it seldom involves the cornea. In contrast to most other types of conjunctivitis, pain is a common symptom. The skin of the eyelids and face is also involved.

Pasteurella tularensis, Mycobacterium tuberculosis, and Treponema pallidum produce unilateral conjunctival nodules which tend to ulcerate and are associated with a palpable preauricular lymph node on the affected side. There is moderate localized injection and minimal discharge. These are extremely rare.

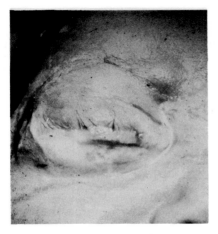

Fig 6-2. Gonorrheal conjunctivitis. Profuse purulent exudate. (Courtesy of P. Thygeson.)

Fig 6-3. Lancet-shaped Diplococcus pneumoniae in conjunctival smear from patient with purulent conjunctivitis. (Photo by Ben Goldfeller.)

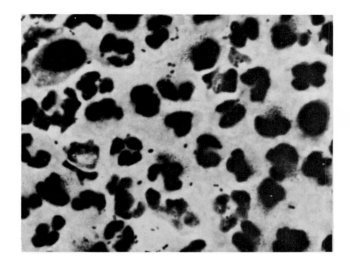

B. Laboratory Findings: In most cases of bacterial conjunctivitis the organisms can be identified by a stained smear of conjunctival scrapings. Cultures are necessary only if the diagnosis is in doubt or if antibiotic sensitivity studies are desired.

Complications and Sequelae

Chronic marginal blepharitis may occur if staphylococcal conjunctivitis is not cured.

Corneal ulceration may result from infection with Neisseria gonorrhoeae, Corynebacterium diphtheriae, or the Koch-Weeks bacillus. Toxic iritis may result from the presence in the anterior chamber of the soluble toxin produced by N gonorrhoeae. Conjunctival membrane formation is typical of diphtheritic and streptococcal conjunctivitis and may lead to obliteration of the lower fornices and corneal scarring.

Treatment

A. Pyogenic Organisms: Sulfonamide therapy should be tried first. Apply sulfacetamide sodium (Sodium Sulamyd®) or sulfisoxazole diethanolamine (Gantrisin Diethanolamine®) 4 times daily. If the conjunctivitis does not respond within 3 days, one of the tetracyclines or erythromycin should be applied in ointment form 5 times daily during the acute phase, decreasing the frequency of application gradually as the process subsides. Proteus vulgaris infection requires specific treatment with neomycin eye ointment 5 times daily. Saline or water irrigations of the conjunctival sac may be used as indicated. Instruction of the patient concerning personal hygiene to prevent spread of the disease is important.

For gonococcal conjunctivitis, systemic penicillin therapy is indicated in addition to local treatment with penicillin ointment, 1000 units/gm.

B. Morax-Axenfeld Bacillus: This organism is sensitive to local sulfonamides and antibiotics.

Course and Prognosis

Conjunctivitis caused by purulent organisms is almost always self-limited. Untreated, it lasts about 10-14 days; if properly treated, it lasts 1-3 days. The exceptions are streptococcal conjunctivitis, which may enter a chronic phase, and gonococcal conjunctivitis, which, when untreated, can cause corneal perforation and endophthalmitis.

VIRAL CONJUNCTIVITIS

Viral conjunctivitis is common. Many different viruses can cause conjunctivitis; some types are severe and debilitating, whereas others are relatively minor and self-limited.

ADENOVIRUS INFECTION

Pharyngoconjunctival Fever

Pharyngoconjunctival fever is characterized by fever of 101-104° F, sore throat, and a follicular conjunctivitis in one or both eyes. Bilateral or (less commonly) unilateral conjunctival discharge is minimal and the corneas are clear. A slight transient superficial keratitis may occur. Preauricular lymphadenopathy may be present. Any of the symptoms may occur singly.

Pharyngoconjunctival fever is caused by type 3 or, less commonly, type 7 of the adenovirus group. The virus can be recognized on tissue culture of conjunctival scrapings by its cytotropic effect on HeLa cells. The diagnosis can also be made serologically by demonstrating a rising titer of neutralizing antibody to the virus during the disease. However, clinical diagnosis is more practical, and laboratory studies are seldom necessary.

This condition is more common in children than adults. Transmission is often traceable to contaminated water in swimming pools.

No specific treatment is available. Sulfonamide ophthalmic ointment should be prescribed locally to prevent secondary bacterial infection. The conjunctivitis is self-limited, usually lasting about 10 days.

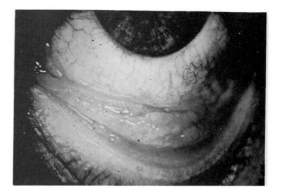

Fig 6-4. Acute follicular conjunctivitis due to adenovirus type 3. (Courtesy of P. Thygeson.)

Epidemic Keratoconjunctivitis

The virus of epidemic keratoconjunctivitis has been identified as type 8 of the adenovirus group. The disease is characterized clinically by unilateral injection, moderate pain, and tearing. There is no purulent discharge, but conjunctival inflammation is pronounced and a large preauricular lymph node is always present. A conjunctival membrane sometimes forms (Fig 6-5). Corneal infiltrates, which distinguish the disease from other types of conjunctivitis, occur in 50% of cases. They are round, centrally located and subepithelial, and usually appear 6-10 days after the onset of the conjunctival inflammation. Corneal sensitivity is not affected. There are no bacteria in the conjunctival smear, but mononuclear cells are numerous. The virus can be identified by serologic methods from material taken from the conjunctival surface. The virus tends to stick to fingers and instruments and will grow in many eye solutions. The physician should wash his hands between examinations and take precautions to prevent the spread of the virus by contamination of instruments. The tonometer footplate should be cleaned with a sterile solution after every use; after use on a red eye, tonometers should be sterilized in flame or in a special hot air tonometer sterilizer. (Epidemic keratoconjunctivitis is the only known serious eye disease transmitted during the course of tonometry.)

Epidemic keratoconjunctivitis in adults is strictly a local disease. In children there may be systemic symptoms of viral infection, eg, fever and sore throat.

Treatment consists of instillation of sulfonamide ointment 4 times daily to prevent secondary bacterial invasion. The acute symptoms disappear in 2-3 weeks, and the conjunctiva and cornea gradually return to normal during the next several weeks. Most patients have enough ocular discomfort to prevent them from working for 2-3 weeks after the onset of symptoms.

HERPES SIMPLEX CONJUNCTIVITIS

Conjunctivitis due to infection with herpes simplex virus is an uncommon infection characterized by unilateral injection, irritation, and mild photophobia. It occurs only in primary (first attack) herpes simplex, usually in association with herpes simplex keratitis. The upper and lower conjunctivas are red, an enlarged preauricular node is present, and vesicular lesions appear on the lids. Polymorphonuclear leukocytes are present in the conjunctival smear. No bacteria are found. The virus can be isolated by scratching a rabbit's cornea with an instrument contaminated with conjunctival exudate or by tissue culture on an egg membrane. The pathologic signs of inflammation are not characteristic.

Treatment is with idoxuridine ointment 4 times daily and sulfonamide locally as necessary to prevent secondary bacterial infection. The use of steroids is contraindicated since they have the effect of aggravating herpes simplex infections. Uncomplicated cases clear in 7-10 days.

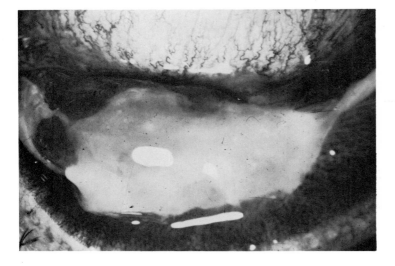

Fig 6-5. Epidemic keratoconjunctivitis. Thick white membrane in lower palpebral conjunctiva. (Courtesy of P. Thygeson.)

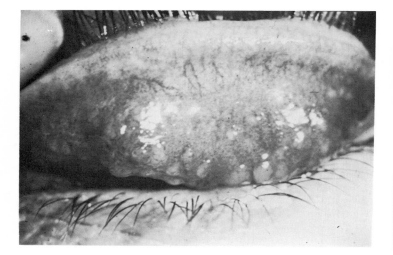

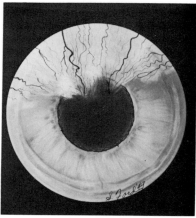

Fig 6-6. **Trachoma, stage II b.** Papillae and follicles in upper tarsal conjunctiva. (Courtesy of P. Thygeson.)

Fig 6-7. **Trachomatous pannus.** (Courtesy of P. Thygeson.)

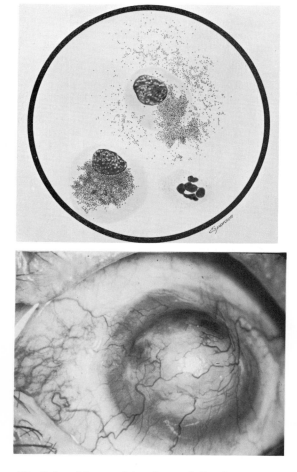

Fig 6-8. Cytoplasmic inclusion body in conjunctival epithelial cells in trachoma. Ruptured inclusion at right. Polymorphonuclear neutrophil (typical in conjunctival scrapings of trachoma) below. (Courtesy of P. Thygeson and C. Dawson.)

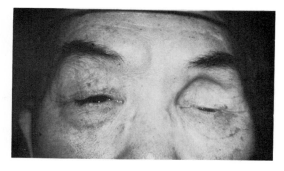

Fig 6-9. **Advanced trachoma following corneal ulceration.** (Courtesy of P. Thygeson.)

Fig 6-10. **Ptosis with an "S" shaped curve of lids associated with chronic trachoma.** (Courtesy of P. Thygeson.)

NEWCASTLE DISEASE CONJUNCTIVITIS

Newcastle disease conjunctivitis is a rare disorder characterized by pain, injection, tearing, and blurring of vision. It is usually unilateral and characteristically occurs following the handling of live Newcastle virus used in inoculating chickens, or after handling infected birds. The superior and inferior palpebral conjunctivas show a marked follicular reaction, and there may be associated superficial corneal opacities and lid edema. Conjunctival discharge is minimal. Fever and headache are usually present also. There are numerous mononuclear cells but no bacteria in the conjunctival smear. The virus of Newcastle disease can be isolated, but this is not necessary if the diagnosis can be made on clinical grounds.

Treatment consists of instillation of sulfonamide ointment 4 times daily to prevent secondary bacterial infection. The disease runs its course in 10-14 days. There are no complications.

MOLLUSCUM CONTAGIOSUM

In conjunctivitis due to molluscum contagiosum there is a recurrent follicular unilateral conjunctival inflammation secondary to one or more molluscum nodules on either the upper or lower lid, or both. No bacteria are present in the conjunctival smear. Diagnosis is made by excisional biopsy. Excision of the nodules results in cure.

CONJUNCTIVITIS DUE TO CHLAMYDIAE*

TRACHOMA

Trachoma is the most common human disease of any kind; approximately 500,000,000 people suffer from it. It affects all races, but is not found in American Negroes, Eskimos,

---

*The chlamydiae are obligate intracellular parasites which cause trachoma, inclusion conjunctivitis, LGV, and psittacosis. The term "TRIC" is no longer being used. Chlamydiae are probably bacteria lacking some important metabolic properties which restrict them to an intracellular existence.

or American Seminole Indians. It is rampant in poor economic areas where bathing facilities are usually inadequate and is consequently extremely common in China and India. It is endemic in the countries bordering the Mediterranean, particularly Egypt. Trachoma is rare in the USA except among the Southwestern American Indian population, in whom it is still prevalent. Trachoma is always bilateral.

Trachoma has a special affinity for the eye and may also affect the genitourinary tract epithelium. Spread is by direct contact. Parents commonly transfer the disease to their children, who may have the disease for many years (sometimes for life). Family contacts should be investigated and treated.

The agent lives in the conjunctival and corneal epithelium and produces a soluble toxin which passes into the subepithelial area, causing a lymphocytic reaction which terminates in necrosis and cicatrization of the palpebral conjunctiva, particularly over the upper tarsi. During the active stage there is follicular and papillary hypertrophy of the superficial conjunctiva. The same pathologic process involves the cornea to varying degrees. The upper limbus is always involved, and scarring of the entire cornea occurs in severe cases.

Clinical Findings

Mild itching and irritation are the principal symptoms. If the process continues, blurring of vision and increasing discomfort will occur. Some people harbor the disease for a lifetime without severe distress as long as secondary bacterial infection does not occur.

The progress of the disease has been divided into 4 stages by MacCallan: In stage I (incipient trachoma), immature follicles are present, particularly in the upper tarsal conjunctiva, and there is incipient pannus at 12 o'clock. Stage II (established trachoma) is divided into type (a), in which follicular hypertrophy is predominant, and type (b), in which papillary hypertrophy is predominant ("acute trachoma"). Stage III is characterized by early conjunctival scarring, visible clinically as fine white lines, in the subepithelial areas of the conjunctiva, and increase in size of the corneal pannus. In stage IV there is smooth scarring of the tarsal conjunctiva and the vascular pannus becomes inactive.

All of the signs of trachoma are much more severe in the upper than the lower conjunctiva. Pannus appears early in the disease, but may be visible in the initial stages only upon magnification with the loupe or slit lamp. A marked trachomatous pannus in the 12 o'clock position is shown in Fig 6-7.

Smears of conjunctival epithelial scrapings stained with Giemsa's stain show inclusion bodies in the epithelial cells (Fig 6-8) in a small percentage of mild chronic cases and in a high percentage of cases of acute and subacute trachoma. There is a polymorphonuclear exudate in the early stages. Leber cells (large macrophages containing necrotic material) are diagnostic but not always present. They are found in material expressed from the conjunctival follicles.

The agent of trachoma (Chlamydia trachomatis) can be easily grown in the yolk sac of the developing chick embryo. The results of large-scale trials of vaccine in several countries have been equivocal.

Differential Diagnosis

Inclusion conjunctivitis is differentiated by the absence of pannus and scarring and the greater inflammatory reaction in the lower rather than in the upper palpebral conjunctiva.

Vernal conjunctivitis produces cobblestone papillae and eosinophils on the smear. Neither of these signs is present in trachoma.

Complications and Sequelae

Secondary bacterial conjunctivitis increases the hazard of corneal ulceration. If this occurs, corneal scarring is more severe. Without corneal ulceration, blindness does not usually occur in trachoma.

Entropion of the upper and lower lids due to the scarred tarsi, with consequent trichiasis, causes constant corneal irritation unless the entropion is corrected. Xerosis may occur as a result of scarring of the lacrimal gland and ducts. Ptosis and dacryocystitis are occasional complications.

Treatment

Treatment should be started on the basis of clinical findings without waiting for laboratory confirmation. Medical treatment consists of a 3-week course of oral sulfonamide, eg, trisulfapyrimidines, 4 gm daily (adult dosage), observing the patient closely for signs of toxicity. If toxicity develops or the patient is sensitive to sulfonamides, give one of the tetracyclines, 250 mg 4 times daily for 3 weeks. (**Caution:** Do not give tetracyclines during pregnancy or to young children, and do not use old preparations.) Oral therapy acts by releasing the drug in the tears.

Topical therapy is much less satisfactory than oral sulfonamides or tetracyclines. When used, it consists of instilling erythromycin or tetracycline ointment 4 times daily.

Hygienic measures are of great importance both in prevention and treatment.

Corneal scarring may require corneal transplantation. Entropion and trichiasis require plastic surgery to evert the lids. Dacry-

ocystectomy may be required if a scarred lacrimal drainage system becomes a problem due to secondary infection.

Course and Prognosis

Without treatment, some degree of permanent corneal and conjunctival scarring is inevitable. The prognosis is excellent when treatment is given early. About 20,000,000 people in the world are blind as a result of trachoma.

INCLUSION CONJUNCTIVITIS
(Inclusion Blennorrhea)

Inclusion conjunctivitis is an uncommon infection characterized clinically by bilateral conjunctival redness and a profuse exudate. Since there is a reservoir of the virus in the genitourinary tract (male urethra and female cervix), the disease is most common in newborns. Transmission in adults is also now established as being from the genitourinary tract to the eye, so in this sense it is a venereal disease. The causative agent is now called Chlamydia oculogenitalis. Eye-to-eye transmission is rare. In adults there are numerous papillae and follicles in the tarsal conjunctivas, more pronounced in the lower. Since the newborn conjunctiva does not form follicles, the appearance of the reddened conjunctivas in newborns is nonspecific. There are no bacteria in the smears, but numerous basophilic inclusion bodies are found in the conjunctival epithelial cells. Pathologically, there are many papillae and a dense cellular infiltration in the subepithelial tissues.

Inclusion conjunctivitis is at times mistaken for trachoma. Like trachoma, it is characterized by many conjunctival follicles and papillae, and on stained conjunctival smears the inclusion bodies are indistinguishable. However, the corneal changes are much different. In most cases of adult inclusion conjunctivitis, only epithelial keratitis develops. Subepithelial opacities may occur which are similar to those seen in epidemic keratoconjunctivitis. In long-standing cases (weeks to months) there may be a micropannus but never any corneal scarring. In trachoma, the upper tarsal conjunctiva is more involved than the lower.

In babies, 1% tetracycline drops in oil instilled 5-6 times daily for 2-3 weeks is very effective. In adults, the local treatment is best supplemented by tetracycline, 1-1.5 gm daily orally for 2-3 weeks. Recurrences are rare. There are no complications, and with treatment the disease can be cured in one week. If not treated, inclusion conjunctivitis persists 3 months to one year. There is never any visual loss. In 15% of patients, otitis media develops on the affected side.

LYMPHOGRANULOMA VENEREUM CONJUNCTIVITIS

Conjunctivitis is a rare manifestation of systemic lymphogranuloma venereum. The eye is red and puffy. There is moderate unilateral conjunctival injection, slight conjunctival discharge, and extreme edema of the upper and lower lids. The preauricular, parotid, and submaxillary lymph glands are enlarged on the affected side. Chlamydia lymphogranulomatis may be recovered by inoculating mouse brains or tissue cultures with conjunctival scrapings. The Frei test is positive.

Treatment is with a broad-spectrum antibiotic locally and systemically for 3-4 weeks. The response is good.

ALLERGIC CONJUNCTIVITIS

CONJUNCTIVITIS ASSOCIATED WITH HAY FEVER

A mild nonspecific conjunctival inflammation is commonly associated with hay fever (allergic rhinitis). Clinical findings include itching, mild photophobia, and mild injection of the palpebral and bulbar conjunctivas, plus a scanty ropy discharge. Occasional eosinophils are found in smears of the conjunctival scrapings. There are no conjunctival papillae or follicles.

Treatment consists of instillation of local steroids during the acute phase. Cold compresses may be applied to relieve symptoms. The response to treatment is good, but recurrences are common.

VERNAL CONJUNCTIVITIS

Vernal conjunctivitis is an uncommon bilateral allergic disease which usually begins in the prepubertal years and lasts 5-10 years.

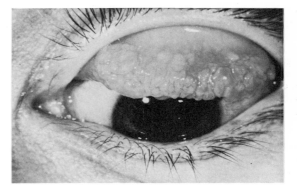

Fig 6-11. Vernal conjunctivitis. "Cobblestone" papillae in superior tarsal conjunctiva. (Courtesy of P. Thygeson.)

The specific allergen is not known. People with vernal conjunctivitis often become allergic to other things, particularly grass pollens. This type of conjunctivitis is less common in temperate than in warm climates and is almost nonexistent in cold climates.

Clinical Findings

Symptoms are always more severe in spring and summer. The patient complains of extreme itching. There are many giant papillae in the palpebral conjunctiva, particularly the upper (Fig 6-11), which give a typical cobblestone appearance. A stringy conjunctival discharge and a milky conjunctival pseudomembrane are frequently present. If there is papillary hypertrophy in the region of the corneoscleral junction, the condition is known as **limbal vernal conjunctivitis.** Many eosinophils are found in a smear of the conjunctival exudate stained with Giemsa's stain. Between attacks, mast cells are found on the stained conjunctival smear but no eosinophils.

Complications and Sequelae

Slight to total pannus is an unusual complication. Superficial corneal ulcers may form with subsequent scarring. A diffuse epithelial keratitis occasionally occurs.

Treatment

Instill corticosteroid solution, 2 drops every 2 hours during the day in the acute phase, and apply cold water compresses for 20 minutes 4 times daily. The patient must be observed closely for the complications of the treatment even more than of the disease since treatment may have to be continued for weeks or months. Herpes simplex keratitis, cataract, and glaucoma are the most likely complications, fungal overgrowth a less common complication of local corticosteroid therapy.

Desensitization to grass pollens helps in a small percentage of cases.

A cool climate is beneficial, or sleeping in a cool air-conditioned room.

Course and Prognosis

Recurrences are common, particularly in the spring. The episodes are more easily combated since the advent of corticosteroid therapy. The papillae eventually disappear completely, leaving no scars.

PHLYCTENULAR KERATOCONJUNCTIVITIS

Phlyctenular keratoconjunctivitis is associated with malnutrition, tuberculosis, or both. It is extremely common among Eskimo children in Alaska. The essential lesion, the phlyctenule, is a concentration of lymphocytes at the limbus which occurs as an allergic reaction to the tubercle bacillus or, in rare cases, to other organisms causing granulomatous infections (eg, Coccidioides immitis).

Photophobia is intense. The phlyctenules occur typically in the limbal areas of both eyes, but may be seen in the cornea itself. They are red, elevated, and wedge-shaped, with the apex toward the central cornea, and vary widely in number and size.

Slight to complete corneal scarring may develop (Fig 6-12). Salzmann's nodular dystrophy is a frequent complication (see p 86).

Instill a corticosteroid suspension, 2 drops in each eye every 2 hours, during the acute phase. Desensitization procedures are indicated with tuberculin if the patient is tuberculin-positive. Treat pulmonary tuberculosis if present. A well balanced diet is highly important. Secondary bacterial infection must be controlled. If the corneal scarring becomes marked, corneal transplant is indicated.

Recurrences are common if the basic causes are not eliminated.

CHEMICAL CONJUNCTIVITIS

Chemical conjunctivitis is a fairly common ocular condition, particularly as an occupational hazard among men. Any irritating substance which enters the conjunctival sac may cause conjunctivitis. Some common irritants are soap, fertilizers, deodorants, hair sprays, tobacco, acids and alkalies, and irritating drugs intentionally or unintentionally used by physicians. Silver nitrate instilled in infants' eyes at birth as an anti-infective agent is a common cause of chemical conjunctivitis in newborns (see p 72). In certain sections of the world, smog has become the commonest cause of mild chemical conjunctivitis. The specific irritant in smog has not been positively identified, and the treatment is nonspecific. There are no permanent ocular effects.

Acids precipitate the proteins in the tissues and so produce their effect immediately;

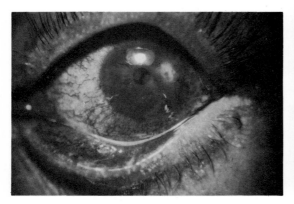

Fig 6-12. Post-phlyctenulosis. Vascularized scar in temporal portion of left cornea.

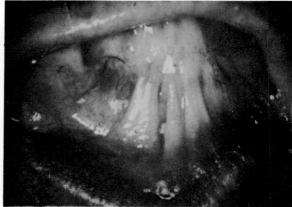

Fig 6-13. Severe symblepharon following an alkali burn of conjunctiva and cornea. (Courtesy of J. Crawford and S. Aiken.)

but proteins are not precipitated by alkalies, which tend to linger in the conjunctival tissues and continue to inflict damage over a period of hours to days.

Pain, injection, photophobia, and blepharospasm are the main symptoms. A history of exposure can usually be elicited. Adhesion between the bulbar and palpebral conjunctivas (symblepharon) and corneal leukoma are more likely to occur if the offending agent is an alkali.

Immediate irrigation of the conjunctival sac with water or saline solution is most important. Do not use chemical antidotes. Steroid solution, at least 2 drops every hour during the acute phase, will decrease inflammation and fibrosis. General symptomatic measures include cold compresses for 20 minutes every hour; atropine, 1%, 2 drops twice daily; and systemic analgesics as indicated. Corneal transplant may be required for corneal scarring, and a conjunctival plastic operation for symblepharon.

If the proper treatment is started immediately, the prognosis is good. If treatment is delayed, permanent conjunctival and corneal scarring may result.

FUNGAL CONJUNCTIVITIS

CANDIDIASIS
(Ocular Candidiasis, Thrush of Eye)

Candida albicans is a rare cause of conjunctivitis. The conjunctivitis is always secondary to infection of other mucous membranes of the body. Clinically, one sees a thin gray membrane involving the upper and lower palpebral conjunctivas. Pathologically, there is nonspecific inflammatory reaction in the subepithelial tissues and necrosis of the conjunctival epithelium. The ocular condition clears with the disappearance of the candidal infection elsewhere in the body. Corneal ulcer may occur.

The antifungal drug of choice is amphotericin B (Fungizone®), 0.15% solution, 2 drops in each eye every 1-2 hours night and day depending on the severity of the ulcer.

LEPTOTRICHOSIS

This is a fairly common, low-grade, nodular, unilateral conjunctivitis due to infection with Leptotrichia buccalis. It is more common in children and in those who come in close contact with cats, which harbor the organism in their mouths. The excised conjunctival nodule shows the general picture of necrosis. There are numerous macrophages containing chromatin.

Symptoms and signs consist of slight injection and irritation, a moderately large nodule on the upper or lower tarsal conjunctiva, an enlarged preauricular node on the affected side, and low-grade fever for several weeks. The surrounding bulbar and palpebral conjunctiva is only slightly infected.

Pathologic examination is necessary to differentiate this condition in its nodular form from a granuloma following an infected chalazion; other causes of nodular conjunctivitis, such as tularemia, syphilis, and tuberculosis, can be diagnosed by their tendency to ulcerate.

Treatment consists of excision of the conjunctival nodule, followed by instillation of a sulfonamide 4 times a day. Close contact with cats must be avoided.

Untreated, the disease lasts about 3 months. The nodule disappears completely, leaving no scar.

CONJUNCTIVITIS DUE TO ANIMAL PARASITES

NEMATODES
(Roundworms)

Onchocerca Volvulus

Ocular infestation with this parasite is a major cause of blindness ("river blindness") in Africa and Central America. It invades the skin of the neck and scalp, causing tumors; from these tumors the parasite migrates to the cornea, uveal tract, and retina as well as the conjunctiva. The scalp nodules should be excised. Chemotherapy with diethylcarbamazine (Hetrazan®) should be tried. Without treatment, the prognosis is grave.

Loa Loa (Filaria Loa, "Eye Worm")

Infestation of the conjunctiva and lids with this parasite is occasionally seen in the natives of tropical West Africa and in missionaries returning to the USA. The anterior chamber and vitreous may be invaded, but Loa loa rarely migrates to the retina. Systemic chemotherapy with diethylcarbamazine (Hetrazan®) is the treatment of choice.

Wuchereria Bancrofti

This parasite may enter the conjunctiva and lids, producing extreme edema similar to the elephantiasis seen elsewhere in the body. If the parasite invades the anterior chamber, the eye may be destroyed.

Thelazia Californiensis and Thelazia Callipaeda

The natural habitat of this roundworm is in herbivorous animals, but accidental infection of the human conjunctival sac and lacrimal apparatus may occur. Three cases have been reported in the USA. Thelazia californiensis causes a nonpurulent conjunctivitis, but its counterpart, Thelazia callipaeda (Oriental eye worm), penetrates and causes blindness.

Trichinella Spiralis

This parasite occasionally localizes in the extraocular muscles and produces conjunctival and lid edema. The worm does not enter the eyeball. The associated eosinophilia, fever, and muscular pain are helpful in the diagnosis.

Ascaris Lumbricoides (Butcher's Conjunctivitis)

Ascaris larvas cause a rare type of violent toxic conjunctivitis. The worms are spread by accidental contamination to butchers and persons performing postmortem examinations. It is postulated that the poison exuded by the larvas has a direct action on the conjunctival vessels. The reaction varies in intensity, but it typically produces extreme chemosis and lid edema. Treatment is by mechanical removal of the organism.

TREMATODES
(Flukes)

Schistosoma Haematobium

This parasitic disease is endemic in Egypt and produces granulomatous conjunctival lesions. The diagnosis is by biopsy and microscopic examination. Treatment consists of excision of the conjunctival granulomas.

CESTODES
(Tapeworms)

Taenia Solium

This parasite occasionally causes conjunctivitis but more frequently invades the retina, choroid, or vitreous to produce ocular cysticercosis. Infection is relatively common in Mexico and South America. Mechanical removal of the parasite from the eye is sometimes possible.

ARTHROPODS

Phthirus Pubis (Pediculus Pubis, Pubic Louse)

These parasites and their eggs form nits which attach themselves to the lashes or to the eyebrows and produce an irritating conjunctivitis. Chemicals are often recommended for treatment, but mechanical removal is usually necessary. Family contacts should be investigated and treated.

Ocular Myiasis

Conjunctival infestation with fly larvas occurs frequently in the tropics but is rare in the USA. Several species of flies have been incriminated. Larvas invade the conjunctival sac and produce a nonspecific inflammatory reaction. If they spread throughout the eye and orbit, the inflammatory reaction and eventual necrosis become severe. Destruction of the orbital contents and bony walls of the orbit with invasion of the meninges may occur.

Extreme itching and irritation are the cardinal symptoms. The conjunctivas are red and excoriated. Numerous elongated white larvas are seen, especially in the fornices.

Treatment consists of mechanical removal of the larvas after first instilling cocaine (10%), which has a paralyzing effect upon them. If the larvas can be removed when they are few in number, the course of the disease is automatically terminated. If they are allowed to multiply, the prognosis is extremely poor inasmuch as they invade the tissues out of reach of any form of treatment. In such cases, destruction of the bony orbital wall and its contents frequently occurs.

CONJUNCTIVITIS OF UNKNOWN ETIOLOGY

CHRONIC FOLLICULAR CONJUNCTIVITIS
(Orphan's Conjunctivitis)

This is a transmissible, mild bilateral disease of childhood characterized by numerous follicles in the upper and lower palpebral conjunctivas. There is a scanty conjunctival discharge and minimal inflammation. There are no complications. Treatment is ineffective. The average duration of the disease is 2-3 years.

A variation of chronic follicular conjunctivitis is drug-induced follicular conjunctivitis due to prolonged administration of miotics (especially physostigmine and isoflurophate) in glaucoma therapy.

CONJUNCTIVAL FOLLICULOSIS

Conjunctival folliculosis is a fairly common benign, bilateral, noninflammatory disorder characterized by follicular hypertrophy of the palpebral conjunctivas. It is more common in children. Symptoms are minimal. The follicles are more numerous in the lower palpebral conjunctivas. The complete lack of inflammation and the inferior involvement differentiate it from chronic follicular conjunctivitis. There are no complications.

No treatment is available. The disease runs its course in about 2-3 years.

OCULAR ROSACEA

Ocular rosacea is an uncommon complication of facial rosacea. It usually manifests itself as a blepharoconjunctivitis. Small gray nodules may be present on the bulbar conjunctiva. Pathologically, these consist of lymphocytes and epithelioid cells. The patient complains of mild injection and irritation. Marginal corneal ulceration is sometimes associated. Phlyctenular keratoconjunctivitis is differentiated from ocular rosacea by the presence of extreme photophobia, the absence of facial rosacea, and the favorable response to cortisone. If marginal corneal ulceration occurs, vascular infiltrates may follow and persist. Secondary staphylococcal conjunctivitis is a frequent complication.

Treatment of ocular rosacea consists of elimination of foods which cause dilatation of the facial vessels and treatment of the secondary staphylococcal infection, if present. Systemic and local steroids should be tried.

The disease is chronic, recurrences are common, and the response to treatment is generally poor. If the cornea is not involved, the visual prognosis is good. The corneal lesions tend to recur and progress, and vision grows steadily worse over a period of years if the cornea is affected.

KERATOCONJUNCTIVITIS SICCA

Keratoconjunctivitis sicca is an uncommon chronic bilateral conjunctivitis of unknown cause which occurs characteristically in postmenopausal women, often as part of Sjögren's syndrome (see Chapter 18). It is rarely seen in young women, or in men at any age. The symptoms are usually more severe than the inflammatory signs would suggest, and treatment is seldom more than symptomatic.

Pathologic examination reveals cellular infiltration of the conjunctiva, mild keratinization of the conjunctival and corneal epithelium, and degenerative changes in the lacrimal gland.

The patient complains of dry eyes and mouth, constant ocular irritation, slightly blurred vision, and a stringy, sticky discharge. Physical examination reveals a nonspecific diffuse inflammation of the conjunctiva (particularly the bulbar conjunctiva), filamentary keratitis, and a scanty, stringy, mucoid conjunctival discharge. Visual acuity is slightly diminished. Lacrimal secretion is decreased, as may be demonstrated by observing the low degree of wetting when filter papers are inserted into the conjunctival sacs (Schirmer test; see p 26).

Microscopic examination of the conjunctival and corneal scrapings reveals keratinization of the epithelium and considerable mucus but no leukocytes. The electrophoretic pattern of the tears shows decreased or absent lysozyme.

Major complications seldom occur. Corneal keratinization may be severe enough to impair vision.

Artificial tears containing methocel are helpful in most patients.

The condition usually lasts a lifetime with minor remissions and exacerbations.

BENIGN MUCOUS MEMBRANE PEMPHIGOID
(Ocular Pemphigus)

This is a rare form of bilateral conjunctivitis which may occur in a purely ophthalmic form but is usually associated with pemphigoid lesions of the nose, throat, and skin. It is believed to be due to a virus, but laboratory confirmation is lacking. The chronic form is much more common than the acute. Pathologically there is cicatrization of the conjunctiva, particularly in the lower fornix, and an irregular pannus. The patient complains of pain, irritation, and blurring of vision. There is a thick, ropy conjunctival exudate and shrinkage of the fornices, particularly the lower fornix. Vesicles and bullae are rare. The secretory ducts from the lacrimal and accessory lacrimal glands are eventually obliterated, and the lack of tears aggravates any corneal pathology.

In the early stages ocular pemphigus is differentiated from trachoma by the presence of a low-grade conjunctival eosinophilia, which is never seen in trachoma. Trachoma involves the upper cornea and palpebral conjunctivas, whereas the reverse is true of pemphigus.

No specific treatment is available. Sulfonamide ointment should be used to reduce the irritation.

The course is prolonged, and the prognosis is poor. Blindness due to complete corneal scarring is the usual end result.

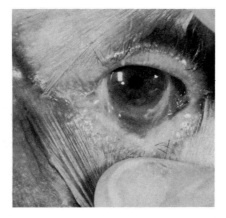

Fig 6-14. Benign mucous membrane pemphigoid. (Courtesy of M. Quickert.)

ERYTHEMA MULTIFORME BULLOSUM

Bilateral conjunctivitis is a common complication of erythema multiforme. It may simulate bacterial conjunctivitis or produce extensive conjunctival membranes which ultimately invade the corneas and canaliculi. Erythema multiforme, along with epidemic keratoconjunctivitis, is one of the 2 most common causes of membranous conjunctivitis. Pain and photophobia are common symptoms. The typical skin and mucous membrane lesions differentiate it from pemphigus. Secondary bacterial infection is rare.

Both local and systemic steroids are helpful in shortening the course of the disease and in preventing permanent scarring of the conjunctivas, corneas, and canaliculi.

The course is prolonged, and recurrences are common. Recovery may be complete, or blindness may occur as a result of corneal scarring.

DERMATITIS HERPETIFORMIS AND EPIDERMOLYSIS BULLOSA

These 2 uncommon skin conditions are occasionally complicated by membranous conjunctivitis with subsequent shrinkage of the conjunctiva. Dermatitis herpetiformis does not ordinarily affect the cornea, but epidermolysis bullosa sometimes produces severe corneal ulceration with subsequent scarring. Dermatitis herpetiformis may produce conjunctival cicatrization, closing the ducts from the lacrimal gland and resulting in xerosis.

No specific treatment is available for either condition.

ERYTHEMA NODOSUM

Bulbar conjunctival nodules are occasionally seen in association with erythema nodosum. The conjunctival nodules disappear simultaneously with the cutaneous lesions.

PSORIASIS

This skin disease may be complicated by a bacterial type of conjunctivitis which may produce conjunctival membranes plus numerous subepithelial corneal infiltrates often followed by corneal ulceration. The conjunctival and corneal lesions vary with the skin lesions and are not affected by specific treatment. There are no serious permanent ocular effects.

REITER'S DISEASE

A mild, nonspecific, bilateral conjunctivitis is present as a part of the syndrome of urethritis, polyarthritis, conjunctivitis, and fever. Reiter's disease occurs only in young men. There is no relation to gonorrhea. No specific organisms have definitely been established as causes, but PPLO (Eaton agent) and TRIC agent have been isolated in a few cases. The conjunctivitis is sometimes complicated by iritis (anterior uveitis), is not affected by treatment, and clears in 2 to 3 weeks, usually before the general symptoms disappear.

SUPERIOR LIMBIC KERATOCONJUNCTIVITIS

This is an unusual bilateral papillary keratoconjunctivitis involving the upper tarsus. It is characterized by hyperemia, punctate keratitis, filaments, a micropannus, and thickening of the epithelium. When scrapings are examined microscopically, keratinization of the epithelial cells is the only finding.

Treating the area occasionally with 1% silver nitrate helps relieve symptoms in some patients, but in general the treatment is unsatisfactory.

DEGENERATIVE DISEASES OF THE CONJUNCTIVA

PINGUECULA

Pinguecula is extremely common in adults. It is manifested by a yellow nodule on either side of the cornea (more commonly on the nasal side) in the area of the lid fissure. The nodules rarely grow, but inflammation is common. Microscopically, they consist of hyaline and yellow elastic tissue. No treatment is indicated.

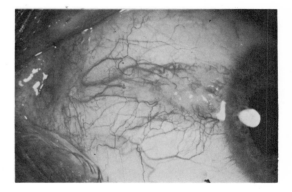

Fig 6-15. Pinguecula. (Courtesy of A. Rosenberg.)

PTERYGIUM

Pterygium is a fleshy, bilateral, triangular encroachment of a pinguecula onto the cornea. It always occurs nasally. Pterygiums are often erroneously referred to by patients as cataracts.

Pterygium is thought to be an irritative phenomenon, as it is common in farmers and others who spend a large part of their lives out of doors in sunny, dusty, or sandy windblown areas. The pathologic findings in the conjunctiva are the same as those of pinguecula. In the cornea there is replacement of the epithelium and Bowman's membrane by the hyaline and elastic tissue.

If the pterygium is enlarging, or produces a cosmetic blemish or visual disturbance, it should be removed surgically, taking care to remove a small portion of superficial clear cornea beyond the area of corneal encroachment.

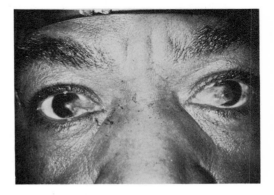

Fig 6-16. Bilateral pterygiums, advanced. (Courtesy of A. Rosenberg.)

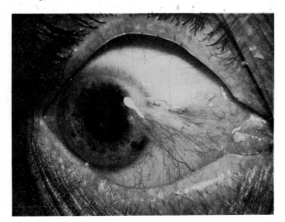

Fig 6-17. Pterygium, right eye.
(Photo by Diane Beeston.)

LYMPHANGIECTASIS

Lymphangiectasis is characterized by small, clear, tortuous, localized dilatations in the conjunctiva. They are merely dilated lymph vessels, and no treatment is indicated unless they are irritating or cosmetically objectionable, in which case they can be cauterized or excised.

LITHIASIS

Conjunctival lithiasis is characterized by small white areas of calcareous deposits in the palpebral conjunctiva. They can be excised if they irritate the cornea.

MISCELLANEOUS DISORDERS OF THE CONJUNCTIVA

SUBCONJUNCTIVAL HEMORRHAGE

This common disorder may occur spontaneously, usually in only one eye, in any age group. Because of the sudden onset and bright red appearance, the patient is usually alarmed. The hemorrhage is caused by the rupture of a small conjunctival vessel, sometimes preceded by a bout of severe coughing or sneezing.

There is no treatment, and the hemorrhage usually absorbs in about 2-3 weeks. The best treatment is reassurance.

In rare instances the hemorrhages are bilateral or recurrent, in which case blood dyscrasias should be ruled out.

OPHTHALMIA NEONATORUM

Ophthalmia neonatorum is any inflammation or infection of the conjunctiva in the newborn. Various types have already been discussed. The most common forms are chemical (silver nitrate) conjunctivitis and staphylococcal, pneumococcal, gonococcal, and inclusion conjunctivitis.

The time of onset is an important factor in diagnosis. Conjunctivitis appearing during the first 24 hours is probably due to silver nitrate. Conjunctivitis which has its onset during the 2nd-5th days is probably due to staphylococci, pneumococci, or gonococci. Inclusion conjunctivitis appears in 5-10 days after birth.

Diagnosis is confirmed by microscopic examination of stained material from a smear of the conjunctival scrapings. Cultures should be taken if the specific cause is in doubt.

Silver nitrate conjunctivitis is treated with sulfonamide and steroid ointments or drops.

Prevention
Bacterial conjunctivitis in newborn infants may be prevented by instilling silver nitrate solution (1%) into the conjunctival sac of each eye immediately after birth. Inadvertent instillation of more concentrated silver nitrate solutions will cause significant permanent corneal scarring, and even the 1% solution frequently causes chemical conjunctivitis; for this reason many ophthalmologists recommend that penicillin may be employed instead. However, penicillin prophylaxis may favor the emergence of penicillin-resistant strains of staphylococci in the nursery. Silver nitrate prophylaxis is legally required in many states and is the only method of prophylaxis approved by the FDA.

Bibliography

Abboud, I. A. , & L. S. Hanna: Ocular fungus. Brit J Ophth **54**:477-83, 1970.

Allansmith, M. , & D. Hutchison: Immunoglobulins in the conjunctiva. Immunology **12**:225-30, 1967.

Allansmith, M. R. , & G. R. O'Connor: Immunoglobulins: Structure, function and relation to the eye. Survey Ophth **14**:367-401, 1970.

Barsam, P. C. : Specific prophylaxis of gonorrheal ophthalmia neonatorum. A review. New England J Med **274**:731-4, 1966.

Bietti, G. B. , & others: Results of large-scale vaccination against trachoma in East Africa (Ethiopia), 1960-65. Am J Ophth **61**:1010-29, 1966.

Collier, L. H. , Duke-Elder, S. , & B. R. Jones: Experimental trachoma produced by cultured virus. Part II. Brit J Ophth **44**:65-88, 1960.

Conference on Trachoma and Allied Diseases. Am J Ophth **63**:1027-657, 1967.

Dawson, C. R. : Epidemic Koch-Weeks conjunctivitis and trachoma in the Coachella Valley of California. Am J Ophth **49**:801-8, 1960.

Dawson, C. , & others: Infection due to adenovirus type 8 in the United States. II. Community-wide infection with adenovirus type 8. New England J Med **268**:1034-7, 1963.

Drug and Therapeutic Information, Inc. : Prophylaxis of gonococcal ophthalmia. Medical Letter **12**:38, 1970.

Gordon, D. M. : Gentamicin sulfate in external eye infections. Am J Ophth **69**:300-6, 1970.

Kazdan, J. J. , Schachter, J. , & M. Okumoto: Inclusion conjunctivitis. Am J Ophth **64**:116-24, 1967.

Mordhorst, C. H. , & C. Dawson: Sequelae of neonatal inclusion conjunctivitis and associated disease in parents. Am J Ophth **71**:861-7, 1971.

Nakhla, L. S. , Al-Hussaini, M. K. , & A. A. W. Shokeir: Acute bacterial conjunctivitis. Brit J Ophth **54**:540-7, 1970.

Neumann, E. , & others: A review of four hundred cases of vernal conjunctivitis. Am J Ophth **47**:166-71, 1959.

Ostler, H. B. , & others: Reiter's syndrome. Am J Ophth **71**:986-91, 1971.

Sexton, R. R. : Eyelids, lacrimal apparatus, and conjunctiva. Annual Review. Arch Ophth **83**:379-96, 1971.

T'ang Fei-Fan, & others: Studies on the etiology of trachoma with special reference to isolation of the virus in chick embryo. Chinese MJ **75**:429-46, 1957.

Thygeson, P. : Published writings of Phillips Thygeson. Am J Ophth (Thygeson Proceedings) **34**:5-6, 1951.

Thygeson, P. : Trachoma Manual and Atlas. U. S. Department of Health, Education, and Welfare, 1958.

Thygeson, P. : Viral infections of the eye and adnexa. Survey Ophth **3**:568-83, 1958.

Thygeson, P. : Trachoma Virus. Chap. 23, pp. 640-55, in: Diagnostic Procedures for Viral and Rickettsial Diseases, 3rd ed. American Public Health Association, 1964.

Thygeson, P. : Historical review of oculogenital disease. Am J Ophth **71**:975-85, 1971.

Thygeson, P. , & C. R. Dawson: Trachoma and follicular conjunctivitis in children. Arch Ophth **75**:3-12, 1966.

Thygeson, P. , & S. J. Kimura: Chronic conjunctivitis. Tr Am Acad Ophth **67**:494-517, 1963.

7...
Cornea and Sclera

I. CORNEA

Anatomy and Functions

The cornea is a transparent and avascular tissue comparable in size and structure to the crystal in a small wrist watch. At the scleral junction (limbus) there is a circumferential depression, the scleral sulcus.

The cornea functions as a refracting and protective "window" membrane through which light rays pass en route to the retina. It has a refractive power equivalent to a +43 diopter lens.

The average adult cornea is 1 mm thick and 11.5 mm in diameter. The 5 distinct layers of the cornea are, from anterior to posterior: epithelium (continuous with the bulbar conjunctival epithelium), Bowman's membrane, stroma, Descemet's membrane, and the endothelium. The epithelium has 5-6 cell layers,

the endothelium only one. The epithelium is a reliable barrier against corneal infection and usually must be traumatized before an infectious agent can gain a foothold in the corneal stroma. Bowman's membrane is a clear, structureless (ie, homogeneous, acellular) layer which is a modified portion of the superficial stroma. Descemet's membrane is a clear elastic membrane which can easily be detached from the stroma; although on gross examination it appears to be structureless, microscopic examination shows Descemet's membrane to contain many fibers. The corneal stroma consists of lamellas and accounts for about 90% of the corneal thickness. Each lamellar fiber is transparent, 1μ thick and 15μ wide, and as long as the diameter of the cornea. The stromal lamellas are parallel to the corneal surface but do intertwine. Each contains a flattened cell nucleus.

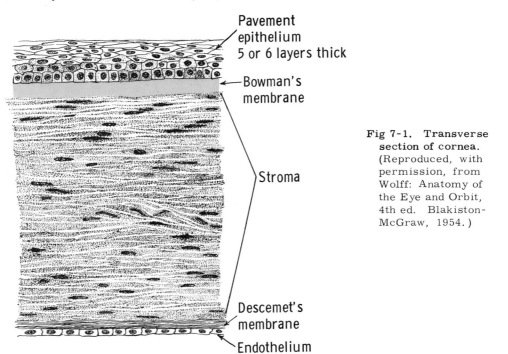

Pavement epithelium 5 or 6 layers thick

Bowman's membrane

Stroma

Descemet's membrane

Endothelium

Fig 7-1. Transverse section of cornea. (Reproduced, with permission, from Wolff: Anatomy of the Eye and Orbit, 4th ed. Blakiston-McGraw, 1954.)

The blood supply to the cornea is derived from the limbal vessels. The cornea has a rich nerve supply from the 5th cranial nerve. The superficial corneal layers contain about 70 sensory nerve fibers, which accounts for the severe pain that results from seemingly minor irritative phenomena.

The **transparency** of the cornea is due to its uniform structure, avascularity, and deturgescence. Deturgescence, the only physiologic variable related to transparency, is believed to depend upon the fact that the osmotic pressure of the tears and aqueous is greater than that of the cornea, which tends to draw out in 2 directions the water that enters the cornea through the perilimbal capillaries. If the endothelium is damaged, aqueous enters the cornea and transparency is lost.

The penetration of drugs through the cornea seems to depend upon phase solubility. The epithelium will allow the passage of fat-soluble substances, and the stroma allows the passage of water-soluble substances. Therefore, in order for a drug to penetrate the cornea, it must be both fat-soluble and water-soluble.

Physiology of Symptoms

Since the cornea has many pain fibers, most superficial corneal lesions such as a corneal foreign body, corneal abrasion, or phlyctenule will cause pain and photophobia. The pain is augmented considerably by the movement of the lids over the cornea, particularly the upper lid. Since the cornea serves as the window of the eye and refracts light rays, corneal lesions cause some degree of blurred vision; blurring is greater if the lesion is centrally located. Since there are no blood vessels or mucus glands in the cornea, there is no discharge except in the case of a purulent bacterial ulcer.

The physician examines for corneal disease by inspection of the cornea under adequate illumination. Examination is often facilitated by first instilling a local anesthetic to relieve the pain and occasionally by instilling fluorescein to outline a corneal lesion which might not otherwise be easily visualized. The loupe and slit lamp are useful but not essential aids in the examination of the cornea; adequate illumination can be furnished by a hand flashlight.

It is important to elicit a history of trauma, since foreign body and erosion are 2 of the most common corneal disorders. The patient should be asked about previous corneal diseases to rule out a recurrent corneal erosion. Local medications should be investigated to rule out steroid therapy, which frequently predisposes to the development of herpes simplex keratitis.

Laboratory investigation of ulcerated corneal lesions is of great importance since if specific therapy is not instituted immediately the cornea may be destroyed in 24 hours. Stained smears should be examined while the patient waits.

Diseases of the cornea are extremely serious since improper management can result in permanent visual impairment ranging from slight blurring to total blindness. Most of the disabling complications of corneal diseases can be prevented by prompt and accurate diagnosis and appropriate treatment.

CORNEAL ULCERS

Scarring or perforation due to corneal ulceration is a major cause of blindness throughout the world. Most forms are amenable to therapy, but visual impairment can be avoided only if appropriate treatment is instituted promptly; in some cases this means within a matter of hours after onset. Corneal ulceration has long been recognized as a distinct clinical entity, but the specific diagnosis and management of its various types present problems which bear analysis.

Classification

Corneal ulceration will be discussed here according to the type of ulcer produced by the following agents:

A. Bacteria: (The most common, in order of frequency.*)
   - Diplococcus pneumoniae (pneumococcus)
   - Streptococcus hemolyticus (beta-hemolytic streptococcus)
   - Pseudomonas aeruginosa (Bacillus pyocyaneus)
   - Moraxella liquefaciens (Diplobacillus of Petit)
   - Klebsiella pneumoniae (Friedländer's bacillus)

B. Viruses:
   - Herpes simplex virus
   - Variola virus (rarely)
   - Vaccinia virus (rarely)

C. Fungi:
   - Candida (Monilia) albicans
   - Aspergillus

---

*Staphylococcus aureus and Escherichia coli, 2 common pathogens, only rarely cause corneal ulceration; their lack of affinity for the cornea is not understood.

Nocardia
Cephalosporum
Mucor
Candida parapsilosis (C. parakrusei)

D. Hypersensitivity Reactions:
   To staphylococci (marginal ulcer)
   To unknown allergens or toxins
       (ring ulcer)
   To tuberculoprotein and, rarely,
       other bacterial proteins (phlycten-
       ular keratoconjunctivitis)

E. Vitamin Deficiency: Avitaminosis A
   (xerophthalmia)

F. Fifth nerve lesions (neurotrophic
   ulcers)

G. Exposure

H. Unknown cause (Mooren's ulcer, or
   "chronic serpiginous ulcer")

BACTERIAL CORNEAL ULCERS

Pneumococcal Ulcer (Acute Serpiginous Ulcer)

The pneumococcus (Diplococcus pneumoniae) is the commonest bacterial cause of
corneal ulcer. Typically it produces a gray,
fairly well circumscribed ulcer (Fig 7-2),
with a marked tendency to spread centrally if
it begins near the limbus. This creeping effect gave rise to the name "acute serpiginous
ulcer," a synonym for pneumococcal ulcer.

Hypopyon is a frequent development; nearly
always sterile, it is a result of the passage of
a bacterial toxin through Descemet's membrane into the anterior chamber.

Pneumococcal ulceration usually follows
corneal trauma and is consequently very common among coal miners. It is particularly
likely to develop if the patient has a chronic
pneumococcal dacryocystitis. Purulent material from the infected tear sac pours into the
conjunctival sac; if the corneal epithelium is
not intact, the organism enters the corneal
substance and begins to multiply. It is curious that conjunctivitis seldom occurs in association with pneumococcal dacryocystitis.

Since the pneumococcus is sensitive to
both sulfonamides and antibiotics, local therapy
is usually effective. If untreated, the cornea
may perforate and the eye may be lost. Concurrent dacryocystitis, if present, should also
be treated.

Streptococcal Ulcer

The ulcer produced by Streptococcus
hemolyticus has no creeping tendency but is
otherwise identical with the pueumococcal ulcer in appearance, course, and response to
treatment.

Pseudomonas Ulcer

The corneal ulceration caused by Pseudomonas aeruginosa characteristically starts in
a small area, usually in the center, and
spreads rapidly, frequently causing perforation of the cornea and loss of the eye within
48 hours. It often follows some minor corneal
injury which has been examined with the aid of
a Pseudomonas-contaminated fluorescein solu-

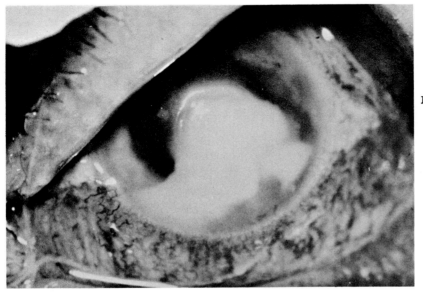

Fig 7-2. Pneumococcal
   corneal ulcer with
   hypopyon.

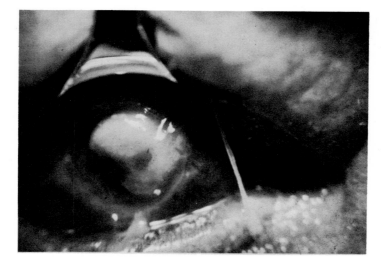

Fig 7-3. Pseudomonas corneal ulcer of right eye. Eviseration was done.

tion. The organism usually produces a bluish-green pigment which is pathognomonic of Ps aeruginosa infection.

Three features of Pseudomonas corneal ulceration deserve emphasis: (1) Ps aeruginosa thrives in fluorescein solution and to a lesser extent in physostigmine solution. These solutions can only be safely used if they are autoclaved at frequent intervals (once a week), since there are no reliable antibacterial preservatives available for them. For this reason the use of sterile fluorescein papers moistened with the patient's tears (or sterile individual dropper units) is strongly advocated as a substitute for fluorescein solution. (2) Since the organism flourishes better on the cornea than on any known culture medium, it can cause rapid destruction of the cornea. Early diagnosis and vigorous treatment are therefore absolutely essential. (3) Polymyxin is the only antibiotic consistently active against Ps aeruginosa; however, since some strains are also sensitive to streptomycin, both drugs should always be administered.

Ps aeruginosa eye infections may occur in premature infants. If these infections are not properly treated, systemic dissemination and death may ensue.

Polymyxin B sulfate is supplied in soluble 25 mg tablets for solution (1 mg = 10,000 units) and in vials containing 50 ml (500,000 units) for injection. Instill 2 drops of a solution containing 10,000 units/ml in saline every 15 minutes around the clock; polymyxin-bacitracin (Poly-

sporin®) ointment is instilled every 2 hours after irrigation with saline solution. (The bacitracin is used for its effect against gram-positive invaders.) A 1000 ml bottle of sterile saline solution can be installed at the bedside on an intravenous standard, with an eye dropper or dull needle attached to the end of the tubing.

In addition, inject gentamicin, 30 mg in 1 ml subconjunctivally daily. The pain associated with the subconjunctival injections may be sufficient to require strong analgesics.

Colistin (Coly-Mycin®) is similar in anti-Pseudomonas effectiveness to polymyxin, and the tissue toxicity of the 2 drugs appears to be the same.

Diplobacillus of Petit Ulcer

Moraxella liquefaciens causes an indolent ulcer, usually centrally located and very slowly progressive. It is ordinarily superficial and unlikely to perforate the cornea. Many of its victims are alcoholics.

Topical treatment with sodium sulfacetamide (Sodium Sulamyd®), sulfisoxazole (Gantrisin®), or broad-spectrum antibiotics is effective.

Friedländer's Bacillus Ulcer

The rare ulcer caused by Klebsiella pneumoniae develops after trauma, is centrally located, progresses slowly, and rarely causes hypopyon. Treatment is with tetracyclines and streptomycin.

VIRAL CORNEAL ULCERS

Herpes Simplex Keratitis (Dendritic Keratitis)

Corneal ulceration caused by herpes simplex virus is fairly common, almost always unilateral, and may affect any age group. The patient usually complains of mild irritation and photophobia, and, if the central cornea is affected, of blurred vision. A history of recent upper respiratory infection with "cold sores" about the face can often be elicited.

The commonest finding is of one or more dendritic ulcers on the corneal surface (Fig 7-5). These are composed of clear vesicles in the corneal epithelium; when the vesicles rupture, the area stains green with fluorescein. Although the dendritic figure is its most characteristic manifestation, herpes simplex keratitis may appear in a number of other forms (Fig 7-6).

Herpes simplex virus can be cultivated by transferring direct scrapings from the corneal ulcer to the chorioallantoic membrane of a developing chick embryo. The dendritic figure is reproducible on the rabbit cornea by scratch inoculation of its surface with scrapings from the corneal ulcer. The virus also produces a typical cytopathic effect on HeLa cell cultures.

Hypopyon is an occasional complication of herpes simplex keratitis. It is usually sterile, a toxic reaction to secondary infection in about two-thirds of cases but to herpes simplex virus itself in one-third. There is no specific treatment for the hypopyon, but it may resolve spontaneously.

Disciform keratitis (see Fig 7-6) is a fairly frequent complication, particularly if iodine has been used to cauterize the initial lesion or if steroids have been used early. There is no specific treatment, but the prognosis is usually good if there is no vessel encroachment from the limbus. Vascularization inevitably produces a permanent scar and permanent visual loss. Occasionally a disciform lesion becomes necrotic centrally, and this in turn leads to hypopyon formation, perforation, or both.

Corneal perforation rarely occurs unless steroids have been used or antibiotics prolonged unduly. If perforation is imminent, immediate corneal transplantation or a thin conjunctival flap is indicated.

The therapeutic objective is to remove the virus-containing corneal epithelium without disturbing Bowman's membrane and the corneal stroma. Infected epithelium is much more loosely attached to Bowman's membrane than healthy epithelium, and is thus easily removed. The safest way to remove it is with a small, tightly wound sterile cotton applicator or a sterile spatula or chalazion curet. Chemical cauterization with tincture of iodine or ether is commonly used but has no advantage over simple mechanical removal of the epithelium and introduces the risk of chemical keratitis. Homatropine, 5%, is instilled to relieve the photophobia. A pressure bandage is applied to hold the lid against the cornea. If sterile instruments have been used there should be no need to instill an antibacterial agent. However, the patient should be observed on the following day to be certain that a secondary bacterial infection has not developed. The pressure bandage is changed daily until the epithelium regenerates.

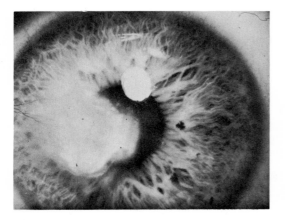

Fig 7-4. Corneal scar caused by recurrent herpes simplex keratitis. (Courtesy of A. Rosenberg.)

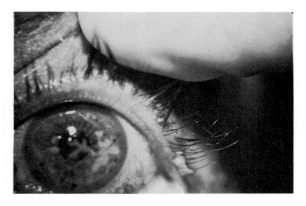

Fig 7-5. Dendritic figures seen in herpes simplex keratitis.

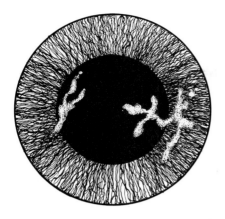

Dendritic

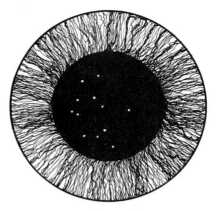

Epithelial Punctate

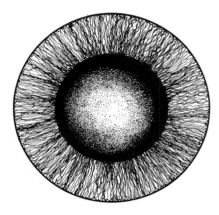

Disciform

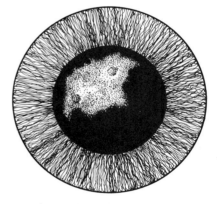

Geographic

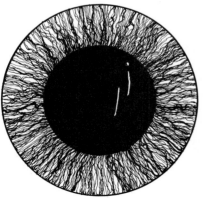

Linear

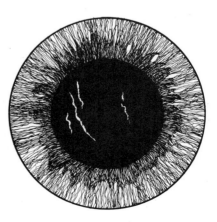

Filamentous

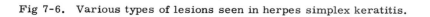

Fig 7-6. Various types of lesions seen in herpes simplex keratitis.

Idoxuridine (IDU; Dendrid®, Herplex®, Stoxil®) is quite effective in the treatment of acute cases. It has no effect on chronic herpes simplex keratitis; does not prevent recurrences; and does not protect against the harmful effects of steroids. It is instilled locally as 0.1% solution or ointment every hour day and night for 3 days and then gradually withdrawn over a period of 3-4 more days. Resistant strains of herpes simplex virus have appeared.

Corticosteroid therapy is contraindicated at all stages of the disease. Corticosteroids increase the activity of the virus, most likely by immunosuppression and by enhancing the action of collagenase (produced by damaged corneal epithelial cells) on the corneal stroma. Before the corticosteroids came into common use, herpes simplex virus infection never caused corneal perforation.

Secondary fungal infection may be another complication of local steroid therapy or of unduly prolonged broad-spectrum antibiotic treatment of corneal ulcers of any type.

When herpetic ulcer is diagnosed early and treated promptly, the prognosis is good. Recurrences are common, however, and there are several "trigger mechanisms" which tend to induce them. The most common of these are fever, colds, exposure to sun, psychic stress, trauma, and menstruation. After the initial attack (primary herpes), the patient develops circulating antibodies in the blood which remain at a constant level throughout life. The antibodies do not prevent recurrences but do modify the cutaneous and conjunctival manifestations of the disease (unfortunately not the corneal manifestation), so that recurrences affecting these tissues are much less severe than the primary attack. If the primary attack is ocular, the conjunctiva is affected as well as the cornea (primary herpetic keratoconjunctivitis); but in any recurrence that affects the eye, whether it follows an initial ocular or an initial cutaneous attack, the conjunctiva is usually spared. There are no reliable methods of preventing recurrences.

Variola Virus Ulcer

Corneal ulcers due to variola virus still occur in areas of the world where smallpox is endemic. Conjunctivitis is frequently present.

Vaccinia Virus Ulcer

Corneal ulcers due to vaccinia virus are occasionally seen as an accidental complication of smallpox vaccination. Prevention of secondary bacterial infection is the only treatment. In accidental vaccinia of the lids, vaccinia immune gamma globulin given IM has been used prophylactically in an effort to prevent spread to the cornea.

FUNGAL CORNEAL ULCERS

The incidence of corneal ulceration due to fungi has been increasing, perhaps as a result of fungal overgrowth from long-term antibiotic and steroid therapy. The organisms find their way into the cornea following damage to the epithelium by trauma or inflammation, eg, herpes simplex ulceration. Most fungal ulcers are gray, indolent, and slowly progressive.

The so-called "satellite phenomenon," a ring of punctate opacities around a denser central ulcer, is an important diagnostic feature of fungal corneal ulcer (Fig 7-7).

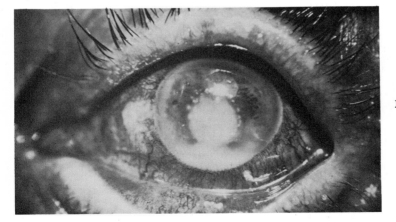

Fig 7-7. Corneal ulcer caused by Candida albicans.

Instillation of amphotericin B (Fungizone®) may be beneficial. As with most corneal ulcers, the best treatment is prevention. Fungi grow in many of the common eye solutions if sterilization procedures are not observed.

CORNEAL ULCERS DUE TO HYPERSENSITIVITY REACTIONS

Marginal Ulcers

Marginal ulcers are by far the commonest corneal ulcers. They are small, unilateral, single or multiple, superficial, round or rectangular ulcers which have a clear space between them and the limbus (Fig 7-8). About 50% are associated with staphylococcal marginal blepharitis; scrapings and cultures taken directly from the ulcers contain no bacteria, and

so they are assumed to be the result of allergic reactions to staphylococcal infection. Many of the remaining 50% are due to food allergies.

Marginal and ring ulcers may also occur in association with conjunctivitis caused by the Koch-Weeks bacillus or Proteus vulgaris. Topical corticosteroid drops are usually curative within 2-3 days. Marginal ulcers tend to recur. Staphylococcal blepharitis, if present, should be vigorously treated.

Ring Ulcers

Ring ulcers are much less common but more destructive than marginal ulcers. The ring ulcer is a unilateral, almost continuous circumferential ulcer just inside the limbus (see Fig 7-9). Smears and cultures from it are negative. In contrast to the marginal ulcer, there is no relationship between ring ulcer and conjunctivitis or blepharitis. There may be an associated systemic disease, however. Two such related conditions are bacillary dysentery and polyarteritis nodosa. In one case of bacillary dysentery, a ring ulcer occurred with the initial attack and recurred coincidentally with the second attack 5 months later. Although it is generally assumed that ring ulcer is a hypersensitivity reaction, the underlying cause can seldom be determined.

Response to local corticosteroid therapy is good.

Phlyctenular Keratoconjunctivitis

This is a disease of malnourished children with systemic tuberculosis and, less frequently, of adults who had had tuberculosis in childhood. For this reason the disease is common among Eskimos and North American Indians. The eye lesions, usually bilateral, are in the

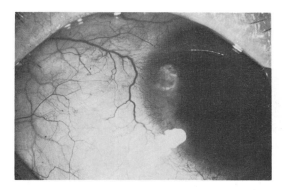

Fig 7-8. Marginal ulcer of temporal cornea, right eye. (Courtesy of P. Thygeson.)

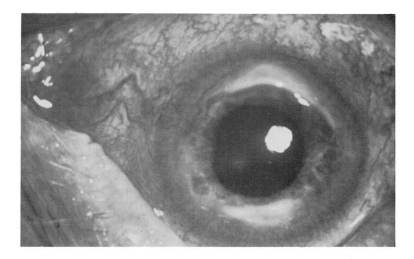

Fig 7-9. Ring ulcer of the cornea. (Courtesy of M. Hogan.)

great majority of cases the result of a sensitivity to tuberculoprotein, which reaches the cornea via the blood stream. In rare instances the agent of the systemic disease may be the staphylococcus, Coccidioides immitis, the agent of lymphogranuloma venereum, or some other pathogen to which the cornea has become hypersensitive. Bacterial conjunctivitis often serves as a trigger mechanism for an attack.

The phlyctenule is the characteristic lesion. It is gray and wedge-shaped, and extends across the limbus onto the cornea. It may be single or multiple. Phlyctenules characteristically involve only the peripheral cornea, but may spread to cover the entire corneal surface. Microscopically one sees many small round cells and dilated blood vessels.

Response to local corticosteroids is dramatic. Systemic steroid therapy is contraindicated since it could cause the dissemination of an existent pulmonary tuberculosis. Equally important in the treatment is a well balanced diet and management of the systemic tuberculosis or other underlying disease.

CORNEAL ULCER
DUE TO VITAMIN A DEFICIENCY

The typical corneal ulcer associated with avitaminosis A is centrally located and bilateral, gray and indolent, with a definite lack of corneal luster in the surrounding area (Fig 7-10). The cornea becomes soft and necrotic (hence the term, "keratomalacia"), and perforation is common. The epithelium of the

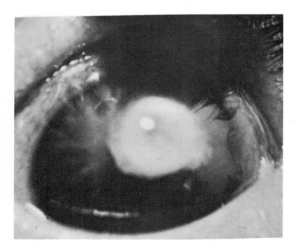

Fig 7-10. Keratomalacia with ulceration associated with xerophthalmia (dietary) in an infant. (Photo by Diane Beeston.)

conjunctiva is keratinized, as evidenced by the presence of a Bitot spot. This is a foamy, wedge-shaped area in the conjunctiva, usually on the temporal side, with the base of the wedge at the limbus and the apex extending toward the lateral canthus. Within the triangle the conjunctiva is furrowed concentrically with the limbus, and dry flaky material can be seen falling from the area into the inferior cul-de-sac. A stained conjunctival scraping from a Bitot spot will show many saprophytic xerosis bacilli (Corynebacterium zerosis; small curved rods) and keratinized epithelial cells.

Avitaminosis A corneal ulceration results from dietary lack of vitamin A or impaired absorption from the gastrointestinal tract and impaired utilization by the body. It may develop in an infant who has a feeding problem; in an adult who is on a restricted or generally inadequate diet; or in any person with a biliary obstruction since bile in the gastrointestinal tract is necessary for the absorption of vitamin A. Lack of vitamin A causes a generalized keratinization of the epithelium throughout the body. The conjunctival and corneal changes together are known as **xerophthalmia**. Since the epithelium of the air passages is affected, many patients, if not treated, will die of pneumonia. Avitaminosis A also causes a generalized retardation of osseous growth. This is extremely important in infants; for example, if the skull bones do not grow and the brain continues to grow, increased intracranial pressure and papilledema can result.

Between 10,000 and 15,000 IU of vitamin A should be administered daily IM (or orally if the absorption rate is known to be normal). Sulfonamide or antibiotic ointment can be used locally in the eye to prevent secondary bacterial infection. The average daily requirement of vitamin A is 1500-5000 IU for children, according to age, and 5000 IU for adults.

NEUROTROPHIC CORNEAL ULCERS

If the trigeminal nerve, which supplies the cornea, is interrupted by trauma, surgery, tumor, inflammation, or in any other way, the cornea loses its sensitivity and one of its best defenses against degeneration, ulceration, and infection. In the early stages of a typical neurotrophic ulcer, fluorescein solution will produce punctate staining of the superficial epithelium. As this process progresses, patchy areas of denudation appear. Occasionally the epithelium may be absent from a large area of the cornea.

The progress of the condition depends on the treatment. Without treatment, the denuded areas become infected. The integrity of the cornea can be maintained as long as the corneal surface is kept moist by wearing a Büller shield,* by suturing the lids together, or by the use of a conjunctival flap. Artificial tears may be of benefit. Under the best conditions, however, the prognosis is poor.

CORNEAL ULCERS DUE TO EXPOSURE

Corneal ulcer due to exposure may develop in any condition in which the cornea is not properly moistened and covered by the eyelids. Examples include exophthalmos from any cause, ectropion, the absence of part of an eyelid as a result of trauma, and inability to close the lids properly, as in Bell's palsy. The 2 factors at work are the drying of the cornea and its exposure to minor trauma. The uncovered cornea is particularly subject to drying during sleeping hours. If an ulcer develops it usually follows minor trauma and occurs in the inferior third of the cornea.

This type of ulcer will be sterile unless it is secondarily infected, and the therapeutic objective is to provide protection and moisture for the entire corneal surface. The method depends upon the underlying condition: a plastic procedure on the eyelids, a Büller shield, or surgical relief of exophthalmos.

MOOREN'S ULCER
(Corneal Ulcer of Unknown Cause)

Mooren's ulcer is a rare disorder which is unilateral in 75% of cases. It starts as an excavated, nonexudative ulcer near the limbus, and slowly progresses to destroy the entire cornea and eventually the eye. Typically it has a raised border at the advancing edge. No microbial agent has ever been isolated. The central cornea is the last area to be destroyed. Mooren's ulcer must be differentiated from excavated marginal ulceration associated with polyarteritis nodosa.

There is no reliable treatment for this extremely destructive process. Delimiting keratotomy with paracentesis repeated daily may be effective, and repeated diathermy of the cornea in front of the advancing border of the lesion has been used to halt the progress of the ulcer.

*The Büller shield is a water-tight cone of exposed x-ray film secured to the surrounding skin with adhesive tape.

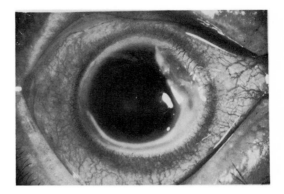

Fig 7-11. Mooren's ulcer. (Courtesy of M. Hogan.)

DEGENERATIVE CORNEAL CONDITIONS

KERATOCONUS

Keratoconus is an uncommon degenerative bilateral disease which is inherited as an autosomal recessive trait. Unilateral cases of unknown cause occur rarely. Symptoms appear in the second decade of life. The disease affects all races. Keratoconus is associated with atopic dermatitis in a significant number of cases. Pathologically there are generalized thinning and anterior protrusion of the central cornea, ruptures in Descemet's membrane, and irregular, superficial linear scars at the apex of the cone which is formed.

Blurred vision is the only symptom. Signs include cone-shaped cornea, indentation of the lower lid by the cornea when the patient looks down, an irregular shadow on retinoscopy, and a distorted corneal reflection with Placido's disk or the keratoscope. The fundi cannot be clearly visualized.

Corneal perforation may occur in advanced cases. When this happens, the eye should be bandaged and the dressing changed daily until a corneal scar seals the wound. Corneal transplant may be necessary.

Contact lenses improve visual acuity in the early stages. A corneal transplant is indicated when the corrected visual acuity decreases to the point where it interferes with the patient's normal activities.

Keratoconus is slowly progressive until the patient becomes blind (between the ages of 20 and 60). If a corneal transplant is done before extreme corneal thinning occurs, the prognosis is excellent; about 80% obtain reading vision.

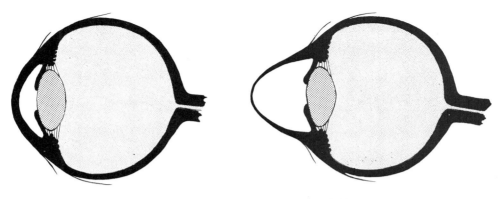

Fig 7-12.   Left: Side view of normal cornea.   Right: Keratoconus.

CORNEAL DYSTROPHY OR DEGENERATION

The corneal dystrophies are a rare group of slowly progressive, bilateral, degenerative disorders which usually appear in the second or third decades of life.   Some are hereditary. Other cases follow ocular inflammatory disease, and some are of unknown cause.

Fatty or Lipoid Degeneration

This disorder may begin in infancy or adulthood.   The cause is not known.   There is a generalized deposition of lipid material within the corneal stroma, replacement of Bowman's membrane by macrophages, and thickening of the epithelium with some infiltration of lipid material.   Clinical findings include blurred vision and haziness and thickening of the cornea, particularly in the central zone.

Symptoms and signs are slowly progressive until useful vision is lost.   Corneal transplant improves vision significantly in most cases.

Marginal Dystrophy

This disorder begins in the later years. The cause is not known.   The corneal stroma is replaced by loose connective tissue; the cornea gradually becomes thinner in the limbal area, most often superiorly, and Descemet's membrane bulges forward.   There are usually no symptoms, but there may be recurrent irritation and injection.   The only complication is rupture of the eyeball at the limbus, and this occurs only rarely.

Because the course of progression is slow and the central cornea is spared, the prognosis is good.

Band Keratopathy

This is a chronic disorder sometimes associated with chronic uveitis due to any cause, uveitis due to Boeck's sarcoid, hypervitaminosis D, or Still's disease in children. There is deposition of calcium salts in the superficial cornea and hyalinization of Bowman's membrane.   Symptoms include irritation, injection, and blurring of vision.   A horizontally placed, whitish rectangular plaque 3-6 mm in diameter is seen extending most of the way across the cornea.   Ulceration and infection may occur.

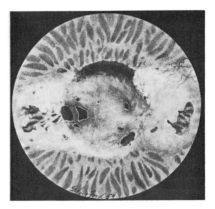

Fig 7-13.   Band keratopathy.
(Courtesy of M. Hogan.)

Zonular dystrophy is the only type of corneal dystrophy in which medical treatment is useful.   Treatment consists of scraping the cornea with a spatula and applying EDTA solution with a cotton applicator to dissolve the calcareous material.   If this is ineffective, corneal transplant will improve visual acuity significantly in about 50% of cases.

CORNEAL TRANSPLANT OPERATION

Corneal transplant (keratoplasty) is indicated for the treatment of corneal opacification. Corneas from young donors are preferred. The donor's eye must be enucleated as soon as possible, since the cornea tends to soften after death. Ideally the cornea should be used immediately, but it may be used up to 24 hours after death if the eye is kept in a sterile container in the cool part of a standard household refrigerator. In recent years many successful lamellar transplants (nonpenetrating transplants of partial thicknesses of cornea) have been performed using corneas stored for months in glycerine or in a frozen state.

Corneal transplants are now being advocated by many ophthalmic surgeons when perforation of a corneal ulcer is imminent. Thin conjunctival flaps are sometimes done preparatory to corneal transplant in these cases.

Technic

A round section of clear cornea from the donor eye is removed with a trephine, which has the same structure and function as a cookie cutter. The same trephine is used to remove the opaque area of the cornea from the recipient eye. The donor cornea is then sutured into place.

Keratoconus offers the most favorable prognosis. Eighty percent of these patients obtain greatly improved visual acuity following a corneal transplant. Corneal transplant for scarring due to other causes is successful in from 30-70% of cases.

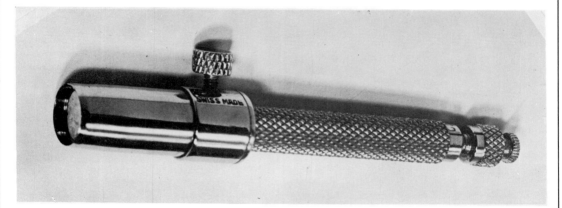

Fig 7-14. Trephine (Franceschetti type; actual size).

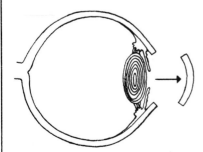

Fig 7-15. Section of cornea removed with trephine.

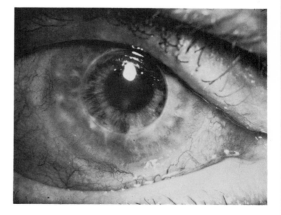

Fig 7-16. Postoperative corneal transplant. (Courtesy of M. Hogan.)

Salzmann's Nodular Dystrophy

This disorder is always preceded by corneal inflammation, particularly phlyctenular keratoconjunctivitis. There is vascularization and degeneration of the superficial cornea which involves the stroma, Bowman's membrane, and epithelium. Symptoms include redness, irritation, and blurring of vision. There is a superficial vascularization, with whitish nodules sometimes occurring in chains interspersed among the blood vessels.

Corneal transplant will significantly improve the visual acuity in about 70% of cases.

Hereditary Corneal Dystrophy

These usually become manifest in the second decade and are slowly progressive over a lifetime. There are 3 types: granular, macular, and reticular. All 3 are characterized by deposition of hyaline material in the superficial lamellas, degeneration of the superficial lamellas and Bowman's membrane, and thickening of the epithelium, particularly in the region above the hyaline deposits in the cornea. Blurred vision is the only symptom. Signs are as follows:

(1) Granular (autosomal dominant): Many whitish, superficial particles in the central corneal area which appear like fragments of stone. (2) Macular (autosomal recessive): A veil-like gray opacity in the superficial cornea which is denser centrally and tends to increase in density with time. (3) Reticular (autosomal dominant): Many white nodules connected by thin white lines are seen in the superficial cornea.

Corneal transplant is successful in over 50% of cases of hereditary corneal dystrophy.

Endothelial and Epithelial Dystrophy (Fuchs's Epithelial Dystrophy)

This disorder begins in the 3rd or 4th decade and is slowly progressive throughout life. The cause is not known. There are hyaline, wart-like deposits on Descemet's membrane, endothelial defects, edema of the corneal stroma, and degeneration of Bowman's membrane and epithelium. Blurred vision is usually the only symptom. The cornea is slightly cloudy initially and becomes progressively more opaque. The surface is rough as a result of the degeneration of the epithelium and Bowman's membrane. Complications include secondary corneal infection and ulceration as a result of breakdown of the protective epithelial barrier. If this occurs, specific antibacterial therapy must be instituted.

Corneal transplant improves vision in about 70% of cases.

ARCUS SENILIS
(Corneal Annulus, Embryotoxon)

Arcus senilis is an extremely common bilateral benign peripheral corneal degeneration which may occur at any age but is far more common in elderly people as part of the aging process. When arcus senilis is present prior to age 50, hypercholesterolemia is usually associated with it.

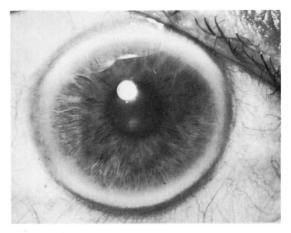

Fig 7-17. Arcus senilis. (Photo by Diane Beeston.)

Pathologically, lipid droplets involve the entire corneal thickness but are more concentrated in the superficial and deep layers, being relatively sparse in the corneal stroma.

There are no symptoms. Clinically, arcus senilis appears as a peripheral, annular, hazy gray ring about 2 mm in width and with a clear space between it and the limbus (Fig 7-17). No treatment is necessary, and there are no complications. Since arcus senilis causes no visual defect, it is not always classified with the corneal dystrophies.

MISCELLANEOUS CORNEAL DISORDERS

SCLEROKERATITIS
(Sclerosing Keratitis)

Sclerokeratitis is an uncommon, unilateral, localized inflammation of the sclera and cornea. The cause is not known but tuberculosis has been implicated. Pathologically, there are many chronic inflammatory cells (small round cells) in the involved portion of both structures. Fibrosis occurs in the later stages. The patient complains of pain, photophobia, and irritation, but there is no discharge. A moderately severe iritis (anterior nongranulomatous uveitis) is usually associated.

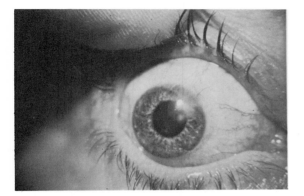

Fig 7-18. Sclerokeratitis. Note fibrovascular scar in upper nasal quadrant of cornea.

No specific treatment is available. The pupil should be kept dilated with atropine, 2%, 2 drops once daily. Warm compresses and local corticosteroid drops are used to relieve the discomfort. Although the process starts as a small area of infiltration, it may progress to total corneal opacification. If it does subside, it usually takes months to years.

SUPERFICIAL PUNCTATE KERATITIS

Superficial punctate keratitis is an uncommon chronic, bilateral disorder of young people (especially women) characterized by discrete epithelial opacities which usually are quite numerous and most common in the pupillary area. The opacities are not visible grossly but can be easily seen with the slit lamp or loupe.

No causative organism has been isolated, but a virus is suspected.

Mild irritation and slight blurring of vision are the only symptoms. The conjunctiva is white. Bulbar hyperemia is occasionally present at the 12 o'clock position.

Epithelial keratitis secondary to staphylococcal blepharoconjunctivitis is differentiated from superficial punctate keratitis by its involvement of the lower third of the cornea. Epithelial keratitis in trachoma is ruled out by its location in the upper third of the cornea and the presence of a pannus. Many other forms of keratitis involving the superficial cornea are unilateral or are eliminated by their histories.

Short-term instillation of corticosteroid drops will often cause disappearance of the opacities, but recurrences are common. The ultimate prognosis, whether the disease is treated or not, is good. Untreated, the disease runs a protracted course of several years.

RECURRENT CORNEAL EROSION

This is a fairly common and serious mechanical corneal disorder which presents some classical signs and symptoms but may be easily missed if the physician does not look for it specifically. The patient is usually awakened during the early morning hours by a pain in the affected eye. The pain is continuous, and the eye becomes red, irritated, and photophobic. If questioned carefully the patient will usually give a history of a previous corneal injury, although it may have occurred several years ago. The eye dries during the night so that the lid adheres to the cornea. When the patient attempts to open his eyes the lid pulls off the epithelium in an area of imperfect healing of a previous injury, resulting in pain and redness.

Instillation of a local anesthetic relieves the symptoms immediately, and fluorescein staining will show the eroded area. This is typically a small area in the lower central cornea.

Treatment consists of a pressure bandage on the eye to promote healing. Mechanical denuding of the corneal epithelium may be necessary. The other eye should be kept closed most of the time to minimize movement of the lid over the affected eye. Bed rest is desirable for 24 hours. The cornea usually heals in 2-3 days. To prevent recurrence and to promote continued healing, it is important for these patients to use a bland ointment (eg, boric acid) at bedtime for several months. In more severe cases, artificial tears are instilled during the day.

Rare instances of bilateral atraumatic dystrophic recurrent corneal erosion with a poor prognosis have also been reported.

INTERSTITIAL KERATITIS DUE TO CONGENITAL SYPHILIS

This self-limited inflammatory disease of the cornea is a late manifestation of congenital syphilis. There has been a sharp decrease in the incidence of the disease in recent years—almost to the point of extinction in some parts of the USA. It occasionally starts unilaterally but almost always becomes bilateral weeks to months later. It affects all races, and is more common in females than males. Symptoms appear between the ages of 5 and 20. Pathologic findings include edema, lymphocytic infiltration, and vascularization of the corneal stroma. Interstitial keratitis may be allergic in nature since Treponema pallidum is not found in the cornea during the acute phase. It may be that organisms enter the cornea at birth and that later in life there is a violent allergic reaction in the cornea to the organisms circulating in the blood stream.

Clinical Findings
A. Symptoms and Signs: Other signs of congenital syphilis may be present, such as saddle nose and Hutchinson's triad (interstitial keratitis, deafness, and notched upper·central incisors). The patient complains of pain, photophobia, and blurring of vision. Physical signs include conjunctival injection, corneal edema, vascularization of the deeper corneal layers, and miosis. There is an associated severe anterior granulomatous uveitis and blepharospasm due to the photophobia. The grayish-pink appearance of the cornea (due to edema and vascularization) which occurs in the acute phase is sometimes referred to as a "salmon patch."

B. Laboratory Findings: Serologic tests for syphilis are positive.

Complications and Sequelae
Corneal scarring occurs if the process has been particularly severe and prolonged. Secondary glaucoma may result from the uveitis.

Treatment
There are no specific measures. Treatment is aimed at preventing the development of posterior synechias, which will occur if the pupil is not dilated. Both eyes should be dilated with frequent instillations of 2% atropine solution and corticosteroid drops. Dark glasses and a darkened room may be necessary if photophobia is severe. Treatment of systemic syphilis should be carried out, even though this usually has little effect on the ocular condition.

Corneal scarring necessitates corneal transplant. Glaucoma must be treated surgically if intractable to local medication.

Course and Prognosis
The disease process itself is not affected by treatment, which is aimed at prevention of complications. It usually lasts several weeks, after which the corneas often clear almost completely, leaving ghost vessels in the corneal stroma.

CORNEAL PIGMENTATION

Pigmentation of the cornea may occur with or without ocular or systemic disease. There are several distinct varieties:

Krukenberg's Spindle
In this common type, brown uveal pigment is deposited bilaterally upon the central endothelial surface in a vertical spindle-shaped fashion. It occurs in a small percentage of people over age 20, usually in myopic women. It can be seen grossly, but is best observed with the loupe or slit lamp. The visual acuity is only slightly affected, and the progression is extremely slow. Pigmentary glaucoma should be ruled out.

Blood Staining
This disorder occurs occasionally as a complication of traumatic hyphema and is due to hemosiderin in the corneal stroma. The cornea is golden brown, and vision is blurred. In most cases the cornea gradually clears in 1-2 years.

Kayser-Fleischer Ring
This is a pigmented ring of variable hue (usually green or brown) 3-4 mm in diameter just inside the limbus. It is a striking sign of hepatolenticular degeneration (Wilson's disease), and is therefore rare. The fine, dense pigment granules collect between the endothelium and Descemet's membrane. Vision is not affected. Electronmicroscopic studies suggest that the pigment is a copper compound. It has been shown clinically that the intensity of the pigmentation can be reduced markedly by the use of chelating agents such as penicillamine.

Stähli's Line

Stähli's line (Hudson's brown line, Hudson-Stähli line) is an uncommon phenomenon which occurs only in elderly persons. It is seen with the slit lamp as a horizontal brown line in the inferior third of the cornea. It does not extend to the limbus on either side. The line probably represents tears in Bowman's membrane. It causes no visual disturbance.

II. SCLERA

The sclera is the fibrous outer protective coating of the eye. It is dense and white and continuous with the cornea anteriorly and with the dural sheath of the optic nerve posteriorly. At the insertion of the rectus muscles it is about 0.3 mm thick; elsewhere it is about 1 mm thick. A few strands of scleral tissue pass over the optic disk. This sievelike structure is known as the lamina cribrosa. Around the optic nerve the sclera is penetrated by the long and short posterior ciliary arteries and the long and short ciliary nerves. Slightly posterior to the equator the 4 vortex veins exit through the sclera, usually one in each quadrant. About 4 mm posterior to the limbus the 4 anterior ciliary arteries and veins penetrate the sclera. Each set penetrates slightly anterior to the insertion of a rectus muscle.

The outer surface of the sclera is covered by a thin layer of fine elastic tissue, the episclera, containing numerous blood vessels which nourish the sclera. The brown pigment layer on the inner surface is the lamina fusca, which is continuous with the sclera and the choroid. On the inner surface at 180° (in a horizontal plane through 9 and 3 o'clock) there is a shallow groove from the optic nerve to the ciliary body in which are embedded the long posterior ciliary artery and the long ciliary nerve. The nerve supply to the sclera is from the ciliary nerves.

Histologically the sclera consists of many dense bands of parallel and interlacing fibrous tissue bundles, each of which is $10\text{-}16\,\mu$ thick and $100\text{-}140\,\mu$ wide. The histologic structure of the sclera is remarkably similar to that of the cornea, which raises the question why the cornea is transparent and the sclera opaque. The apparent physiologic reason is the relative deturgescence of the cornea and the less uniform structure of the sclera as compared with the cornea. The cornea has the ability to absorb a great deal of water, whereupon it becomes opaque. The sclera is almost completely hydrated in its normal state.

EPISCLERITIS

Episcleritis is a common, localized, unilateral disease which usually occurs temporally. The cause is not known, although an allergic background is often present. A small percentage of cases are associated with rheumatoid arthritis, keratoconjunctivitis sicca, or coccidioidomycosis. The patient complains of slight pain, photophobia, tenderness, and redness. The inflammation always spreads by contiguity to the sclera internally and Tenon's capsule and the conjunctiva externally. Conjunctivitis can be ruled out by the absence of a discharge and the localized nature of episcleritis. A mild iritis (anterior nongranulomatous uveitis) is frequently associated. There are no complications, and the inflammation can be resolved in 3 or 4 days by instilling corticosteroid drops 4 times daily. Recurrences are common.

Less frequently, the episcleritis assumes a nodular form (Fig 7-19), with exactly the same signs and symptoms except for the presence of a small inflammatory nodule in the episcleral tissues which is firmly attached to the sclera. Treatment with corticosteroids is less effective than in the usual type of episcleritis, and the disease usually runs a course of several weeks or months.

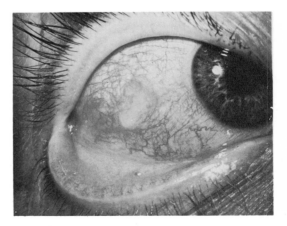

Fig 7-19. Nodular episcleritis, right eye. (Photo by Diane Beeston.)

STAPHYLOMA

Scleral staphylomas are localized, thin, dark blue, bulging areas lined on their inner surfaces with uveal tissue. They may be congenital or may occur following trauma or chronic inflammation which has weakened the scleral wall, and may be single or multiple. Staphylomas are named according to their anatomic location. The following types are recognized: **Intercalary**, between the ciliary body and the cornea; **ciliary**, over the ciliary body (Fig 7-20); **equatorial**, at the anatomic equator; and **posterior**, between the equator and the optic nerve.

In most cases no treatment is available. Small staphylomas are best left alone. In severe cases, the staphyloma gradually enlarges and enucleation is eventually necessary. Scleral transplants have been tried with limited success.

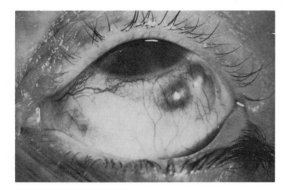

Fig 7-20. Ciliary staphyloma.
(Courtesy of P. Thygeson.)

SCLERITIS

Scleritis is a rare chronic, nonspecific inflammation of the sclera of unknown cause but sometimes associated with systemic collagen disease. It may be diffuse, or localized and nodular. If nodular, there is an elevated dark blue area in the anterior portion of the sclera. In both types there is considerable pain and photophobia, and a severe anterior uveitis is often associated. If the adjacent cornea becomes inflamed it is known as a sclerokeratitis.

Scleritis is resistant to all types of treatment.

HYALINE DEGENERATION

Hyaline degeneration is a fairly frequent finding in the scleras of persons over 60. It is manifested by small round, translucent, gray areas. They are usually about 2-3 mm in diameter, located slightly anterior to the insertion of the rectus muscles. They cause no symptoms or complications.

SCLEROMALACIA PERFORANS

This is a rare scleral disease characterized by the appearance of one or more dehiscences in the sclera in the absence of obvious inflammatory signs. The cause is not known, but severe rheumatoid arthritis is usually associated. The uvea is visible, and may be bulging.

If the sclera becomes necrotic, a conjunctival flap must be performed in order to cover the diseased area with healthy conjunctiva.

Scleromalacia perforans persists indefinitely, and the prognosis is poor (depending upon the extent of the process.

There is no medical treatment and scleral transplant is seldom successful.

• • •

Bibliography

Antine, B.: Histology of congenital hereditary corneal dystrophy. Am J Ophth **69**: 964, 1970.

Ashton, N., & C. Cook: Mechanisms of corneal vascularization. Brit J Ophth **37**:193-209, 1953.

Brown, S. I.: The pathogenesis and treatment of collagenase-induced diseases of the cornea. Tr Am Acad Ophth **74**:375-83, 1970.

Brown, S. I., Weller, C. A., & S. Akiya: Pathogenesis of ulcers of the alkali-burned cornea. Arch Ophth **83**:205-8, 1970.

Burns, R. P.: Pseudomonas aeruginosa keratitis: Mixed infections of the eye. Am J Ophth **67**:257-62, 1969.

Charney, S. M., & M. Goldenberg: Idiopathic band keratopathy. Arch Ophth **75**:505-7, 1966.

Choyce, D. P.: Diagnosis and management of ocular leprosy. Brit J Ophth **53**:217-23, 1969.

Cogan, D. G.: Applied anatomy and physiology of the cornea. Tr Am Acad Ophth **55**:329-403, 1951.

Council on Drugs, AMA: Evaluation of idoxuridine (IDU). JAMA **190**:535-6, 1964.

Dawson, C., & others: Infections due to adenovirus type 8 in the United States. II. Community-wide infection with adenovirus type 8. New England J Med **268**:1034-7, 1963.

Dawson, C. R., & others: Adenovirus type 8 keratoconjunctivitis in the United States. Am J Ophth **69**:473-80, 1970.

De Voe, A. G.: Management of chronic corneal ulcers. South MJ **62**:1175, 1969.

De Voe, A. G.: The management of endothelial dystrophy of the cornea. Am J Ophth **61**:1084-9, 1966.

Donaldson, D. D.: Atlas of External Diseases of the Eye. Vol. III: The Cornea and Sclera. Mosby, 1971.

Edelhauser, H. F., Schultz, R. O., & D. L. Van Horn: Experimental herpes simplex keratitis. Am J Ophth **68**:458-66, 1969.

Golden, B., Fingerman, L. H., & H. F. Allen: Pseudomonas corneal ulcers in contact lens wearers. Arch Ophth **85**:543-7, 1971.

Goldman, J. N., Dohlman, C. H., & B. A. Krabitt: The basement membrane of the human cornea in recurrent epithelial erosion syndrome. Tr Am Acad Ophth **73**:471, 1969.

Hessburg, P. C.: Management of Pseudomonas keratitis. Survey Ophth **14**:43-54, 1969.

Hogan, M. J., & G. Bietti: Hereditary deep dystrophy of the cornea (polymorphous). Am J Ophth **68**:777-88, 1969.

Hughes, W. F.: Treatment of herpes simplex keratitis. Am J Ophth **67**:313-28, 1969.

Karseras, A. G., & D. C. Price: Central crystalline corneal dystrophy. Brit J Ophth **54**:659-62, 1970.

Kaufman, H. E.: Management of herpetic keratitis with IDU. Ann Ophth **1**:199, 1970.

Kaufman, H. E., Brown, D. C., & E. D. Ellison: Herpes virus in the lacrimal gland, conjunctiva, and cornea of man. A chronic infection. Am J Ophth **65**:32-6, 1968.

Kaufman, H. E., & R. M. Wood: Mycotic keratitis. Am J Ophth **59**:993-1000, 1965.

Laibson, P. R.: Cornea and sclera. Annual review. Arch Ophth **83**:738-61, 1971.

Lowe, R. F.: Recurrent erosion of the cornea. Brit J Ophth **54**:805-9, 1970.

Naumann, G., Green, W. R., & L. E. Zimmerman: Mycotic keratitis: A histopathologic study of 73 cases. Am J Ophth **64**:668-82, 1967.

Picetti, B., & M. Fine: Keratoplasty in children. Am J Ophth **61**:1344-9, 1966.

Ruedemann, A. D., Jr.: Clinical course of keratoconus. Tr Am Acad Ophth **74**:384-98, 1970.

Sato, K., & others: Pseudomonas corneal ulcers. J Clin Ophth **19**:655-9, 1965.

Sen, D. K.: Surgery of pterygium. Brit J Ophth **54**:606-8, 1970.

Sen, K.: Keratomalacia: Causes, diagnosis, treatment, and prevention. J Indian MA **35**:17-20, 1954.

Slansky, H. H., & C. H. Dohlman: Collagenase and the cornea. Survey Ophth **14**:402-16, 1970.

Smolin, G., & M. Okumoto: Herpes simplex keratitis. Arch Ophth **83**:746-51, 1970.

Smolin, G., & M. Okumoto: Potentiation of Candida albicans keratitis by antilymphocyte serum and corticosteroids. Am J Ophth **68**:675-82, 1969.

Symposium on direct fungal infection of the eye. Organized by B. R. Jones, presented at the Oxford Ophthalmological Congress, 1969. Reprinted from Trans Ophthal Soc UK, Vol. 89, 1969.

Taylor, R. P.: Fornix-based conjunctival flap in the treatment of corneal ulcers. Am J Ophth **67**:754-6, 1969.

Thygeson, P.: Clinical and laboratory observations on superficial punctate keratitis. Am J Ophth **61**:1344-9, 1960.

Tschetter, R. T.: Lipid analysis of the human cornea with and without arcus senilis. Arch Ophth **76**:403-5, 1966.

Vaughan, D. G., Jr.: Corneal ulcers. Survey Ophth **3**:203-15, 1958.

8 . . .

Uveal Tract

The uveal tract is composed of 3 parts: the iris, the ciliary body, and the choroid. It is the middle vascular layer of the eye, protected externally by the cornea and sclera. It contributes to the blood supply of the retina.

Anatomy of the Iris

The iris is the anterior extension of the ciliary body. It presents a relatively flat surface with a round aperture in the middle called the pupil. It forms the posterior wall of the anterior chamber and the anterior wall of the posterior chamber. The pupil varies in size and has the same form and function as the aperture of a camera lens. The iris is in contact with the lens and the aqueous posteriorly and the aqueous anteriorly. It has 2 zones on its anterior surface, the ciliary and pupillary zones. The sphincter and dilator muscles, which serve to constrict and dilate the pupil, are in the iris stroma.

Because of their thick walls, normal iris arterioles have the histologic appearance of being quite sclerotic. The 2 posterior layers of epithelium are heavily pigmented and represent the anterior extension of the pigmented epithelium of the retina plus the retina proper. The blood supply is from the major circle of the iris (see p 6). The nerve supply is described on p 135.

When the iris is cut, as in doing a small peripheral iridectomy for acute angle-closure glaucoma, it seldom bleeds, and the wound remains permanently with no tendency to heal. Pain fibers are present, as shown by the pain caused by traction on the iris during surgery.

Anatomy of the Ciliary Body

The ciliary body is a roughly triangular structure which extends forward from the anterior termination of the choroid to the root of the iris, a distance of about 6 mm. Grossly

Ora serrata   Zonules   Ciliary process   Pars plana

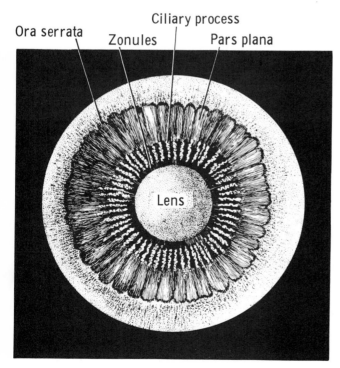

Lens

Fig 8-1. **Posterior view of ciliary body, zonules, lens, and ora serrata.** (Redrawn and reproduced, with permission, from Wolff: Anatomy of the Eye and Orbit, 4th ed. Blakiston-McGraw, 1954.)

it consists of 2 zones: the corona ciliaris, the corrugated anterior 2 mm; and the pars plana, the smoother and flatter posterior 4 mm. The surface of the corona ciliaris consists of many elevations and depressions; the white elevations are the white ciliary processes. The intervening depressions are dark (Fig 8-1).

There are 2 layers of ciliary epithelium, the external pigmented and the internal nonpigmented, both of which continue as pigmented layers over the posterior surface of the iris. The pigmented epithelium represents the forward extension of the pigmented epithelium of the retina. It is absent at the tips of the ciliary processes (hence their white appearance), but is heaped up in the valleys, which accounts for the dark appearance of these areas (Fig 8-1). The nonpigmented epithelium, with the exception of the pigmented epithelium of the internal limiting membrane of the retina, is continuous with the entire retina.

The ciliary muscle consists of longitudinal, radial, and circular portions. Its function is to contract and relax the zonular fibers. This results in decreased or increased tension on the capsule of the lens, which allows the lens to become more convex or less convex for near (accommodation) or far vision, respectively. The ciliary processes themselves are composed mainly of veins which drain through the vortex veins.

The pars plana consists of a thin layer of ciliary muscle and vessels covered by ciliary epithelium. The zonular fibers, which hold the lens in place, originate in the valleys between the ciliary processes (see Fig 8-1). The blood vessels to the ciliary body come from the major circle of the iris (see p 6). The sensory nerve supply is through the ciliary nerves.

Anatomy of the Choroid

The choroid (the posterior portion of the uveal tract and the middle coat of the eye) lies between the retina and the sclera. It is largely composed of blood vessels. The choroidal vessels are bounded by Bruch's membrane internally and the suprachoroid externally. The suprachoroid is composed of a thin layer of laminated protoplasmic plaques containing nuclei. Bruch's membrane is a structureless membrane which consists of 2 sheaths: an outer elastic sheath and an inner cuticular sheath.

The lumens of the blood vessels decrease the deeper they are located in the choroid. There are 3 layers of blood vessels: large, medium, and small. The innermost layer of small blood vessels is known as the choriocapillaris and consists of large capillaries which nourish the outer portion of the retina. Most of the large vessels consist of veins. These coalesce and leave the eye as the 4 vortex veins, one in each of the 4 posterior quadrants. The vessel layers of the choroid also contain some elastic fibers and chromatophores.

The choroid is firmly attached to the margin of the optic nerve posteriorly and extends to the ora serrata anteriorly, where it joins the ciliary body.

Functions of Uveal Structures

The function of the iris is to control the amount of light which enters the eye. This occurs by reflex constriction of the pupil under the stimulus of light and dilatation of the pupil in darkness. The ciliary body forms the root of the iris and serves, through the zonular fibers, to govern the size of the lens in accommodation. Aqueous humor is secreted by the ciliary processes into the posterior chamber. The choroid consists of abundant blood vessels; its function is to nourish the outer portion of the underlying retina.

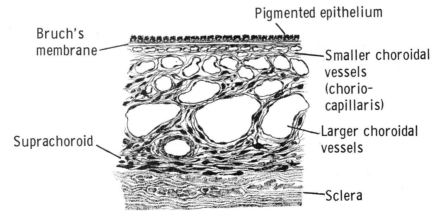

Fig 8-2. Cross-section of choroid. (Redrawn and reproduced, with permission, from Wolff: Anatomy of the Eye and Orbit, 4th ed. Blakiston-McGraw, 1954.)

Physiology of Symptoms

Symptoms of uveal tract disorders depend upon the site of the disease process. For example, since there are pain fibers in the iris, the patient with iritis will complain of moderate pain and photophobia. Inflammation of the iris as such does not cause blurring of vision unless the process is severe or advanced enough to cause clouding of the aqueous, cornea, or lens. Choroidal disease itself does not cause pain or blurred vision. Because of the close contact of the choroid with the retina, choroidal disease almost always affects the retina (eg, chorioretinitis). If the macular area of the retina is involved, central vision will be impaired.

The vitreous may also become cloudy as a result of posterior uveitis. The impairment of vision is in proportion to the density of vitreus opacity, and is reversible as the inflammation subsides and the vitreous haze clears.

The physician examines for disease of the anterior uveal tract with the flashlight and loupe or slit lamp, and disease of the posterior uveal tract with the ophthalmoscope.

UVEITIS*

Inflammation of the uveal tract has many causes and may involve one or all 3 portions simultaneously. The most frequent form of uveitis is acute anterior uveitis (iritis), usually unilateral and characterized by a history of pain, photophobia, and blurring of vision; a red eye (circumcorneal flush) without purulent discharge; and a small pupil. It is important to make the diagnosis early and to dilate the pupil to prevent the formation of permanent posterior synechias.

Inflammatory disorders of the uveal tract, usually unilateral, are common principally in the young and middle age groups. In most cases the cause is not known. In posterior uveitis the retina is almost always secondarily affected. This is known as chorioretinitis.

Two major types of uveitis may be distinguished upon clinical as well as pathologic

---

*"Uveitis" is a general term for inflammatory disorders of the uveal tract. "Anterior uveitis" is the preferred general term for iritis and iridocyclitis. "Posterior uveitis" is the preferred term for choroiditis and chorioretinitis. The term "iritis," used above, means acute anterior nongranulomatous uveitis.

grounds: nongranulomatous (more common) and granulomatous.† Because pathogenic organisms have not been found in the nongranulomatous type and because it responds to steroid therapy, it is thought to be a sensitivity phenomenon. Granulomatous uveitis usually follows active microbial invasion of the tissues by the causative organism (eg, Mycobacterium tuberculosis or Toxoplasma gondii). However, these pathogens are rarely recovered, and a definite etiologic diagnosis is seldom possible. The etiologic possibilities can often be narrowed to a few probable causes by clinical and laboratory examination.

Nongranulomatous uveitis occurs only in the anterior portion of the tract, ie, the iris and ciliary body. There is an inflammatory reaction, as evidenced by the cellular infiltration of lymphocytes and plasma cells in significant numbers and an occasional mononuclear cell. In severe cases a large fibrin clot or a hypopyon may form in the anterior chamber.

Granulomatous uveitis may involve any portion of the uveal tract but has a predilection for the posterior area. Nodular collections of epithelioid cells and giant cells surrounded by lymphocytes are present in the affected areas. Inflammatory deposits on the posterior surface of the cornea are composed mainly of epithelioid cells and pigment. It is possible to make a specific etiologic diagnosis histologically in an enucleated eye by identifying the pseudocyst of toxoplasmosis, the acid-fast bacillus of tuberculosis, the spirochete of syphilis, the distinctive granulomatous appearance of sarcoidosis and sympathetic ophthalmia, and a few other rare specific causes.

Clinical Findings

A. Symptoms and Signs: In the nongranulomatous form, the onset is characteristically acute, with pain, injection, photophobia, and blurred vision. There is a circumcorneal flush caused by dilated limbal blood vessels. Fine white deposits (keratic precipitates, "KP's") on the posterior surface of the cornea can be seen with the slit lamp or with a loupe. The pupil is small, and there may be a collection of fibrin with cells in the anterior chamber. If posterior synechias are present, the pupil will be irregular in shape and the light reflex will be absent. Posterior uveitis is generally classified as granulomatous.

---

†The clinical differentiation of the 2 types is not always clear. In some clinics this classification has been discarded in favor of an anatomic differentiation into 3 types: anterior, posterior, and pan-uveitis.

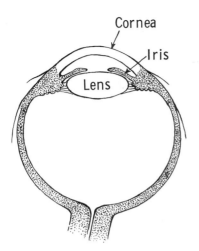

Fig 8-3. Normal anterior chamber.

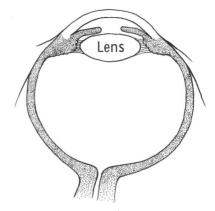

Fig 8-4. Anterior synechias (adhesions).
The peripheral iris adheres to the cornea.

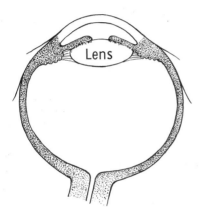

Fig 8-5. Posterior synechias. The
iris adheres to the lens.

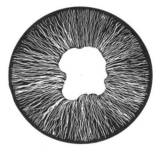
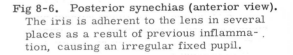

Fig 8-6. Posterior synechias (anterior view).
The iris is adherent to the lens in several
places as a result of previous inflammation, causing an irregular fixed pupil.

The patient should be asked about previous episodes of arthritis and possible exposure
to toxoplasmosis, histoplasmosis, tuberculosis, and syphilis. The remote possibility
of a focus of infection elsewhere in the body
should also be investigated.

In granulomatous uveitis (may cause anterior uveitis, posterior uveitis, or both), the
onset is usually insidious. Vision gradually
becomes blurred and the affected eye becomes
diffusely red with circumcorneal flush. Pain
is minimal, and photophobia is less marked
than in the nongranulomatous form. The pupil
is often constricted and becomes irregular as
posterior synechias form. Large gray "mut-
ton-fat" KP's on the posterior surface of the
cornea may be seen with the slit lamp. Flare
and cells are seen in the anterior chamber,
and nodules consisting of clusters of white

cells are seen on the iris (Koeppe nodules).
These nodules are the equivalent of the mutton-
fat KP's.

Fresh active lesions of the choroid appear
as yellowish-white patches seen hazily with the
ophthalmoscope through the cloudy vitreous.
Such posterior cases are generally classified
as granulomatous disease. Because of the
intimate relationship of the choroid and retina,
the retina is nearly always involved also (chorioretinitis). As healing progresses, the vitreous haze lessens and pigmentation occurs
gradually at the edges of the yellowish-white
spots. In the healed stage, there is usually
considerable pigment deposition. If the macula has not been involved, recovery of central
vision is complete. The patient is usually not
aware of the scotoma in the peripheral field
corresponding to the scarred area.

Table 8-1. Differentiation of granulomatous and nongranulomatous uveitis.

	Nongranulomatous	Granulomatous
Onset	Acute	Insidious
Pain	Marked	None or minimal
Photophobia	Marked	Slight
Blurred vision	Marked	Marked
Circumcorneal flush	Marked	Slight
Keratic precipitates	Fine white	Large gray ("mutton-fat")
Pupil	Small and irregular	Small and irregular (variable)
Posterior synechias	Sometimes	Sometimes
Anterior chamber	Flare predominates	Cells predominate
Iris nodules	Absent	Sometimes
Vitreous haze	Absent	Sometimes
Site	Anterior tract	Posterior tract (variable)
Course	Acute	Chronic
Prognosis	Good	Fair to poor
Recurrence	Common	Sometimes

B. Laboratory Findings: Extensive laboratory investigation is usually not indicated in anterior uveitis, particularly if it is nongranulomatous or is readily responsive to nonspecific treatment. In persistent nonresponsive anterior or posterior uveitis, an attempt should be made to arrive at an etiologic diagnosis. Skin tests for tuberculosis, histoplasmosis, and toxoplasmosis may be helpful, as well as complement fixation tests and methylene blue dye tests (toxoplasmosis). On the basis of these tests and the clinical appearance, it is possible to make an etiologic diagnosis.

Differential Diagnosis

In conjunctivitis, vision is not blurred, pupillary responses are normal, a discharge is present, and there is no pain, photophobia, or ciliary injection.

In acute glaucoma the pupil is dilated, there are no posterior synechias, and the cornea is steamy.

After repeated attacks, nongranulomatous uveitis may acquire the characteristics of granulomatous uveitis. In recent years there has been less emphasis on this differentiation, and some authorities are disregarding it completely. Nevertheless, to the clinician the differentiation is still of value as a guide to treatment and prognosis.

Complications and Sequelae

Anterior uveitis may produce peripheral anterior synechias, which impede aqueous outflow at the anterior chamber angle and cause glaucoma. Posterior synechias can cause glaucoma by impeding the flow of aqueous from the posterior to the anterior chamber. Early and constant pupillary dilatation lessens the likelihood of both kinds of synech-

ias. Interference with lens metabolism may cause cataract. Retinal detachment occasionally occurs as a result of traction on the retina by vitreous strands.

Treatment

A. Nongranulomatous Uveitis: Symptomatic measures include warm compresses for 10 minutes 3-4 times a day, systemic analgesics as necessary for pain, and dark glasses for photophobia. The pupil must be kept dilated with atropine, 2%, 2 drops at least twice daily. Local steroid drops are usually quite effective for their anti-inflammatory action. In severe and unresponsive cases, systemic steroids are given also.

B. Granulomatous Uveitis: If the process includes the anterior segment, pupillary dilatation with atropine, 2%, is indicated. Since it is often possible to make a tentative or likely etiologic diagnosis, an attempt with specific therapy is indicated as outlined in Table 8-2.

C. Treatment of Complications: Glaucoma is the most common complication. Treatment of the uveitis is of primary importance, particularly dilating the pupil with atropine (not constricting the pupil, as with all forms of primary glaucoma). Carbonic anhydrase inhibitors often effectively reduce intraocular tension by depressing aqueous production. Epinephrine also lowers intraocular pressure by reducing ciliary body secretion of aqueous.

Cataract frequently develops in chronic uveitis. The eye tolerates removal of such cataracts very poorly; but if vision is poor enough, cataract surgery may be essential. Retinal detachment is also very difficult to treat successfully surgically when it occurs in association with uveitis.

Table 8-2. Treatment of granulomatous uveitis.

	Anti-infective Chemotherapy	Use of Corticosteroids
Toxoplasmosis	Give pyrimethamine (Daraprim®), 150 mg orally as loading dose followed by 25 mg twice daily for 4 weeks, in combination with trisulfapyrimidines (sulfadiazine, sulfamerazine, and sulfamethazine, 0.167 gm of each per tablet), 4 gm orally as loading dose followed by 1 gm 4 times daily for 4 weeks. If a fall in the white or platelet count occurs during therapy, give folinic acid (leucovorin), 1 ml IM twice weekly.	If the response is not favorable after one month, continue anti-infective therapy and give systemic steroids, eg, prednisolone, 40-80 mg every other day for 4-6 weeks,* to protect the macula. Steroids may activate the organisms of toxoplasmosis and tuberculosis, but are given as a calculated risk to control the inflammatory response when it threatens vision.
Tuberculosis	Isoniazid, 100 mg 3 times daily, and aminosalicylic acid (PAS), 4 gm 3 times daily after meals. If PAS is not tolerated, give streptomycin, 1 gm IM twice weekly. Continue treatment for 4-6 months.	If a favorable response does not occur in 6 weeks, continue antimycobacterial therapy and give systemic steroids, eg, prednisolone, 40-80 mg every other day for 2 months.*
Sarcoidosis	Treat with local corticosteroids and mydriatics and, during active stages, with systemic corticosteroids such as prednisolone, 40-80 mg every other day.* Give supplemental potassium chloride, 2 gm 3 times daily. The usual contraindications to systemic steroid therapy apply.	
Sympathetic ophthalmia	Treat with local steroids and mydriatics and systemic steroids in high doses, eg, prednisolone, 40-120 mg every other day.* The usual contraindications to systemic steroid therapy apply, and the drugs may be needed in higher doses and for a longer time. Therefore, management of the side effects is often more difficult.	

*Administration every other day has been advocated to minimize the effects of stress and make drug withdrawal easier and safer.

Course and Prognosis

With treatment, an attack of nongranulomatous uveitis usually lasts a few days to weeks. Recurrences are common.

Granulomatous uveitis lasts months to years, sometimes with remissions and exacerbations, and may cause permanent damage with marked visual loss despite the best available treatment. The prognosis for a focal peripheral chorioretinal lesion is considerably better, often healing well with no significant visual loss.

SPECIFIC TYPES OF UVEITIS
(Uveitis Syndromes)

UVEITIS ASSOCIATED WITH JOINT DISEASE

About 20% of children with **rheumatoid arthritis (Still's disease)** develop a chronic bilateral nongranulomatous iridocyclitis. Females are far more commonly affected than males (12:1). The average age at which the uveitis is detected is 5$\frac{1}{2}$ years. In most cases the onset is insidious, the disease being discovered only when the child is noted to have heterochromia of the iris, a difference in the size or shape of the pupil, or the onset of strabismus. There is no correlation between the onset of the arthritis and of the uveitis. The uveitis may precede the arthritis by 3-10 years. The knee is the most common joint involved. The cardinal signs of the disease are calcific band keratopathy, cells and flare in the anterior chamber, small to medium-sized white keratic precipitates with or without flecks of fibrin on the endothelium, posterior synechiae, often progressing to seclusion of the pupil, complicated cataract, variable secondary glaucoma, and macular edema.

Corticosteroids and mydriatics are of value, especially in acute exacerbations, but their long-range effect seems merely to delay the inevitable, ie, severe visual impairment or phthisis bulbi. The prognosis is very poor because of the relentless and progressive character of the disease which leads to serious complications.

Iridocyclitis occurring in association with adult peripheral rheumatoid arthritis is strictly coincidental. The adult group is more likely to develop scleritis and sclero-uveitis. It is unfortunate that the associated cells and flare in the aqueous humor that accompany the scle-

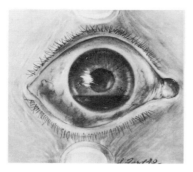

Fig 8-7. Blood in the anterior chamber (hyphema) associated with rheumatoid iridocyclitis. (Courtesy of M. Hogan.)

ritis have been misinterpreted in the past as "iridocyclitis."

About 10-60% of patients with **Marie-Strümpell ankylosing spondylitis** develop an anterior uveitis. There is a marked preponderance in males. The uveitis presents as a mild to fairly severe nongranulomatous type of iridocyclitis with moderate to severe ciliary injection, pain, blurred vision, and photophobia. It is usually recurrent and eventually may lead to permanent damage if not adequately treated.

Ocular examination shows ciliary injection, moderate cells and flare in the anterior chamber, and fine white keratic precipitates located mostly on the inferior cornea. Posterior synechiae, peripheral anterior synechiae, cataracts, and glaucoma are common complications after hyperacute attacks of inflammation. Macular edema occurs in 1% of cases with severe anterior iridocyclitis, which, if persistent, leads to cystoid degeneration and loss of central vision.

Confirmation of the diagnosis is by x-rays of the lumbosacral spine. In about 50% of patients with ankylosing spondylitis, the clinical signs and symptoms may all be absent so that the diagnosis may be made only by the radiologist.

HETEROCHROMIC UVEITIS
(Fuchs's Heterochromic Cyclitis)

This disease of unknown etiology accounts for about 3% of all cases of uveitis. It is essentially a quiet cyclitis associated with depigmentation of the iris in the affected eye. Pathologically, the iris and ciliary body show moderate atrophy, diffuse fibrosis, patchy depigmentation of the pigment layer, and diffuse infiltration of lymphocytes and plasma cells.

Involvement is typically unilateral but may be bilateral, and the eyes are of different colors.

The onset is insidious in the 3rd or 4th decade. The lighter-colored eye is usually affected, and there is no redness, pain, or photophobia; the patient is often unaware of the disorder until cataract formation results in blurred vision.

With the slit lamp (or loupe) one sees fine white deposits on the posterior corneal surface, flare and cells in the anterior chamber, and a slightly atrophic iris. Anterior vitreous floaters may be evident with the ophthalmoscope or slit lamp.

Cataract develops within a few years in about 15% of cases. Glaucoma occurs in 10-15% of cases. No treatment affects the course of this type of uveitis. It is not necessary to dilate the pupil, as this is one type of uveitis in which posterior synechias do not form. The disease does not subside spontaneously, but the visual prognosis is good since the cataract can be removed safely despite the low-grade active uveitis. This disease is believed to be degenerative rather than inflammatory because there are no posterior synechias, corticosteroid therapy has no effect, and the eyes are remarkably tolerant to cataract surgery.

LENS-INDUCED UVEITIS

There are no data at present to substantiate the implication that lens material per se is toxic, so that the term phacotoxic uveitis should no longer be considered as a type of lens-induced uveitis. The terms phacogenic or lens-induced uveitis are more appropriate when referring to an autoimmune disease secondary to lens antigen. The classical case of lens-induced uveitis occurs when the lens develops a hypermature cataract. The lens capsule leaks and lens material passes into the anterior chamber, causing an inflammatory reaction characterized by the accumulation of plasma cells, mononuclear phagocytes, and a few polymorphonuclear cells. The eye becomes red and moderately painful; the pupil is small; and vision is markedly reduced (at times to light perception only). Lens-induced uveitis may also occur following traumatic cataracts.

Endophthalmitis phaco-anaphylactica, the term used for the more severe form of lens-induced uveitis, occurs following an extracapsular lens extraction when the same operation has already been performed on the fellow eye and the patient has been sensitized to his own lens material. Many polymorphonuclear leukocytes and mononuclear phagocytes appear in the anterior chamber. The eye becomes red and painful, and vision is blurred. Since most of the lens material has already been removed, treatment is conservative, consisting of corticosteroids locally and systemically plus atropine drops to keep the pupil dilated. If this is ineffective, the cataract incision must be opened and the anterior chamber irrigated.

Glaucoma is a common complication of lens-induced uveitis. Treatment consists of lens extraction after intraocular tension has been brought under control. If this is done, both the uveitis and the glaucoma are cured, and the visual prognosis is good if the process has not been present for more than 1-2 weeks.

SYMPATHETIC OPHTHALMIA
(Sympathetic Uveitis)

Sympathetic ophthalmia is a rare but devastating granulomatous bilateral uveitis which comes on 10 days to many years following a perforating eye injury in the region of the ciliary body, or following retained foreign body. The cause is not known, but the disease is probably related to hypersensitivity to uveal pigment. It very rarely occurs following uncomplicated intraocular surgery for cataract or glaucoma.

The injured (exciting) eye becomes inflamed first and the fellow (sympathizing) eye second. Pathologically, there is a diffuse granulomatous uveitis. The epithelioid cells, together with giant cells and lymphocytes, form noncaseating tubercles. From the uveal tract the inflammatory process spreads to the optic nerve and to the pia and arachnoid surrounding the optic nerve.

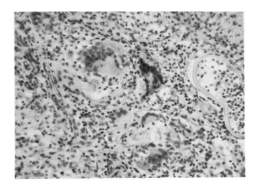

Fig 8-8. **Microscopic section of giant cells and lymphocytes in sympathetic ophthalmia involving the choroid.** (Courtesy of R. Carriker.)

The patient complains of photophobia, redness, and blurring of vision. If a history of trauma is obtained, look for a scar representing the wound of entry in the exciting eye. With the slit lamp or loupe one sees KP's and a flare in the anterior chamber of both eyes. Iris nodules may be present.

Sympathetic ophthalmia is differentiated from tuberculous uveitis by the history of trauma or ocular surgery, and is bilateral, diffuse, and acute rather than unilateral, localized, and chronic, as tuberculous uveitis tends to be. The tubercles of tuberculous uveitis caseate, whereas the granulomas of sympathetic ophthalmia do not. Lens-induced uveitis is bilateral, and there is no history of injury.

The recommended treatment of a severely injured eye (eg, a penetrating injury through the sclera, ciliary body, and lens, with loss of vitreous) is immediate enucleation to prevent sympathetic ophthalmia, and every effort must be made to secure the patient's reasoned consent to the operation. If enucleation can be performed within 10 days after injury, there is almost no chance that sympathetic ophthalmia will develop. However, when the inflammation in the sympathizing eye is advanced, it is wise not to enucleate the injured eye since it may eventually prove to be the better of 2 very bad eyes.

If inflammation has appeared in the sympathizing eye, begin treatment immediately with corticosteroids locally and systemically plus atropine locally. Continue corticosteroids for at least a year.

Without treatment, the disease progresses slowly but relentlessly over a period of months or years to complete bilateral blindness.

TUBERCULOUS UVEITIS

Tuberculosis causes a granulomatous type of uveitis. Tuberculous uveitis is diagnosed clinically far more often than the disease can be proved by positive identification of tubercle bacilli in the tissues. Although the infection is said to be transmitted from a primary focus elsewhere in the body, uveal tuberculosis is rare in patients with active pulmonary tuberculosis.

Tuberculous uveitis may be diffuse but is characteristically localized in the form of a severe caseating granulomatous chorioretinitis. The tubercle itself consists of giant cells and epithelioid cells. Caseation necrosis commonly occurs.

The patient complains of blurred vision, and the eye is moderately injected. If the anterior segment is involved, iris nodules and "mutton fat" KP's are visible on slit lamp examination. If the choroid and retina are primarily affected, one can see a localized yellowish mass partially obscured by a hazy vitreous.

The nodules and the localized nature of tuberculous uveitis help to make a clinical differentiation from sympathetic ophthalmia, and the caseation necrosis differentiates it pathologically from sympathetic ophthalmia and Boeck's sarcoid.

The pupil should be kept dilated with atropine, 2%, 2 drops 2-3 times daily. Antituberculosis drugs should be prescribed systemically if a reasonably certain clinical diagnosis can be made. (See Table 8-2.)

After a prolonged course of several months, the disease usually resolves, leaving permanently damaged tissues and blurred vision due to scarring of the retina.

SARCOIDOSIS
(Boeck's Sarcoid)

Sarcoidosis is a chronic granulomatous disease of unknown cause characterized by multiple cutaneous and subcutaneous nodules with similar invasions in the viscera and bones and periodic exacerbations and remissions. The onset is usually in the third decade. The tissue reaction is much less severe than in tuberculous uveitis, and caseation does not occur. The tuberculin skin test is usually negative or only faintly positive. When the parotid glands are involved, the disease is called uveoparotid fever (Heerfordt's disease); when the lacrimal glands are involved, it is called Mikulicz's syndrome.

Thirty percent of cases are complicated by chronic bilateral anterior uveitis, whereas posterior uveitis is far less common. Anterior uveitis is nodular, and in prolonged cases may lead to severe visual impairment due to cataract and secondary glaucoma. Posterior uveitis is characterized by multiple whitish-yellow retinal exudates and perivasculitis.

Corticosteroid therapy (see Table 8-2) given early in the disease may be effective, but recurrences are common and the long-term visual prognosis is poor.

TOXOPLASMIC UVEITIS

Toxoplasmosis is primarily an inflammation of the CNS caused by Toxoplasma gondii, a protozoan parasite. In congenital toxoplasmosis, chorioretinitis is almost invariably present. Toxoplasmosis occurring in later life does not usually involve the eye in the acute stage, but chorioretinitis frequently occurs in the chronic form.

The disease is more common in tropical countries.* Pathologically there is a granulomatous chorioretinitis. The retina is characteristically necrotic, and Toxoplasma organisms are found in the retinal tissues. The clinical picture is variable, but typically there is a chorioretinal lesion or lesions, usually in the macular area, which in the early stages appear as elevated white masses partially obscured by a hazy vitreous. In the later stages, a punched-out pigmented chorioretinal lesion develops through which the sclera is clearly visible. The methylene blue dye test on the patient's serum is positive, ie, antibodies in the serum prevent the dye from staining Toxoplasma organisms.

Although the pathology of the chorioretinitis is essentially the same, there are 2 distinct clinical types of ocular toxoplasmosis: congenital and acquired. The congenital type is due to intra-uterine infection. As in the acquired (adult) type, the chorioretinitis is usually confined to the macular area. The inflammatory process is more severe in congenital than in acquired toxoplasmosis, and is frequently bilateral. Cerebral involvement, with radiopaque calcification and mental deficiency, is present in 10% of cases of the congenital type.

Acquired ocular toxoplasmosis is usually milder than congenital toxoplasmosis. It may appear at any age, is often unilateral, and frequently occurs in the absence of CNS involvement. The patient complains of blurred vision if the macula is involved.

For treatment, see Table 8-2.

The chorioretinitis progresses to a healed stage, leaving a scarred retina and choroid. If the macula has been involved, loss of central vision is permanent.

---

*The cat is the definitive host of Toxoplasma gondii. It is a coccidian undergoing typical schizogonic cycles and gametogony in the intestinal epithelial cells of the cat. Intermediate hosts such as rodents, birds, or man become infected by ingestion of the oocysts passed in cat feces. Additional means of transmission among intermediate hosts occurs by carnivorism with ingestion of trophozoites or cysts present mainly in brain and muscle tissue.

HISTOPLASMOSIS

In some areas of the USA where histoplasmosis is endemic (eg, Cincinnati, Baltimore), the diagnosis of chorioretinitis due to histoplasmosis is being made with increasing frequency. The macular lesion begins as a small area of edema and is indistinguishable from central serous retinopathy. The patient must have a positive skin test to histoplasmin and must also demonstrate "histo" spots in the peripheral retina. These spots are small, irregularly round or oval, depigmented areas, sometimes with a fine pigmented border. They are smaller and have less pigment than the usual healed chorioretinal lesion. The macular lesion may progress to a hemorrhagic stage, finally healing with considerable macular scarring and visual loss, or macular edema may subside with little or no scarring. Vitreous haze does not occur.

It has been postulated that, in areas where histoplasmosis is endemic, many persons develop a benign form of asymptomatic peripheral chorioretinitis. These lesions soon heal, leaving "histo" spots. This exposure sensitizes the choroid. A later antigenic insult to the choroid results in the observed macular changes. This hypothesis has not been verified, and as yet the parasite has never been identified in the choroid on histologic section.

Many types of treatment have been advocated, including systemic steroids, amphotericin B (Fungizone®), antihistamines, and intradermal desensitization with histoplasmin. The results have been questionable in all cases.

• • •

Bibliography

Asbury, T.: The status of presumed ocular histoplasmosis, including a report of a survey. Trans Amer Ophth Soc 64:371-400, 1966.

Coles, R.S.: Uveitis. A review. Survey Ophth 5:355-404, 1960.

Coles, R.S.: Uveitis associated with systemic disease. Survey Ophth, Part I, 8:377-92, and Part II, 8:479-506, 1963.

Foerster, H.W.: Pathology of granulomatous uveitis. Survey Ophth 4:283-326, 1959.

Frenkel, J.K., Dubey, J.P., & N.L. Miller: Toxoplasma gondii in cats: Fecal stages identified as coccidian oocysts. Science 167:893-6, 1970.

Hogan, M.J., Kimura, S.J., & G.R. O'Connor: Ocular toxoplasmosis. Arch Ophth 72:592-600, 1964.

Irvine, S.R., & A.R. Irvine, Jr.: Lens induced uveitis and glaucoma. Am J Ophth 35:177-86, 370, 375, and 489-99, 1952.

Kazdan, J.J., McCulloch, J.C., & J.S. Crawford: Uveitis in children. Canad MAJ 96:385-91, 1967.

Kimura, S.J., & others: Uveitis and joint diseases. Arch Ophth 77:309-17, 1967.

Kimura, S.J., & W.M. Caygill (editors): Differential Diagnostic Problems of Posterior Uveitis. Lea & Febiger, 1966.

Leopold, I.H.: Drug therapy in uveitis. The XVII Annual Francis I. Proctor Lecture. Am J Ophth 56:709-24, 1963.

Maumenee, A.E.: Clinical entities in "uveitis": An approach to the study of intraocular inflammation. Am J Ophth 69:1-27, 1970.

Maumenee, A.E. (editor): Uveitis. Symposium by the Council for Research in Glaucoma and Allied Diseases. Survey Ophth 4:217-423, 1957.

Maumenee, A.E., & A.M. Silverstein (editors): Immunopathology of Uveitis. Williams & Wilkins, 1964.

Morse, P.H., & J.R. Duke: Sympathetic ophthalmitis. Am J Ophth 68:508-12, 1969.

Schlaegel, T.F., Jr.: Essentials of Uveitis. Little, Brown, 1969.

Schlaegel, T.F., Jr.: The uvea. Annual review. Arch Ophth 85:524-35, 1971.

Sugar, H.S.: Heterochromia iridis with special consideration of its relation to cyclitic disease. Am J Ophth 60:1-18, 1965.

Van Metre, T.E., Jr., Knox, D.L., & A.E. Maumenee: Specific ocular uveal lesions in patients with evidence of histoplasmosis and toxoplasmosis. South MJ 58:479-86, 1965.

Wirostko, E., & H.F. Spalter: Lens induced uveitis. Arch Ophth 78:1-7, 1967.

9 . . .

Retina

Anatomy and Function

The retina, the most essential part of the eye, is equivalent in function to the film in a camera; all the other structures of the eye exist only to nourish and protect the retina and to focus light rays upon it.

The retina is attached to the underlying choroid at the optic nerve border posteriorly and at the ora serrata anteriorly; between these 2 points it is in contact with but not attached to the choroid. It covers the entire inner aspect of the eyeball posterior to the ora serrata.

The retina averages 0.4 mm in thickness and is thinner in the region of the macula and ora serrata. At the posterior pole of the globe it leaves the eye as the optic nerve. It is composed of highly developed inelastic nerve tissue. When detached it appears gray, but normally it is transparent. Histologically, the retina consists of 10 distinct layers (Fig 9-2).

A marked variation in the structure of the retina is present in the region of the macula lutea. The macula is round, and has the same diameter as the optic disk. Its center is 3.5 mm temporal to and 0.5 mm below the optic disk. It is depressed, and thus reflects light from the ophthalmoscope in the manner of a concave mirror. The macular periphery contains many ganglion cells.

In the center of the macula lutea is the fovea centralis, which is composed only of cones. It is extremely thin and avascular. The peripheral or extramacular retina contains all of the normal layers of the retina and includes both rods and cones, the rods being much more numerous than the cones. The macula is nourished by the choroidal vessels only, whereas the peripheral retina has a double blood supply, the inner two-thirds being nourished by branches of the central retinal artery and the outer one-third by the choriocapillaris.

The ora serrata is the junction of the retina and ciliary body. In an average-sized eye it is 8 mm posterior to the limbus.

Physiology

The cones of the fovea centralis are used for detailed vision (eg, in reading or distinguishing distant objects) and color perception. The rods are used to detect movement and for night vision. Thus, as an automobile approaches an intersection at night, the driver's peripheral retinal rods will first detect a car approaching from a side street; he will then turn his eyes so that the foveal cones may discern the details of the vehicle.

The visual cells have light-sensitive molecules, which consist of retinal (the alcohol corresponding to the aldehyde, vitamin A) adherent to a large protein (opsin). The opsin in the rods differs from that in the cones, but the retinal is the same. When light enters the eye, it isomerizes the retinal from its 11-cis shape to its all-trans shape so that it can no longer remain adherent to the opsin. The 2 molecules separate, and this somehow causes visual excitation. The free, all-trans retinal is metabolized to its 11-cis isomer and rejoined to the opsin, or it may be stored as vitamin A. According to need, the vitamin A will be converted to 11-cis retinal and joined once more to the opsin.

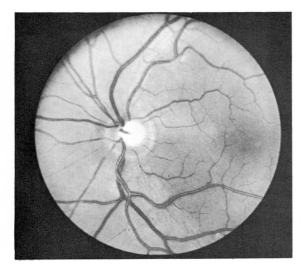

Fig 9-1. Ophthalmoscopic view of a normal retina. Note deep physiologic cup. (Courtesy of Stacey Mettier, Jr.)

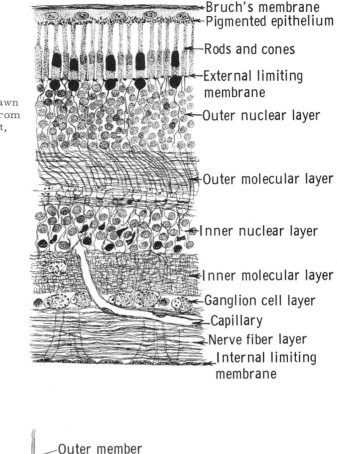

Bruch's membrane
Pigmented epithelium
Rods and cones
External limiting membrane
Outer nuclear layer
Outer molecular layer
Inner nuclear layer
Inner molecular layer
Ganglion cell layer
Capillary
Nerve fiber layer
Internal limiting membrane

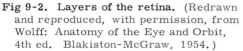

Fig 9-2. Layers of the retina. (Redrawn and reproduced, with permission, from Wolff: Anatomy of the Eye and Orbit, 4th ed. Blakiston-McGraw, 1954.)

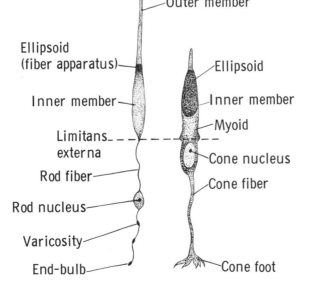

Outer member
Ellipsoid (fiber apparatus)
Ellipsoid
Inner member
Inner member
Myoid
Limitans externa
Cone nucleus
Rod fiber
Cone fiber
Rod nucleus
Varicosity
End-bulb
Cone foot

Fig 9-3. Rod (left) and cone (right). (From Wolff: ibid.)

Physiology of Symptoms

The retina is designed to receive visual images and transfer them to the brain. It contains no pain fibers. When the retina is normal and there are no uncorrected refractive errors, the images received will be sharply in focus. Most disorders of the retina will cause blurred vision. If the macular area is diseased, the patient's central visual acuity will be affected and he will have difficulty reading and discerning objects in the distance (eg, street signs). If the peripheral portion of the retina is diseased, side vision is impaired but the patient will continue to read well. In extreme cases of contracted peripheral visual fields the patient can read the finest print but will bump into large objects such as chairs and desks when passing through a strange room.

There is no pain with retinal disease, and the eye does not become red or inflamed. The physician diagnoses retinal disease by the history, by testing the visual acuity and visual fields, and by ophthalmoscopy.

DEGENERATIVE DISEASES INVOLVING THE RETINA

DRUSEN

Drusen are common bilateral retinal lesions, degenerative in nature and of unknown cause, which manifest themselves ophthalmoscopically as small, light-colored dots that may become shiny with age due to calcification. They may be found in the macular area at any age but are much more common in older people. Pathologically, they consist of hyaline deposits upon Bruch's membrane. Drusen may also occur on the optic disk, causing pseudopapilledema.

Drusen cause no visual loss. Macular degeneration occurs occasionally as an independent process but is not considered to be a complication of drusen.

There is no treatment, and the visual prognosis is excellent.

ANGIOID STREAKS

Angioid streaking is an uncommon bilateral process of unknown cause which is associated with degeneration of the elastic portion of Bruch's membrane. The onset is in early and middle life. Pathologically, there are rents in Bruch's membrane with proliferation of the pigmented epithelium over them. With the ophthalmoscope one sees deep brown streaks which simulate blood vessels. The streaks are usually concentric with the optic disk, with a spoke-like pattern.

Angioid streaks need not be confused with other conditions. Macular degeneration is present in 50% of cases. Pseudoxanthoma elasticum is commonly associated; Paget's disease less often.

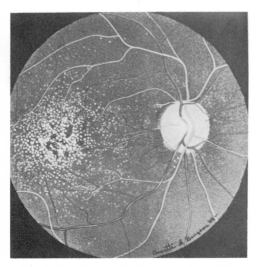

Fig 9-4. Drusen in the macula. (Reproduced, with permission, from Wilmer: Atlas Fundus Oculi. Macmillan, 1934.)

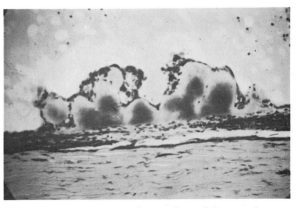

Fig 9-5. Microscopic section of drusen (excrescences of Bruch's membrane). Retina not shown. (Courtesy of M. Hogan.)

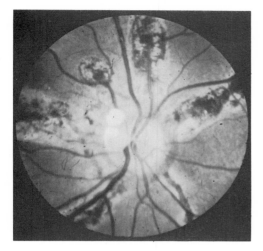

Fig 9-6. Retinal photograph showing
angioid streaks in retina. (Courtesy
of M. Hogan and S. Aiken.)

No treatment is available. The visual prognosis is good if macular degeneration does not
occur.

CIRCINATE DEGENERATION
OF THE RETINA

This relatively common degenerative disorder of the macula, usually bilateral, occurs
primarily in the older age groups. Pathologically, there is cystoid degeneration of the retina and the cystic spaces are filled with hyaline

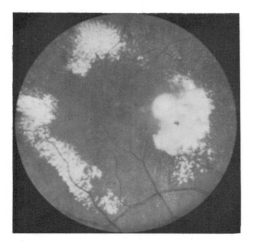

Fig 9-7. Circinate retinopathy. (Courtesy of A. Irvine, Jr.)

and lipid materials, particularly in the nuclear
layers of the retina around the macular region.
Ophthalmoscopically, the macular area is surrounded by a girdle of white to yellow spots.
The normal macular reflection is lost, and
macular degeneration eventually occurs. Macular hemorrhages are not common.

Blurred vision and loss of central vision
are present as a result of macular degeneration. Peripheral vision is retained inasmuch
as the remainder of the retina continues to
function. No treatment is available.

DISCIFORM DEGENERATION
OF THE MACULA
(Kuhnt-Junius Disease)

Disciform macular degeneration is so
named because of its discoid ophthalmoscopic
appearance. It is common in older people
but may occur in persons under 40 (juvenile
type). Pathologically, there is degeneration
of the elastic membrane of Bruch, which permits extravasation of serum, plasma, or whole
blood between Bruch's membrane and the pigmented epithelium. If whole blood is extrava-
sated, organization occurs and, after several
weeks, a solid fibrotic mass involving the retina and choroid results. If serum is extrava-
sated, as commonly happens in the juvenile
type, resolution may occur without fibrosis or
permanent retinal damage.

Central vision is blurred. In the early
stages there is an elevated red, solid-appear-
ing mass in the macular area in one or sometimes both eyes. This later becomes an elevated white mass which is usually round and
fairly well circumscribed. The optic nerve
and the remainder of the retina are usually
normal. In the juvenile type the retina in the
macular area is only slightly elevated and appears somewhat edematous.

Malignant melanoma involving the macula
may be difficult to differentiate from disciform
degeneration. It is sometimes necessary to
wait weeks or months to see if growth occurs
or if the characteristic pigment of malignant
melanoma appears. Unfortunately, eyes have
been enucleated on the basis of a clinical diagnosis of malignant melanoma of the macular
area which upon pathologic examination showed
only disciform degeneration.

No treatment is available. In the juvenile
type the vision may rarely return to normal in
a matter of weeks or months. In the older age
groups there is usually complete loss of central
vision, but peripheral vision is maintained
throughout life. Both eyes are seldom affected
simultaneously, but the fellow eye eventually

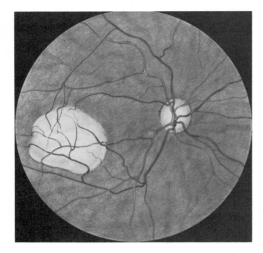

Fig 9-8. Healed disciform macular degeneration (drawing). (Courtesy of F. Cordes.)

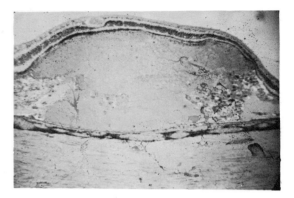

Fig 9-9. Microscopic section, disciform macular degeneration. (Courtesy of M. Hogan.)

follows the same course in the majority of cases.

HEREDODEGENERATION OF THE MACULA

This bilateral, degenerative, abiotrophic, dominant hereditary disorder may begin at any age. Macular heredodegeneration which has its onset under the age of 40 is usually arbitrarily designated as juvenile. Pathologically, retinal elements are absent in the macular area, and proliferation of the pigmented epithelium is apparent. The choroid and Bruch's membrane are not affected.

Ophthalmoscopically, there is loss of the normal macular reflection. In the early stages the macula appears granular; later it assumes a "moth-eaten" appearance, and small hemor-

rhages are occasionally present. Heredodegeneration is differentiated from disciform macular degeneration by its lack of elevation.

Central vision is usually lost, but peripheral vision is retained since the remainder of the retina continues to function in a normal manner. Other coincidental defects in the retina or the CNS may occur concomitantly (eg, peripheral retinal degeneration, optic atrophy).

The onset is insidious and the progress slow. No treatment is available.

PERIPHERAL CYSTOID DEGENERATION OF THE RETINA

Microcystic degeneration of the peripheral retina is almost universally present after age 8. Pathologically, there is a breakdown in the nu-

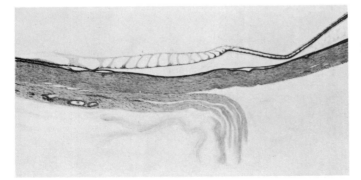

Fig 9-10. Peripheral cystic degeneration of the retina. (Reproduced, with permission, from Arruga: Detachment of the Retina. Salvat, 1936.)

clear layers near the ora serrata which extends posteriorly to a variable degree as a system of confluent microtunnels within the retina. Ophthalmoscopically, the affected retina has a "moth-eaten" appearance, most marked anteriorly, where the spaces are larger; and least noticeable posteriorly, where the degeneration blends with normal retina. Because of the peripheral location of the degeneration, it does not affect the visual field. It is asymptomatic and usually harmless.

RETINOSCHISIS

Retinoschisis is an exaggerated manifestation of cystic degeneration, a splitting of the retina that simulates retinal detachment. It is present in about 10% of the adult population. Ophthalmoscopically, it is characterized by a shallow elevation of the inner surface of the peripheral retina. It is often so subtle that it can only be seen with the help of scleral depression, or it may be extensive and bullous in both eyes, especially in the inferior temporal quadrants.

Bullous retinoschisis must be distinguished from atrophied detached retina. It has a smooth, immobile surface, a regular outline, and a very thin inner wall with a dappled appearance. The external wall of the retinoschisis is a mottled grayish membrane in contact with the pigmented structures.

Though usually harmless and asymptomatic, retinoschisis may extend posteriorly to the macula and affect visual acuity. The internal and external walls of the cavity are prone to hole formation; on occasion, a combination of holes in both walls gives the effect of a through and through retinal hole and can cause a retinal detachment.

Because retinoschisis does not usually threaten vision, it is ordinarily best not to attempt treatment. If it is progressive, photocoagulation is indicated to contain the process.

PAVING STONE
DEGENERATION OF THE RETINA

Paving stone degeneration of the retina is a striking, common (but harmless and asymptomatic) degeneration of the retina and pigmented epithelium. It increases with age, affecting approximately 30% of persons at 60 years of age. Pathologically, it consists of a discrete loss of pigmented epithelium rods and cones and external limiting membrane, with the formation of a mild adhesion between the residual

retina and Bruch's membrane. Ophthalmoscopically, it is characterized by discrete, yellowish-white, rounded lesions of variable size up to 1 disk diameter. They are frequently multiple and bilateral; usually below the horizontal meridian; and almost exclusively confined to the peripheral retina.

LATTICE DEGENERATION
OF THE RETINA

Lattice degeneration of the retina affects about 5% of the general population over the age of 10. Pathologically, it is characterized by excavation of the inner surface of the retina and the formation of a strong vitreoretinal adhesion with variable sclerosis and pigmented epithelium disturbance. It is located at or near the equator. It varies in size from one-half to several disk diameters, and is often multiple. Its manifestations are many, and stem from a variable combination of retinal sclerosis and pigmentation. All gradations are common, from a subtle disarray of pigment and mild sclerosis of retinal vessels within the lesion on the one hand, to gross hyperpigmentation and marked sclerosis on the other.

Lattice degeneration is usually asymptomatic and harmless and goes unsuspected. However, the thinning which occurs can cause retinal detachment, especially in young people.

No treatment is usually required. However, if the patient has had retinal detachment in one or both eyes, areas of lattice degeneration should be sealed by photocoagulation, cryogenic coagulation, or diathermy.

MACULAR CYSTIC DEGENERATION

Macular cysts occur occasionally in older persons. They are usually unilateral and degenerative. Cystic degeneration of the macula may also occur following trauma, glaucoma, sclerosis of the choroidal and retinal vessels, and long-standing retinal detachment. The essential pathologic change consists of the presence of fluid-filled cystic spaces, particularly in the outer plexiform layer and most especially in Henle's fiber layer in the region of the fovea. Eventually, the internal limiting membrane of the retina ruptures and a macular hole results.

Central vision is blurred if the cyst is large enough to involve the fovea directly or if a macular hole occurs. Blindness does not result, however, if the remainder of the retina continues to function normally. These patients are not prone to retinal detachment.

RETINITIS PIGMENTOSA

Retinitis pigmentosa is a genetically determined, abiotrophic degenerative disease which has its onset between 6 and 12 years of age. It is more common among men than women (3:2); is almost always bilateral; and is most often inherited as an autosomal recessive characteristic (although many published pedigrees show autosomal dominant inheritance also). There are few pedigrees showing sex-linked inheritance, although these cases are the most severe. Retinitis pigmentosa usually occurs as a single entity, but it may be part of the Laurence-Moon-Biedl syndrome (blindness, obesity, mental retardation, hypogenitalism, and polydactyly) and, rarely, other syndromes.

Pathologic findings include bilateral degeneration of the retina (especially the rods), migration of pigment into the retina, obliterative sclerosis of the vessels, and atrophy of the optic nerve. The choroid is normal.

Night blindness is the first symptom. This is followed by a gradually progressive constriction of the peripheral fields and eventually blurred vision. Ophthalmoscopically, the retinal arterioles are narrowed, the disks pale yellow, and pigment deposits are present throughout the retina, particularly in the mid-periphery. Macular degeneration occurs in the late stages. High myopia, cataract, and glaucoma are occasionally present also. In rare cases there is an absence of pigment (retinitis pigmentosa sine pigmento).

No treatment is available. Cataract and glaucoma are treated by the usual measures.

The peripheral field gradually constricts in each eye over a period of years until at the age of 50 or 60 only a 3-5° central field (gun barrel vision) remains. In most cases these patients retain reading vision until death, although as a result of their poor peripheral vision they move in strange areas with difficulty (particularly at night). In a small percentage of cases, total blindness results.

VASCULAR DISEASES OF THE RETINA

OCCLUSION OF THE CENTRAL RETINAL VEIN

Thrombosis of the central retinal vein is an uncommon unilateral condition which is seen in older people when the central retinal vein or any of its branches becomes occluded. This usually occurs at the level of the lamina cribrosa, by proliferation of the endothelial

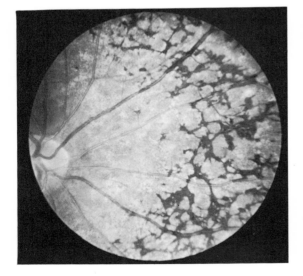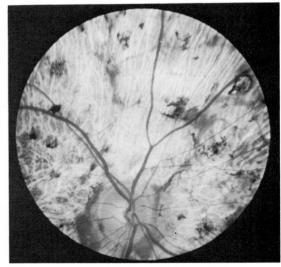

Fig 9-11. Retinitis pigmentosa. Left: Typical "bone spicule" arrangement of pigmentary changes. **Right:** Clumped, scattered pigment, attenuated arteries, and choroidal sclerosis. (Photos by L. Arlinghaus.)

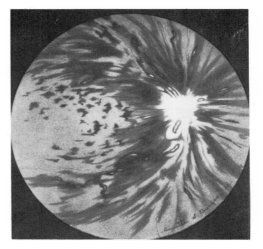

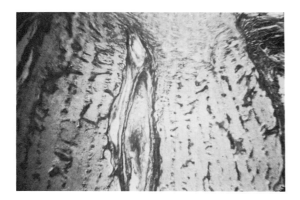

Fig 9-12. Microscopic section showing thrombus in the central retinal vein. (Courtesy of M. Hogan and L. Garron.)

Fig 9-13. Thrombosis of the central retinal vein (drawing). (Reproduced, with permission, from Wilmer: Atlas Fundus Oculi. Macmillan, 1934.)

surface or sclerosis of the adjoining central retinal artery, and spreads to the vein by contiguity. In the retina itself the arterioles and veins have a common wall at arteriovenous crossings. Multiple hemorrhages are scattered throughout the retina, and all vessels, including those of the iris, are dilated and engorged.

Loss of central vision in the affected eye is sudden and painless. Ophthalmoscopically, multiple hemorrhages are visible throughout the retina, particularly in the region of the optic disk where it appears as though the area has been "slapped with a red paint brush." A branch of the central retinal vein occasionally becomes occluded at a point where an artery crosses the vein, in which case hemorrhages are localized to this sector of the retina. Visual acuity is markedly decreased if a macular hemorrhage occurs, but the peripheral vision is relatively good.

Differentiation from other disorders is usually not difficult. In metastatic tumor to the optic disk the hemorrhages are less marked throughout the retina and the surface of the optic nerve head is irregularly elevated. Retinal hemorrhages associated with anemia are more circumscribed than those which occur with occlusion of the central retinal vein, and the area of the optic disk is relatively free of hemorrhage. Diabetic retinopathy is bilateral and can be distinguished by the waxy exudates which accompany it. Hypertensive retinopathy, also bilateral, can be differentiated by the characteristic narrowing of the arterioles and cotton wool exudates.

Secondary optic atrophy and glaucoma often develop in cases of complete occlusion of the central retinal vein, usually within 6 months after onset. Late vitreous hemorrhage due to subsequent vitreous traction on the new retinal vessels may mar an otherwise good recovery from a branch occlusion. It may be treated and even successfully prevented by closing the new vessels by photocoagulation.

All types of treatment, including short-term and long-term anticoagulant therapy, have proved to be valueless. If glaucoma develops it is usually intractable, and enucleation or retrobulbar injection of alcohol is indicated to relieve the pain.

About 20% of patients with occlusion of the central retinal vein regain at least 20/30 visual acuity in the affected eye. The over-all prognosis is grave; about half ultimately have less than 20/200 visual acuity. The prognosis for the other eye is excellent.

OCCLUSION OF THE
CENTRAL RETINAL ARTERY

This uncommon unilateral disorder occurs only in older people. Occlusion may be the result of thrombin formation on a preexisting plaque, or a subintimal hemorrhage with resultant displacement of the plaque or an embolus. Spasm of the artery is often a complicating factor. There is a sudden, painless, complete loss of vision in the affected eye. Oph-

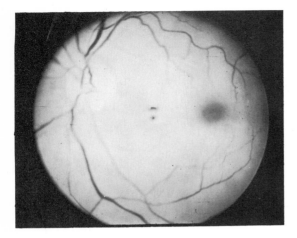

Fig 9-14. Twenty-four hours after closure of
the central retinal artery, left eye. The
disk is pale; the macula is edematous and
ischemic. The fovea appears as a "cherry-
red spot" because of its choroidal blood
supply showing through.

thalmoscopic examination soon after onset reveals segmentation of the blood in the veins and
arterioles as a result of the absence of retinal
blood flow. The disk is pale, and there is
marked retinal edema in the posterior pole.
The choroid is seen at the fovea as a "cherry-
red" spot. If the occlusion is complete, total
light perception is permanently lost and the
pupil will not react directly to light (although
the consensual pupillary light reflex is normal).

If the patient is seen within 30-60 minutes
after onset, an effort should be made to restore
blood flow through the obstructed artery by
vigorous massage of the eyeball or paracentesis of the anterior chamber followed by systemic administration of a rapid-acting vasodilator,
eg, tolazoline (Priscoline®), 75 mg IV. Massage consists of forceful pressure on the globe
for several seconds, sudden release of pressure, and then prompt repetition of the maneu-
ver. Stellate ganglion block may be necessary.

Anterior chamber paracentesis is performed as follows: The conjunctiva should be
grasped by a surgical assistant with small forceps near the limbus at the 6 and 12 o'clock
positions. A puncture incision is then made
at the limbus through the cornea into the anterior chamber, taking care to keep the instrument in the same plane as the iris so as not to
strike the lens and cause a cataract. A No. 11
Bard-Parker blade, keratome, or Graefe knife
may be used. These instruments make a hole
in the cornea and permit the extrusion of aqueous. A No. 25 needle on a 1 ml tuberculin
syringe can also be used, in which case the
aqueous must be aspirated (about 0.2 ml). The

rationale of this procedure is to cause a sudden
decrease in the intraocular pressure so that
the pressure behind the occlusion will force
the thrombus or embolus through the artery.
Vasodilators are administered to relieve arterial spasm if present.

Because the retina can survive hypoxia
longer than brain tissue, the prognosis is not
hopeless if treatment is instituted promptly.
If treatment is delayed for over 30-60 minutes,
the visual prognosis is all but hopeless and the
value of any type of treatment is questionable.

RETINAL DETACHMENT (SEPARATION)

Partial separation of the retina from the
choroid is seen most commonly in elderly persons but can occur at any age with or without
trauma. It is to be remembered that in both
the embryonic and the fully developed eye the
retina and choroid are in apposition but not
anatomically joined except at the optic nerve
border and ora serrata. The superior temporal part of the retina is most commonly affected, but any part or even the entire retina
may become detached.

Etiology
A. Primary Causes:
1. Trauma - About 20% of cases are precipitated by trauma (often minimal) to the head
or eye. Predisposing factors are present in
85-90% of these cases, but severe trauma can
produce retinal detachment even in healthy
eyes.
2. Vitreous strands - These occur as a
complication of chorioretinitis, vitreous or retinal hemorrhages, or as a result of prior surgery or trauma. If they become attached to the
retina they may detach it as they contract.
3. Vitreoretinal factors - The vast majority of retinal detachments are associated with
vitreous collapse due to syneretic degeneration
with consequent vitreous traction on a variety
of retinal lesions, including lattice degeneration, congenital retinal rosettes, and meridional folds.
4. Neoplasms - Malignant melanoma of the
choroid in adults and retinoblastoma or retrolental fibroplasia in infants are the commonest
intraocular tumors producing retinal detachment. These account for about 1% of cases.
5. Idiopathic - Some cases of retinal detachment have no recognizable cause.

B. Predisposing Factors: Aphakia and high
myopia. (About 60% of patients have one or
both of these disorders.)

Pathology

A tear in the retina is the fundamental finding in the absence of tumor. This permits vitreous and a transudate from the choroidal vessels to get behind the retina and separate it from the choroid. Other findings depend upon the nature of the primary or predisposing factors listed above.

Clinical Findings

The patient complains of a sudden onset of ''soot-like'' spots in front of his eyes and of ''lightning flashes'' which persist until in a few days or weeks there is blurred vision. (''A curtain came over my eye.'')

The peripheral fields are constricted, and the visual acuity is decreased if the macula is detached. Ophthalmoscopically, a gray detached area of the retina is seen (see p 112).

Differential Diagnosis

If no retinal tear is found, the eye should be examined to rule out malignant melanoma of the choroid. A tumor can almost always be visualized. If a retinal tear is present, a choroidal tumor is extremely unlikely. Transillumination is an unreliable means of differentiating ocular tumors. Spontaneous choroidal detachment must also be considered.

Complications and Sequelae

Complications rarely occur if the retina is reattached with one surgical procedure. Glaucoma is uncommon even in uncured cases. Uveitis occurs frequently in long-standing retinal detachment. Cataract may develop as a result of the uveitis.

Treatment

Reattachment of the retina can be accomplished only by surgery.

A. Preparation for Surgery: An extensive ophthalmoscopic examination is necessary in order to determine beforehand the number and location of the retinal tears. A diagram of the retina showing the location of the tears should be made for reference during the operation. Until surgery, both eyes should be bandaged and the patient kept at bed rest, positioned so that the retina will have a chance to settle back against the choroid.

B. Surgery: Choroidal exudates are produced in a circular fashion around the retinal tear or tears by passing a partially penetrating diathermy electrode through the area of the sclera which corresponds to the retinal defects. The subretinal fluid is then drained by perforating the sclera and choroid with a sharp suture needle or electrode. Drainage of the subretinal fluid is important so that the retina can settle back against the choroid. The artificially created choroidal exudate then begins to organize, and in a few weeks forms a cicatricial bond involving the retina, choroid, and sclera. Scleral buckling may be necessary in order to shorten the sclera and maintain contact between the choroid and retina.

Cryothermy is also being used effectively in the treatment of retinal detachment and may eventually replace diathermy. A supercooled probe is applied to the sclera to cause an adhesive chorioretinal exudate with minimal scleral damage. This decreased scleral damage (as compared with diathermy) makes the operation less hazardous and, because scar formation is minimal, greatly facilitates reoperation.

C. Photocoagulation: This treatment for retinal detachment consists of directing a strong light from a carbon arc source through the dilated pupil to cause a small choroidal retinal inflammatory exudate. This treatment cannot be used if the retina is elevated more than 1 mm; it is mainly useful in minimal detachment and postoperatively to supplement inadequate diathermy or cryothermy.

The **laser** (light amplification by stimulated emission of radiation) is a form of photocoagulation.

D. Postoperative Care: If the operation is successful, the patient may return to activity status after 2-4 weeks. In the first 3-4 weeks after surgery, the patient is advised to limit his physical activity.

Course and Prognosis

With meticulous care it is possible with the first operation to reattach the retina in about 75% of cases. Another 15% can be cured by a second operation. (Cure rates are greatly decreased if retinal detachment is total, if there are many vitreous strands, or if the detachment is of long standing.) If the retina is still attached 2 months postoperatively, the patient can be assured that there is little chance of a recurrence. Without treatment, retinal detachment almost always becomes total and the patient becomes permanently blind in the affected eye within 6-12 months. Spontaneous reattachment or delimitation of the detachment occurs rarely. Ophthalmoscopic examination of the other eye often reveals one or more retinal tears in the absence of detachment. These can be sealed by photocoagulation.

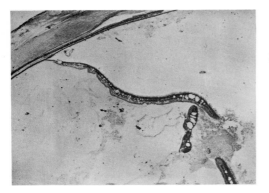

Fig 9-15. Tear in retina causing retinal detachment (microscopic section). Also shows cystic degeneration of retina. (Reproduced, with permission, from Arruga: Detachment of the Retina. Salvat, 1936.)

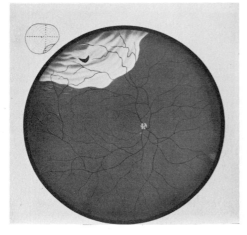

Fig 9-16. Retinal detachment 3 days after onset with crescent-shaped retinal tear. (From Arruga: ibid.)

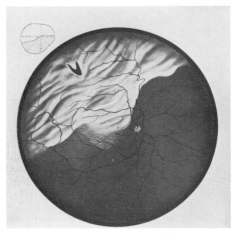

Fig 9-17. Retinal detachment and retinal tear 6 days after onset. (From Arruga: ibid.)

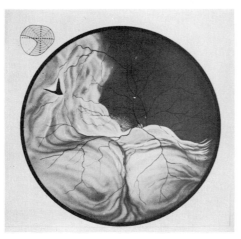

Fig 9-18. Appearance of retinal detachment 40 days after onset. (From Arruga: ibid.)

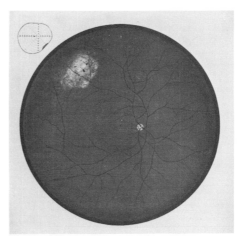

Fig 9-19. Operative cure of retinal detachment. Appearance of retina 2 months after surgical diathermy. (From Arruga: ibid.)

MISCELLANEOUS
DISORDERS OF THE RETINA

SEROUS DETACHMENT
OF THE MACULA

This uncommon disorder may occur at any age after the early teens, and is more common in males. Ten to 15% of cases are bilateral.

The cause is not known, although detachment of the macula may occur in association with aphakia, vitreous detachment, ocular hypotony, acute iritis, ocular tumors, vascular hypertension, and toxoplasmosis.

This disorder was previously called central angiospastic retinopathy. This term is a misnomer since the retina itself is not involved.

The only symptom is a seemingly sudden onset of blurred vision. On ophthalmoscopic examination the macular reflection is absent and the retina in the area of the macula is elevated. The vitreous is clear.

On pathologic examination the retina is seen to be detached from the pigmented epithelium by a collection of serous fluid. There is no retinal edema.*

No treatment is available.

In 90% of cases the macular detachment subsides in weeks or months, but recurrences are fairly common. Macular hemorrhage may occur, with subsequent retinal involvement and scarring (ie, disciform macular degeneration, or Kuhnt-Junius disease) and permanent central visual loss.

RETROLENTAL FIBROPLASIA

Retrolental fibroplasia is a bilateral retinal disease of premature infants characterized by wildly disorganized growth of the fetal retinal tissue. It was first reported in 1942, and caused total blindness in a large number of premature infants until 1954, when the cause was found to be excessive oxygen given to premature infants during the first few weeks of life, causing an abnormal response on the part of the underdeveloped capillary network of the fetal retina. New cases of this disease are rare, and can usually not be explained on the basis of excessive oxygen administration.

_____

*Gass, Maumenee, and others have reported some complex variations that are beyond the scope of this book.

Initially there is edema of the peripheral retina followed by vascular dilatation and tortuosity and peripheral retinal detachment. Fibrous tissue replacement of the retina and total retinal detachment occur later.

In advanced cases the retina is seen as a white retrolental membrane. A few surface vessels are evident on the membrane. The anterior chambers are shallow and the pupillary light reflexes are absent. The lenses are clear, and transillumination is normal. The contracting retrolental tissues draw the ciliary body anteriorly, and the ciliary processes can be seen with the ophthalmoscope in the periphery of the dilated pupils.

Differentiation from persistent hyperplastic vitreous is not difficult since this condition is unilateral. Retinoblastoma has a later onset, does not transilluminate, and the anterior chamber is of normal depth; if bilateral, it is usually much more advanced in one eye.

Glaucoma, uveitis, cataract, and phthisis bulbi may occur months to years after the onset of retrolental fibroplasia. Strabismus and myopia are commonly associated.

Premature infants should receive only the amount of oxygen necessary for survival. Oxygen administration should be controlled by blood gas measurements, not by percentage flow rates. The arterial oxygen concentration should be maintained in the range of 60-80 mm Hg and should never exceed 100 mm Hg. If blood gas measurements are not available, oxygen concentration should be kept below 40% and the infant transferred as soon as possible to a facility where such measurements are available.

Retrolental fibroplasia usually has its onset in the first few days of life and progresses rapidly over a period of weeks to cause blindness. In some early cases there is complete regression in both eyes; less commonly, the disease process regresses in one eye only, which allows the development of normal vision in that eye. Myopia and strabismus are common among those children who retain useful vision. Once blindness occurs, there is no hope for restoration of sight.

EXTERNAL HEMORRHAGIC RETINITIS
(Exudative Retinopathy, Coats's Disease)

Coats's disease is a rare unilateral retinal disorder with hemorrhagic and exudative properties affecting otherwise healthy young boys. Pathologically, there is a retinal mass containing dilated blood vessels, fibrous tissue, cholesterol, inflammatory cells, tissue debris, and blood elements. The choroid is normal.

Poor vision may be detected without any complaint, or the child may present with blurred vision or strabismus. In advanced stages the presenting symptom may be a pale retrolental mass, cataract, or pain. Ophthalmoscopically, the dominant features are progressive accumulations of yellow exudate in and beneath the retina, together with a variable degree of small vessel anomalies such as aneurysms, dilatations, and new vessels. The anomalous small vessels give rise to progressive exudation and hemorrhages. Early obliteration of such vessels by photocoagulation will arrest the downhill course and allow the existing hemorrhages and exudate to absorb with preservation of useful vision. Without treatment, the result is a blind, painful eye that must eventually be enucleated.

COLOR VISION AND COLOR BLINDNESS

As perceived by the human eye, **light** consists of those wavelengths of electromagnetic radiation (approximately 400-700 mμ) which are capable of eliciting retinal response and subsequent visual perception in the human occipital cortex. In other species with different perceptive mechanisms, light may consist of other wavelengths.

Color (hue) is dependent upon the wavelength of the incident light, and objects appear to have color because they refract and reflect light of various wavelengths selectively. Color is a more general term than hue, but the 2 words can be used interchangeably.

Color is dependent upon light intensity in that the cone-dependent mechanism essential to its perception is activated only by relatively high intensities.

Brightness accounts for apparent differences in the intensity of color when the hue remains unchanged. The addition of ''black'' to a given hue produces various ''shades.'' **Saturation** is an index of the purity of a color. If a color is 100% red it is completely saturated, whereas a pink color (eg, red plus white) is an incompletely saturated color.

Theoretically, 3 **primary colors** are required to produce all possible hues in the spectrum. Any 3 colors may be defined as primary provided none of them can be produced by a mixture of the other 2. The idea of red, green, and blue being the primary colors is no longer completely acceptable.

According to the **Young-Helmholtz trichromatic theory of color perception,** there are 3 types of photoreceptors in the human retina employing at least 3 distinct photosensitive pigments. Much research is being carried out in both ultrastructure and photochemistry to elucidate the exact nature of these receptor elements and their pigments.

Color blindness as it is encountered clinically lends strong support to the trichromatic theory of color vision. F.H.C. Marriott states that 8% of men and 0.4% of women are colorblind. He classifies them as follows:

(1) **Dichromats:** Persons having bivariant rather than trivariant color vision. They are divided into 3 groups: **Protanopes,** or redblind subjects, are insensitive to deep red light. **Deuteranopes** confuse shades of red, green, and yellow. **Tritanopes** are blue-blind subjects who confuse blue and green shades and, generally, orange and pink shades.

(2) **Rod monochromats:** Rod monochromatism is a very rare foveal disorder in which there is a complete lack of cone function. It is always associated with photophobia and nystagmus.

(3) **Cone monochromats:** The incidence of cone monochromatism is 1:1,000,000 or less. It may be due to a combination of tritanopia and protanopia or deuteranopia.

(4) **Anomalous trichromats: Protans** have similar but milder defects than occur in true protanopia; **deutans** have similar but milder defects than occur in true deuteranopia; and **tritans** have similar but milder defects than occur in true tritanopia.

The more common types of color blindness are inherited by the sex-linked route. Acquired causes of color blindness include retinal disease or poisoning which may affect color vision in a limited area of the visual field.

Treatment is of no value.

Detection of color blindness is described on p 33. Because of the obvious relationship to choice of occupation, automobile driving, and general understanding of the world, everyone should have a color vision test early in life (eg, age 8-12).

Bibliography

Aaberg, T. J., Blair, C. J., & J. D. Gass: Macular holes. Am J Ophth **69**:555, 1970.

Carr, R. E.: Optics and visual physiology. Annual review. Arch Ophth **84**:238-51, 1970.

Cox, M., Schepens, C., & H. Freeman: Retinal detachment due to ocular contusion. Arch Ophth **76**:678-86, 1966.

Davis, C. T., & R. W. Hollenhorst: Hereditary degeneration of the macula. Am J Ophth **39**:637-42, 1955.

Dobree, J. H.: Simple diabetic retinopathy. Brit J Ophth **54**:1-10, 1970.

Duke-Elder, S., & G. H. Dobree: Diseases of the Retina. System of Ophthalmology, Vol. 10. Mosby, 1967.

Elwyn, H.: Diseases of the Retina, 2nd ed. Blakiston-McGraw, 1953.

Ewald, R. A., & C. L. Ritchey: Sun gazing as the cause of foveomacular retinitis. Am J Ophth **70**:491-7, 1970.

Freeman, H. M., Schepens, C. L., & G. C. Couvillion: Current management of giant retinal breaks. Tr Am Acad Ophth **74**:59, 1970.

Friedenwald, J. S.: Diabetic retinopathy: The Fourth Francis I. Proctor Lecture. Am J Ophth **33**:1187-99, 1950.

Gass, J. D. M.: Pathogenesis of disciform detachment of the neuroepithelium. Am J Ophth **63**:573-711, 1967.

Gass, J. D. M.: Serous detachment of the macula. Am J Ophth **67**:821-41, 1969.

Gass, J. D. M.: Stereoscopic Atlas of Macular Diseases. Mosby, 1970.

Hardenbergh, F. E.: Occlusion of central retinal artery. Arch Ophth **67**:556-61, 1962.

Havener, W. H., & S. Gloeckner: Atlas of Diagnostic Techniques and Treatment of Retinal Detachment. Mosby, 1967.

Hyams, S., & E. Neumann: Peripheral retina in myopia. Brit J Ophth **53**:300-6, 1969.

Kearns, T. P., & R. W. Hollenhorst: Chloroquine retinopathy. Arch Ophth **76**:378-84, 1966.

Kinsey, V. E., & others: Retrolental fibroplasia. Arch Ophth **56**:481-544, 1956.

Klien, B. A.: Diseases of the macula. Basic histopathologic processes in retina, pigment epithelium, and choroid which modify their clinical appearance. Arch Ophth **60**:175-86, 1958.

L'Esperance, F. A., Jr.: The retina and optic nerve. Annual review. Arch Ophth **83**:771-94, 1970.

MacFaul, P. A.: Visual prognosis after solar retinopathy. Brit J Ophth **53**:534-41, 1969.

Maumenee, A. E.: Further advances in the study of the macula. Arch Ophth **78**:151-66, 1967.

Norholm, I.: Central serous retinopathy. Acta Ophth **47**:890, 1969.

Norton, E. W. D.: Present status of cryotherapy in retinal detachment surgery. Tr Am Acad Ophth **73**:1029-34, 1969.

O'Malley, P., & R. Allen: Peripheral cystoid degeneration of the retina. Arch Ophth **77**:769-77, 1967.

Patz, A.: Retrolental fibroplasia. Survey Ophth **14**:1-29, 1969.

Taylor, E., & J. H. Dobree: Proliferative diabetic retinopathy. Brit J Ophth **54**:11-8, 1970.

Vannas, S., & C. Raitta: Retinal venous occlusion. Am J Ophth **62**:874-85, 1966.

Welch, R. B.: A survey of retinal detachment surgeons on the use of cryotherapy or diathermy. Am J Ophth **69**:749-54, 1970.

Young, T.: On the theory of light and colors. Lectures in Natural Philosophy (London) **2**:613, 1807.

Zauberman, H.: Tensile strength of chorioretinal lesions produced by photocoagulation, diathermy, and cryopexy. Brit J Ophth **53**:749-52, 1969.

Zweng, H. C., Little, H. L., & R. R. Peabody: Laser Photocoagulation and Retinal Angiography: With Current Concepts in Retinal and Choroidal Diseases. Mosby, 1969.

10 ...

Lens

Anatomy and Function

The lens is a biconvex, avascular, color-less and almost completely transparent struc-ture, about 4 mm thick and 9 mm in diameter. It is suspended behind the iris by the zonule, which connects it with the ciliary body. Anterior to the lens is the aqueous; posterior to it, the vitreous. The lens capsule (see be-low) is a semipermeable membrane (slightly more permeable than a capillary wall) which will admit water and electrolytes.

A subcapsular epithelium is present ante-riorly (Fig 10-1). The lens nucleus is harder than the cortex. With age, subepithelial la-mellar fibers are continuously produced, so that the lens gradually becomes larger and less elastic throughout life. The nucleus and cortex are made up of long concentric lamellas. The suture lines formed by the end to end join-ing of these lamellar fibers are Y-shaped when viewed with the slit lamp (Fig 10-2). The Y is erect anteriorly and inverted posteriorly.

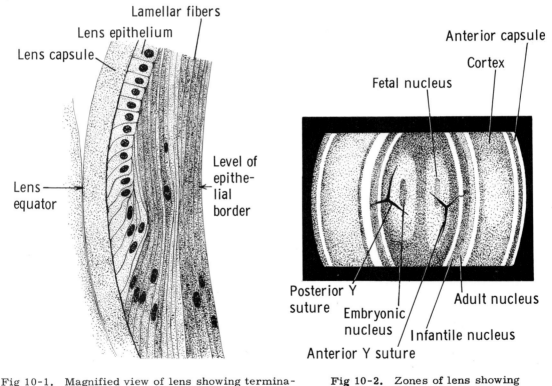

Fig 10-1. Magnified view of lens showing termina-tion of subcapsular epithelium (vertical section). (Redrawn from Duke-Elder: Text-book of Oph-thalmology, Vol. I. Mosby, 1942. Drawing first appeared in Salzmann: Anatomy and His-tology of the Human Eyeball in the Normal State. Chicago Medical, 1912.)

Fig 10-2. Zones of lens showing Y sutures. (From Duke-Elder: ibid.)

Each lamellar fiber contains a flattened nucleus. These nuclei are evident microscopically in the peripheral portion of the lens near the equator and are continuous with the subcapsular epithelium.

The lens is held in place by a suspensory ligament known as the zonule (zonule of Zinn). This is composed of numerous fibrils which arise from the surface of the ciliary body and insert into the lens equator.

The sole function of the lens is to focus light rays upon the retina. In order to focus light from a distant object, the ciliary muscle relaxes, tautening the zonular fibers and reducing the anteroposterior diameter of the lens to its minimal dimension; in this position the refractive power of the lens is minimized, and parallel rays are thus focused upon the retina. In order to focus light from a near object, the ciliary muscle contracts, pulling the choroid forward and releasing the tension on the zonules. The elastic lens capsule then molds the lens into a more spherical body with correspondingly greater refractive power. The physiologic interplay of the ciliary body, zonule, and lens which results in focusing near objects upon the retina is known as **accommodation.** As the lens ages, its accommodative power is gradually reduced.

Composition

The lens consists of about 65% water, about 35% protein (the highest protein content of any tissue of the body), and a trace of minerals common to other body tissues. Potassium is more concentrated in the lens than in most tissues. Ascorbic acid and glutathione are present in both the oxidized and reduced forms.

There are no pain fibers, blood vessels, or nerves in the lens.

Physiology of Symptoms

The only disorders of the lens are opacification and dislocation. Consequently, the patient with an opacity or dislocation of the lens will complain of blurred vision without pain. The physician examines for diseases of the lens by testing the visual acuity and by viewing the lens with an ophthalmoscope, a hand flashlight, or a slit lamp or loupe, preferably through a dilated pupil.

CATARACT

A cataract is a lens opacity. Cataracts vary markedly in degree of density and may be due to a variety of causes but are usually associated with aging. Some degree of cataract

formation is to be expected in persons over age 70. Most are bilateral, although the rate of progression in each eye is seldom equal. Traumatic cataract, congenital cataract, and other types are less common.

Cataractous lenses are characterized by lens edema, protein alteration, necrosis, and disruption of the normal continuity of the lens fibers. In general, lens edema varies directly with the stage of cataract development. The immature (incipient) cataract is only slightly opaque. A completely opaque mature (moderately advanced) cataractous lens is somewhat edematous. If the water content is maximal and the lens capsule is stretched, the cataract is called intumescent (swollen). In the hypermature (far-advanced) cataract, water has escaped from the lens, leaving a relatively dehydrated, very opaque lens and a wrinkled capsule.

Most cataracts are not visible to the casual observer until they become dense enough (mature or hypermature) to cause blindness. However, a cataract in its earliest stages of development can be observed through a well dilated pupil with an ophthalmoscope, loupe, or slit lamp.

The ocular fundus becomes increasingly more difficult to visualize as the lens opacity becomes denser, until the fundus reflection is completely absent. At this stage the cataract is usually mature and the pupil may be white.

The clinical degree of cataract formation, assuming that no other eye disease is present, is judged primarily by the visual acuity. Generally speaking, the decrease in visual acuity is directly proportionate to the density of the cataract. However, some individuals who have clinically significant cataracts when examined with the ophthalmoscope or slit lamp see well enough to carry on with their normal activities. Others have a decrease in visual acuity out of proportion to the degree of lens opacification. This is due to distortion of the image by the partially opaque lens.

Cataract formation is characterized chemically by a reduction in oxygen uptake and an initial increase in water content followed by dehydration. Sodium and calcium content is increased; potassium, ascorbic acid, and protein content is decreased. Glutathione is not present in cataractous lenses. Attempts to accelerate or retard these chemical changes by medical treatment have not been successful, and their causes and implications are not known.

SENILE CATARACT

Senile cataract (Figs 10-3, 10-4) is by far the most common type. Progressively blurred

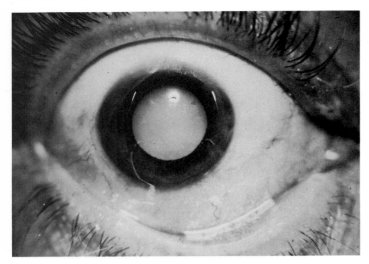

Fig 10-3. Mature senile cataract viewed through a dilated pupil. (Courtesy of A. Rosenberg.)

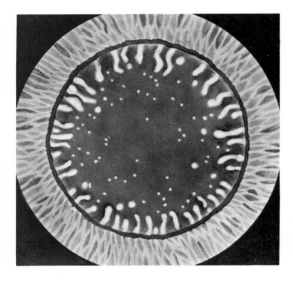

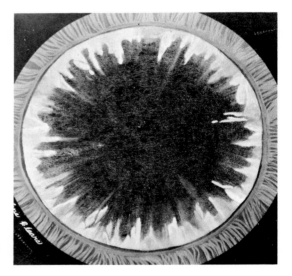

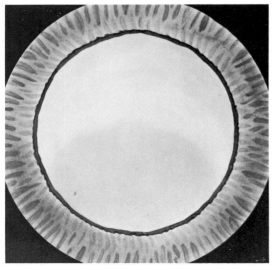

Fig 10-4. Cataract types. Above, left: Senile cataract, "coronary" type: club-shaped peripheral opacities with clear central lens; slowly progressive. Above, right: Senile cataract, "cuneiform" type: peripheral spicules and central clear lens; slowly progressive. Left: Senile cataract, "morgagnian" type (hypermature lens): the entire lens is opaque, and the lens nucleus has fallen inferiorly. (Reproduced, with permission, from Cordes: Cataract Types, 3rd ed. American Academy of Ophthalmology and Otolaryngology, 1954.)

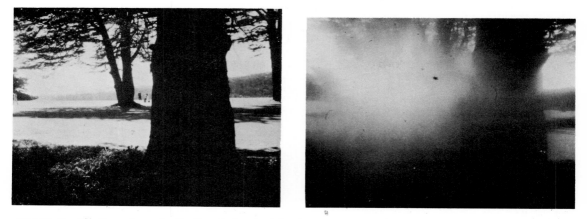

Fig 10-5. Senile cataract. In the photo at right the scene shown at left is reproduced as if seen by a person with a moderately advanced senile cataract (opacity denser centrally). (Courtesy of E. Goodner.)

vision is the only symptom. Paradoxically, although distant vision is blurred in the incipient cataract stage, near vision may be somewhat improved. Consequently, these patients read better without glasses (''second sight''). The artificial myopia is due to the greater convexity of the lens in the incipient stage of cataract formation. Glaucoma and lens-induced uveitis are uncommon complications. There is no medical treatment for cataract. Lens extraction (see pp 122-124) is indicated when visual impairment interferes with the patient's normal activities. If glaucoma secondary to lens swelling (intumescent lens) occurs, surgical extraction of the lens is indicated. Lens-induced uveitis requires surgical extraction of the lens to remove the source of the offending lens products.

Senile cataract is usually slowly progressive over a period of years, and the patient frequently dies before surgery becomes necessary. If surgery is indicated, lens extraction definitely improves the visual acuity in well over 90% of cases. The remainder either have preexisting retinal damage or develop serious postsurgical complications such as glaucoma, retinal detachment, vitreous hemorrhage, infection, or epithelial down-growth into the anterior chamber that prevents significant visual improvement.

Corneal contact lenses have made it possible for the patient who has been operated on for cataract to adjust to his new world of sight much more easily, since the corneal lens allows almost normal vision without the distortion, magnification, and diminished peripheral vision caused by the thick cataract glasses. Corneal lenses are of particular value for the patient who has undergone surgery for unilateral cataract since these patients were unable to obtain binocular visual function until the development of contact lenses.

CONGENITAL CATARACT

Congenital cataracts are common but may not cause significant visual loss. Most are bilateral and are probably genetically determined. They occasionally occur as a consequence of maternal rubella during the first trimester of pregnancy. Only those congenital cataracts that cause a marked loss of vision are discussed here.

The mother notices that the child does not see well during the first few months or years of life. The pupil may be white. The opacities vary greatly in density.

If the cataracts are bilateral, and dense enough so that the retinas are not clearly visible, lens extraction by aspiration should be done in one eye at the age of 6 months to permit normal development of vision and to prevent nystagmus. Surgery on the second eye should be delayed until the child is about 2 years of age since the eye is then larger and easier to operate on.

Months or years following surgery, vitreous strands may develop which upon contraction produce retinal detachment. Retinal detachment may be successfully treated by surgery in more than half of such cases. Recent improved technics of aspiration have materially reduced the incidence of vitreous loss and therefore the late complication of retinal detachment.

Most congenital cataracts are not dense enough to blur the vision significantly and are not progressive. Others progress slowly and may not require surgery until the child is 10-15 years of age.

The visual prognosis for congenital cataract patients requiring surgery is not so good as that for patients with senile cataract. The

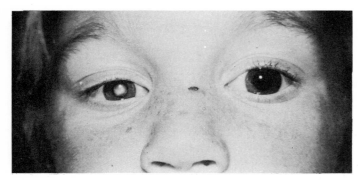

Fig 10-6. Congenital cataract.

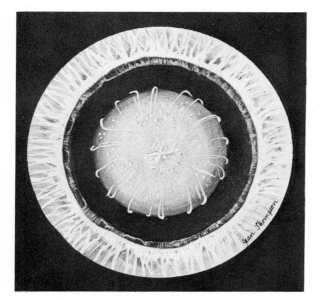

Fig 10-7. Congenital cataract, zonular type. One zone of lens involved. The cortex is relatively clear. (Reproduced, with permission, from Cordes: Cataract Types, 3rd ed. American Academy of Ophthalmology and Otolaryngology, 1954.)

complications of the operation and occasional associated anomalies of the optic nerve or retina lower the degree of useful vision obtainable in this group of patients. Probably no more than 70% of operations for congenital cataract result in significantly and permanently increased visual acuity in the operated eye. Rubella cataract has the worst visual prognosis.

TRAUMATIC CATARACT

Traumatic cataract (Figs 10-8, 10-9, 10-10) is most commonly due to a metallic intraocular foreign body striking the lens. B. B. shot is a frequent cause; less frequent causes include arrows, rocks, over-exposure to heat ("glass-blower's cataract"), x-rays, and radioactive materials. Most traumatic cataracts are preventable. In industry the best safety measure is a good pair of safety goggles.

The lens becomes white soon after the entry of the foreign body since the interruption of the lens capsule allows aqueous and sometimes vitreous to penetrate into the lens structure. The patient is often an industrial worker who gives a history of striking steel upon steel. A minute fragment of a steel hammer, for example, may pass through the cornea and lens at a tremendous rate of speed and lodge in the vitreous where it can usually be seen with the ophthalmoscope.

The patient complains immediately of blurred vision. The eye becomes red, the lens opaque, and there may be an intraocular hemorrhage. If aqueous or vitreous escapes from the eye, the eye becomes extremely soft. Complications include infection, uveitis, retinal detachment, and glaucoma.

The intraocular foreign body must be removed without delay.

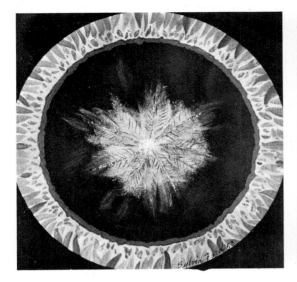

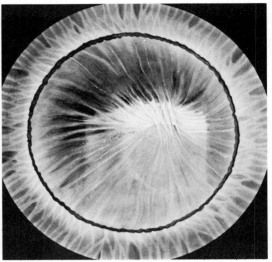

Fig 10-8. Traumatic "star-shaped" cataract in the posterior lens. This is usually due to ocular contusion and is only detectable through a well dilated pupil. (From Cordes: ibid.)

Fig 10-9. Traumatic cataract with wrinkled anterior capsule. (From Cordes: ibid.)

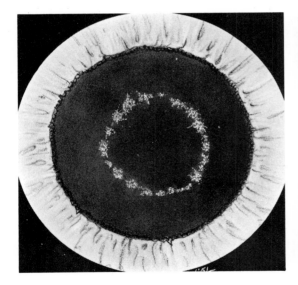

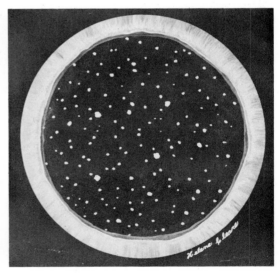

Fig 10-10. "Vossius' ring." Traumatic cataract caused by the imprint of the iris pigment on the anterior surface of the lens. The remainder of the lens is clear, and vision is not impaired. (From Cordes: ibid.)

Fig 10-11. Punctate dot cataract. This type of cataract is sometimes seen as an ocular complication of diabetes mellitus. It may also be congenital. (From Cordes: ibid.)

Antibiotics and corticosteroids should be given systemically and locally over a period of several days to minimize the chance of infection and uveitis. Atropine sulfate, 2%, 2 drops 3 times daily, is recommended to keep the pupil dilated and to prevent the formation of posterior synechias.

The cataract should be removed after the inflammation subsides and it is certain that no further absorption of lens material is taking place. It should be noted that in people under 20 years of age the lens material in a traumatic cataract will often absorb almost completely over a period of months without surgery. A thin membrane may remain, in which case discission (needling) may be necessary to improve vision.

CATARACT SECONDARY TO INTRAOCULAR DISEASE ("Complicated Cataract")

Cataract may develop as a direct effect of intraocular disease upon the physiology of the lens (eg, severe recurrent uveitis). The cataract usually begins in the posterior subcapsular area and eventually involves the entire lens structure. Intraocular diseases commonly associated with the development of cataracts are chronic or recurrent uveitis, glaucoma, retinitis pigmentosa, and retinal detachment.

These cataracts are usually unilateral. The visual prognosis is not as good as in ordinary senile cataract.

CATARACT ASSOCIATED WITH SYSTEMIC DISEASE

Bilateral cataracts may occur in association with the following systemic disorders: Hypoparathyroidism, myotonic dystrophy, atopic dermatitis, galactosemia, and Lowe's, Werner's, and Down's syndromes.

TOXIC CATARACT

Toxic cataract is uncommon. Many cases appeared in the 1930's as a result of ingestion of dinitrophenol, a drug taken to suppress appetite. Other offenders are triparanol (MER/29®) and corticosteroids administered over a long period of time. It has been suggested that echothiophate iodide, a strong miotic now being used in the treatment of glaucoma, may cause cataracts.

AFTER-CATARACT

After-cataract is the term applied to the portion of the lens remaining after an extracapsular cataract extraction or a partially absorbed traumatic cataract. The opacity usually consists of capsular and cortical material.

If vision is reduced, discission of the membrane is the treatment of choice. Since discission is a simple, safe, and usually successful procedure, it may be performed when visual loss is relatively minor (VA 20/50 to 20/60) if this loss is a definite handicap to the patient.

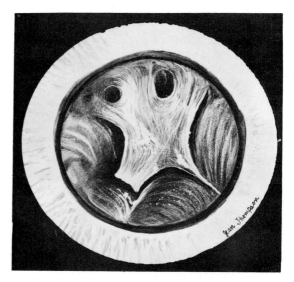

Fig 10-12. "After-cataract." (From Cordes: ibid.)

CATARACT SURGERY

In a cataract operation the lens is removed from the eye (lens extraction). There are 2 principal types of lens extraction, intracapsular and extracapsular. The former consists of removing the lens in toto, ie, within its capsule. In the extracapsular operation the anterior portion of the capsule is first ruptured and removed and the lens cortex and nucleus are expressed from the eye, leaving the posterior capsule behind. This procedure is easier to perform than intracapsular lens extraction, but a secondary membrane forms which requires discission in about 30% of cases.

The intracapsular operation has become the procedure of choice as a standard cataract procedure, but extracapsular extraction is still indicated in some types of congenital and traumatic cataract.

Enzymatic zonulolysis is an important advance in cataract surgery. The technic involves the injection of chymotrypsin, a fibrinolytic and proteolytic enzyme, in strengths not greater than 1:5000, into the anterior chamber of the eye. The material is left in the chamber for 2-3 minutes and the lens is then extracted. This substance has a specific lytic action on the zonules, and so makes possible much easier removal of the cataractous lens. Chymotrypsin can cause temporary postoperative glaucoma associated with poor wound healing and iris prolapse. This unique secondary glaucoma can be prevented by giving acetazolamide (Diamox®) postoperatively. Zonulolysis is used primarily in the younger age group (20-50), in whom the toughness of the zonules creates operative difficulties. The method is contraindicated in patients under 20 (congenital cataract) because up to this age the lens is attached to the vitreous, and intracapsular extraction will surely lead to considerable loss of vitreous and possible destruction of the eye.

Cataract surgery can be performed successfully in many ways. The variables relate mainly to the size of the wound and the actual method of lens delivery. In performing the intracapsular procedure, the time-honored method has been to make a large (160-180°) limbal incision superiorly, grasp the lens with

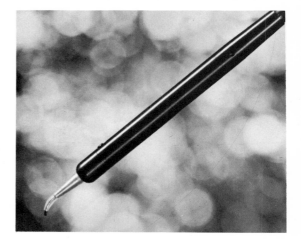

Fig 10-13. Amoils curved cataract cryopencil.
(Courtesy of Keeler Optical Products, Inc.)

a metal capsule forceps, and remove the lens intracapsularly. In recent years, the cryoprobe (Fig 10-13) has become popular as a replacement for the capsule forceps. The cryoprobe affords a firmer attachment to the lens and tends to result in fewer ruptures of the lens capsule. In young (under 30) patients, who have softer (more easily liquefied) cataracts, the **aspiration** technic has proved to be extremely satisfactory and can be done through a tiny limbal incision which does not require suturing. **Phacoemulsification**, utilizing a very small incision, is a new technic which is undergoing clinical trial and may hold promise for patients in the under 50 group with relatively soft cataracts.

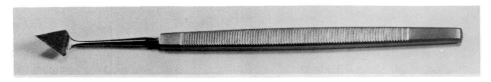

Fig 10-14. Keratome.

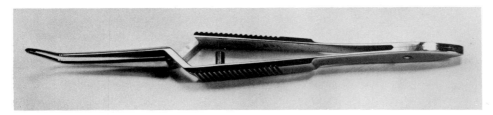

Fig 10-15. Arruga type cross action lens capsule forceps.

Postoperative Care

The patient may be ambulatory on the day of surgery, but is advised to move slowly and cautiously and to avoid straining of any type for at least 3 weeks. The eye is kept bandaged for 10-14 days.

Three to 6 weeks postoperatively the patient can be given a pair of temporary thick, convex cataract glasses. He is advised to wear them initially only when sitting down, as there is considerable visual distortion for him to adjust to. In most cases the patient learns to adjust to a new world where everything is 30% larger by the time his permanent glasses are ordered (7 to 8 weeks postoperatively). If the patient can tolerate contact lenses, visual distortion is eliminated.

DISLOCATED LENS
(Ectopia Lentis)

Partial or complete lens dislocation may be hereditary or may result from trauma.

Hereditary Lens Dislocation

Hereditary lens dislocation is usually bilateral and may be associated with coloboma of the lens, homocystinuria, Marfan's syndrome, and Marchesant's syndrome. The vision is blurred, particularly if the lens is dislocated out of the line of vision. If dislocation is partial, the edge of the lens and the zonular fibers holding it in place can be seen in the pupil. If the lens is completely dislocated into the vitreous it can be seen with the ophthalmoscope.

A partially dislocated lens is often complicated by cataract formation. If so, the cataract may have to be removed, but this should be delayed as long as possible because vitreous loss, predisposing to subsequent retinal detachment, is prone to occur during surgery. If the lens is free in the vitreous it may lead in later life to the development of glaucoma of a type which responds poorly to treatment.

If dislocation is partial and the lens is clear, the visual prognosis is good.

Traumatic Lens Dislocation

Partial or complete traumatic lens dislocation may occur following a contusion injury such as a blow to the eye with a fist. If the dislocation is partial, there may be no symptoms; but if the lens is floating in the vitreous the patient has blurred vision and usually a red eye. **Iridodonesis,** a quivering of the iris when the patient moves his eye, is a common sign of lens dislocation and is due to the lack of lens support. This is present both in partially and completely dislocated lenses, but is more marked in the latter.

Iritis and glaucoma are common complications of dislocated lenses, particularly if dislocation is complete.

If there are no complications, dislocated lenses are best left untreated. If uncontrollable glaucoma occurs, lens extraction must be done despite the poor results of this operation. The technic of choice is **cryoextraction.** In this procedure the lens is touched by a supercooled metal probe. After a few seconds an ice ball forms in the lens, firmly uniting the lens to the instrument. The cataract is then removed by gentle traction on the probe.

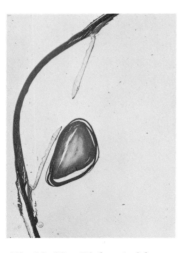

Fig 10-16. Dislocated lens.
(Courtesy of R. Carriker.)

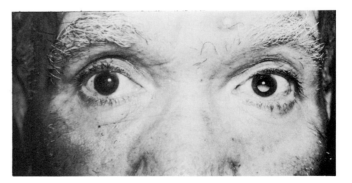

Fig 10-17. Dislocated lens.

• • •

Bibliography

Allen, H. F., & A. B. Mangiaracine: Bacterial endophthalmitis after cataract extraction. Arch Ophth **72**:454-62, 1964.

Becker, B.: The side effects of corticosteroids. Invest Ophth **3**:492-8, 1964.

Bettman, J. W.: Thompson, F., & R. DeBoskey: Cataractogenic effects of steroids. Invest Ophth **2**:101, 1963.

Cordes, F. C.: Cataract Types, 3rd ed. American Academy of Ophthalmology and Otolaryngology, 1954.

De Roetth, A., Jr.: Cryoextraction of cataracts in glaucomatous eyes. Am J Ophth **71**:54-6, 1971.

Freeman, H. M.: The lens and vitreous. Annual review. Arch Ophth **82**:551-66, 1969.

Maumenee, A. E.: Cataract extraction with the cryoprobe. Tr Am Acad Ophth **73**: 1044-6, 1969.

Scheie, H., Rubenstein, R., & R. Kent: Aspiration of congenital cataracts. Am J Ophth **63**:3-8, 1967.

Shaffer, R., & J. Hetherington: Anticholinesterase and cataracts. Am J Ophth **61**: 613-9, 1966.

Spector, A.: Physiological chemistry of the eye. Annual review. Arch Ophth **83**:506-22, 1970.

Troutman, R.: Microsurgery of cataract. Tr Am Acad Ophth **73**:460-2, 1969.

Von Noorden, G. K., Ryan, S. J., & A. E. Maumenee: Management of congenital cataracts. Tr Am Acad Ophth **74**:352-9, 1970.

Williamson, J., & others: Posterior subcapsular cataracts and glaucoma associated with long-term oral corticosteroid therapy. Brit J Ophth **53**:361-72, 1969.

Worthen, D. M., & R. E. Brubaker: An evaluation of cataract cryoextraction. Arch Ophth **79**:8-9, 1968.

11...

Vitreous

Anatomy and Function

The vitreous is a transparent, avascular gelatinous body which comprises two-thirds of the volume and weight of an adult eye. It fills the space between the lens and the optic nerve. It is the longest segment of the intraocular optical pathway, and helps give form to the eye. If the vitreous were aspirated, the eye would collapse.

The outer surface of the vitreous, the hyaloid membrane, is normally in contact with the following structures: the posterior lens capsule, the zonular fibers, the pars plana epithelium, the retina, and the optic nerve head. The vitreous maintains a firm attachment throughout life to the pars plana epithelium and the retina immediately behind the ora serrata. Its attachment to the lens capsule and the optic nerve head, while firm in early life, soon disappears. This is the principal reason that intracapsular cataract extraction without vitreous prolapse or "loss" is possible in adults and not in children. In addition, the vitreous is prone to vitreoretinal adhesions at the site of lattice degeneration of the retina, congenital retinal rosettes, meridional retinal folds, vitreoretinal scars, and new retinal blood vessels as in diabetes and central retinal vein occlusions.

The hyaloid canal, which in the fetus contains the hyaloid artery, passes anteroposteriorly from the lens to the optic nerve head. The hyaloid artery usually disappears soon after birth, but the hyaloid canal (Cloquet's canal) remains throughout life. It is not visible ophthalmoscopically. A rudimentary portion of the hyaloid artery occasionally remains and can be seen floating in the vitreous with its anterior portion attached to the posterior surface of the lens. This point of attachment can be seen as a black dot (Mittendorf's dot) with the ophthalmoscope.

Composition

The vitreous is about 99% water. The remainder consists of a small amount of an insoluble protein called residual protein, a soluble component composed mainly of hyaluronic acid, other proteins, and the usual electrolytes found in plasma and aqueous. The gelatinous structure of the vitreous, unique among body fluids, is believed to be due to the highly organized state of the residual protein.

Aging

With the passage of time the vitreous undergoes a variety of physiochemical changes called syneresis since they are associated with some degree of liquefaction of the gel. The gel usually collapses down or forward. The new position of the posterior vitreous face and the effect of ocular rotations may impose a stress on the retinal vessels to produce many clinical disorders such as vitreous detachment, vitreous hemorrhage, and retinal tear with or without retinal detachment.

VITREOUS DETACHMENT

Bilateral or unilateral detachment of the vitreous from the retina occurs in over half the population over the age of 60. Patients usually complain of "spots," "spiders," "cobwebs," "soot," "lightning flashes," or a "ring" in the field of vision. Very little can usually be seen with the ophthalmoscope, but if the detachment is from the area of the optic disk a dark ring the size of the disk can be seen in the mid-vitreous area. If the vitreous is detached from above, the line of the detachment is hard to see with the ophthalmoscope but can be seen with the slit lamp through a dilated pupil.

There is no treatment for vitreous detachment; the vision is not usually significantly affected, and the prognosis is excellent. However, on occasion it causes hemorrhage due to rupture of normal vessels or new vessels, as in diabetes or closure of the central retinal vein or one of its branches. It may cause retinal tears with or without retinal detachment beginning at the time of vitreous collapse or much later.

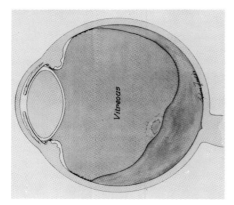

Fig 11-1. Vitreous detachment. Side view through a sectioned eye. (Drawing by Sylvia Ford.)

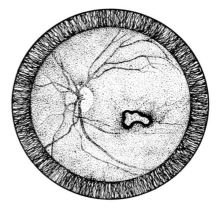

Fig 11-2. Vitreous detachment as seen with the +8 lens of the ophthalmoscope.

SYNCHYSIS SCINTILLANS
(Spintherism)

Synchysis scintillans is an uncommon, usually bilateral condition in which the examiner sees numerous glistening white cholesterol crystals which tend to settle in the lowest part of very fluid vitreous when the eyes are motionless. When the eyes are moved, the crystals spring up in great showers and fly around the vitreous cavity until the movement of the eyes is stopped.

Synchysis scintillans usually has its onset before age 40. There is usually no predisposing disease, but it may follow chronic uveitis. No relationship has been established with elevated blood cholesterol levels or any other systemic abnormality.

There is no blurring of vision, and the patient is unaware of his condition. The visual prognosis is excellent, as the condition does not progress.

ASTEROID HYALOSIS
(Benson's Disease)

Asteroid hyalosis is an uncommon unilateral condition which occurs in otherwise healthy eyes in elderly people. Hundreds of small yellow spheres consisting of calcium soaps are seen in the vitreous. These move when the eyes move but always return to their original positions because they are attached to inter-

lacing fibers. There are no related ocular or systemic diseases. The opacities have little or no effect upon vision and are of no clinical significance.

VITREOUS HEMORRHAGE

Hemorrhage into the vitreous is an uncommon but serious disorder. It is usually due to traumatic rupture of a retinal vessel but may be related to diabetes mellitus, hypertension, perivasculitis, or retinal detachment. One or both eyes may be affected, depending upon the cause.

There is a sudden and complete loss of vision in the affected eye. The fundus reflection is absent, but the anterior chamber, cornea, and lens are clear.

The visual prognosis is guarded no matter what the cause, since the blood often remains in the vitreous for months. If the vitreous clears after a long period the retina will usually have been damaged by prolonged intimate contact with blood elements. **Note:** These patients should be observed periodically, as the hemorrhage occasionally clears dramatically in a few days or weeks to reveal a retinal detachment. **If this happens, vision may be restored by surgical reattachment of the retina. It takes a very small amount of blood in the vitreous to completely obscure the examiner's view of the retina.**

VITREOUS ABSCESS
(Endophthalmitis*)

Vitreous abscess is a rare unilateral infection usually caused by Bacillus subtilis, a common barnyard contaminant. (In most reported cases the organism has been introduced by a penetrating injury.) The vitreous is an excellent culture medium for this organism, and the abscess characteristically progresses rapidly to destroy the eye despite injections of antibiotics into the vitreous. In rarer instances, vitreous abscess is the result of blood-borne infection.

VITREOUS FLOATERS
(Muscae Volitantes)

"Spots before the eyes" is an extremely common condition in older people or in persons with high myopia. The spots may be single or multiple, unilateral or bilateral, and usually move about. Vitreous floaters do not disappear, but they may settle below the line of vision where they are no longer noticed by the patient. The patient should be cautioned that if a single spot develops which enlarges and does not move about, he should return for another examination. If this occurs, tumor or retinal detachment should be suspected.

The exact nature of vitreous floaters is not known. They probably represent a degenerative change in the vitreous.

•   •   •

Bibliography

Freeman, H. M.: The lens and vitreous. Annual review. Arch Ophth **82**:551-66, 1969.

Freeman, H. M., & others: Vitreous surgery. I. An experimental study. II. Instrumentation and technique. Arch Ophth **77**:677-82, 1967.

Luxenberg, M., & D. Sime: Relationship of asteroid hyalosis to diabetes mellitus and plasma lipid levels. Am J Ophth **67**:406-13, 1969.

Pischel, D. K.: Detachment of the vitreous as seen by slitlamp examination. Am J Ophth **36**:1497-507, 1953.

Spector, A.: Physiological chemistry of the eye. Annual review. Arch Ophth **83**:506-22, 1970.

*If all 3 coats of the eye as well as the vitreous are involved by an inflammatory process, the condition is known as panophthalmitis. The line of demarcation between endophthalmitis and panophthalmitis is usually obscure.

12 . . .
Orbit

Anatomy

The bony orbits are the sockets containing the eyeballs and associated structures. The orbital cavity is roughly similar in shape to a truncated pyramid, being composed of 4 walls which converge on the apex posteriorly. The anterior opening is the base of the pyramid, the circumference of which is the orbital margin or rim. The greatest diameter of each orbit lies just within the rim, the overhang serving to protect the eyeball from injury. The periosteum of the orbit is called the periorbita.

There are several openings within and adjacent to the orbits through which pass blood vessels and nerves to supply the eyeball, its muscles, and other nearby structures: (1) the superior and inferior orbital fissures (motor nerves of the ocular muscles; ophthalmic nerve and vein); (2) the supraorbital notch (supraorbital nerves and vessels from the orbit); (3) the optic foramen (optic nerve); and (4) the infraorbital foramen (infraorbital artery and nerve).

The orbits are related to the frontal sinus above, the maxillary sinus below, and the ethmoid and sphenoid sinuses medially.

The lacrimal gland is located laterally beneath the overhang of the superior orbital margin. The supraorbital notch cuts across the margin superiorly at the junction of its medial third and lateral two thirds. This transmits the supraorbital nerves and vessels from within the orbit. A second or frontal notch is sometimes found medial to the supraorbital notch. This transmits the medial frontal branch of the nerve if it has divided within the orbit.

The lateral orbital rim, or zygomatic process, is the strongest part of the orbital rim. Suspensory ligaments, the lateral palpebral tendon (ligament), and check ligaments have their connective tissue attachments to the orbital tubercle in this area.

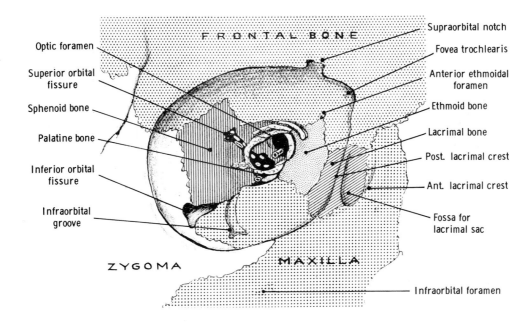

Fig 12-1. Frontal view of right orbit. (Reproduced, with permission, from Kronfeld and McHugh: The Human Eye in Anatomical Transparencies. Bausch & Lomb Press, 1943.)

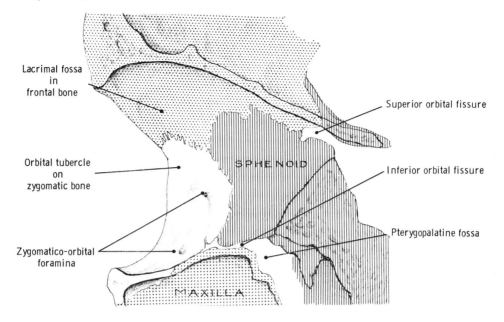

Fig 12-2. Lateral (temporal) wall of orbit. (From Kronfeld and McHugh: ibid.)

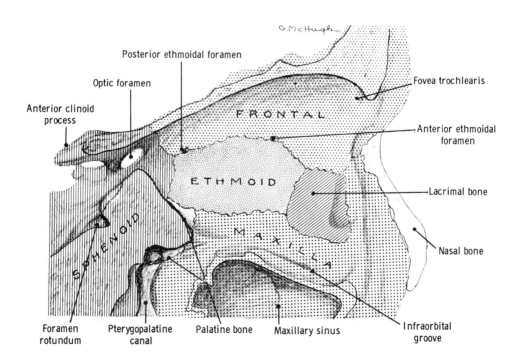

Fig 12-3. Medial (nasal) wall of orbit. (From Kronfeld and McHugh: ibid.)

The volume of the orbit is about 30 ml in adults. The average entrance dimensions are about 35 mm high and 40 mm wide, although there are great racial and individual differences.

A decrease in growth of the orbit occurs if an enucleation is performed in childhood. This may cause significant facial asymmetry.

Contents of the Orbit

The contents of the orbit are the eyeball, the extraocular muscles, connective tissue fascia and ligaments, fat, blood vessels, and nerves. The eyeball occupies only 20% of the orbital volume. It is situated anteriorly in the orbit just within the rim, and is surrounded by its extraocular muscles, fascial attachments, and Tenon's capsule, with an extramuscular fat pad posteriorly. Anteriorly the eyeball lies just beneath the conjunctiva, with which it fuses 3 mm from the limbus. Above the eyeball, in the lacrimal fossa of the frontal bone superiorly and temporally, is the lacrimal gland. The blood vessels and the nerves which supply the eyeball, its muscles, and other nearby structures enter the orbit through its posterior openings and terminate in the structures within the orbit or traverse the orbit to reach the surface (supraorbital and infraorbital structures).

A sheet of connective tissue fascia extending from the orbital rim to the tissue of the lids in the area of the tarsus forms an anterior limiting membrane known as the orbital septum. Tenon's capsule is a connective tissue capsule which surrounds the eyeball. It is continuous with the fascial expansions of the muscle sheaths, which likewise expand peripherally to form check ligaments for these muscles.

Physiology of Symptoms

Owing to the rigid bony structure of the orbit, with only an anterior opening for expansion, any increase in the orbital contents taking place to the side of or behind the eyeball will

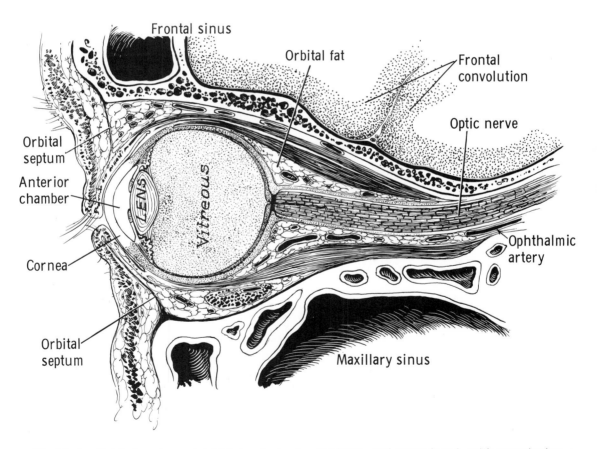

Fig 12-4. Orbital anatomy (right lateral view). (Redrawn and reproduced, with permission, from Wolff: Anatomy of the Eye and Orbit. Blakiston-McGraw, 1954.)

displace that organ. Pressure behind the eyeball will push it forward (proptosis). Pressure on one side will displace the eyeball to the other side.

With the change in position of the eyeball, especially if it takes place rapidly, there may be enough interference with the movement of the eye to cause dissociation of ocular movements and diplopia (double vision). Pain is absent unless there is extreme swelling of the tissues or unless the eyelids are unable to protect the cornea adequately and there is irritation from exposure.

EXOPHTHALMOS
(Proptosis)

Etiology and Classification

Exophthalmos may be due to any of the following factors: (1) a space-occupying lesion in the rigid bony orbit, displacing the only moveable tissue, the eyeball; (2) swelling of the retrobulbar tissues through edema or hemorrhage, pushing the eyeball forward; (3) relaxation of the retracting effect of the extraocular muscles through paralysis or trauma; and (4) the apparent forward displacement (pseudoexophthalmos) seen with lid retraction (Graves' disease) and large eye (myopia, macrophthalmos).

A. Acute Exophthalmos:
1. Emphysema due to rupture of the medial orbital wall, allowing air from the sinus to enter the orbit.
2. Hemorrhage, either traumatic or spontaneous.

B. Pulsating Exophthalmos:
1. Carotid-cavernous sinus fistula.
2. Vascular tumors or aneurysms.
3. Cerebral pulsation due to a defect in the orbital roof.

C. Unilateral Exophthalmos:
1. Inflammatory - Cellulitis, pseudotumor of orbit, abscess, tenonitis, lacrimal gland inflammation, panophthalmitis, cavernous sinus thrombosis (may become bilateral).
2. Vascular - Hemorrhage, traumatic or spontaneous; varicosities, aneurysms.
3. Traumatic - Fracture, hemorrhage, rupture of the extraocular muscles, emphysema from sinuses, aneurysms.
4. Tumors - Primary, from the eye or orbital contents; spread from surrounding structures, metastatic.
5. Cysts - Congenital dermoid, parasitic, mucocele from surrounding sinuses.

6. Relaxation of retractors of eyeball, as with paralysis of the extraocular muscles.
7. General disease - Leukemia, lymphoma.

D. Bilateral Exophthalmos:
1. Endocrine (sometimes begins as unilateral exophthalmos) - Thyrotoxic (hyperthyroid, Graves' disease), thyrotropic (malignant, ophthalmoplegic).
2. Pseudoexophthalmos - Congenital macrophthalmos, high myopia, lid retraction (Graves' disease).

Retraction of the upper lid gives an exaggerated impression of the degree of exophthalmos in thyrotoxicosis. Malignant exophthalmos (also called exophthalmic ophthalmoplegia and hyperophthalmopathic Graves' disease) is a progressive and more severe form which is often triggered by surgical or medical treatment of thyrotoxicosis. Disorders of the pituitary gland have been thought to cause the tissue changes which produce malignant exophthalmos. These changes consist of infiltration of the extraocular muscle tissue with edema fluid and lymphocytes and similar changes in the rest of the orbital contents, forming a firm mass which pushes the eye forward.

Treatment

Thyroid exophthalmos is often greatly improved as soon as the hyperthyroidism is brought under control. Malignant exophthalmos presents a much more difficult therapeutic problem. High doses of systemic corticosteroids are frequently effective in reducing the amount of proptosis. Retrobulbar and subconjunctival corticosteroids may be effective also. If prominence of the eye becomes so great that the lids can no longer protect the cornea, surgical closure of the lids (tarsorrhaphy) must be performed to prevent exposure keratitis. Even this is not possible in many instances, however, in which case decompression of the orbit must be performed using the transcranial, antral, or temporal approach.

Surgical exploration of orbit is indicated in unilateral exophthalmos if there is a palpable mass which can be biopsied; if there are x-ray changes of bone; or if progressive visual loss occurs. If there is no palpable mass, no x-ray changes, and no visual loss or corneal changes, conservative management is indicated. Diplopia alone is not a sufficient indication for exploration of the orbit.

ENOPHTHALMOS

Retraction of the eye into the orbit is a normal change in elderly people which is due to senile atrophy of the orbital fat.   Enophthalmos in early life (before age 25) occurs rarely as part of Horner's syndrome or due to atrophy of the orbital fat following a severe contusion of the eye.

INFLAMMATORY ORBITAL DISEASES

ORBITAL CELLULITIS

Orbital cellulitis is usually caused by pneumococci, streptococci, or staphylococci, the same organisms that cause acute sinusitis. They enter the orbit by direct extension or through the vascular channels between the orbital contents and infected ethmoidal, sphenoidal, maxillary, or frontal sinuses.

Swelling and redness of the eyelids, chemosis, exophthalmos of varying degrees, and dull pain are usually present in mild cases. The onset is often sudden.   More severe involvement may cause greater tenderness upon palpation and more pain as well as headache on rotation of the eyeball.   Occasional intraocular hemorrhage and inflammatory signs are probably due to involvement of the vessels of the retina or choroid.   Constitutional symptoms vary, according to the severity of the infection, from mild fever, malaise, and leukocytosis to high fever and marked debility.   Infection may spread to the cavernous sinuses or meninges.

Orbital cellulitis must be differentiated from tenonitis, orbital periostitis, and cavernous sinus thrombosis.   In children, rhabdomyosarcoma must be ruled out.

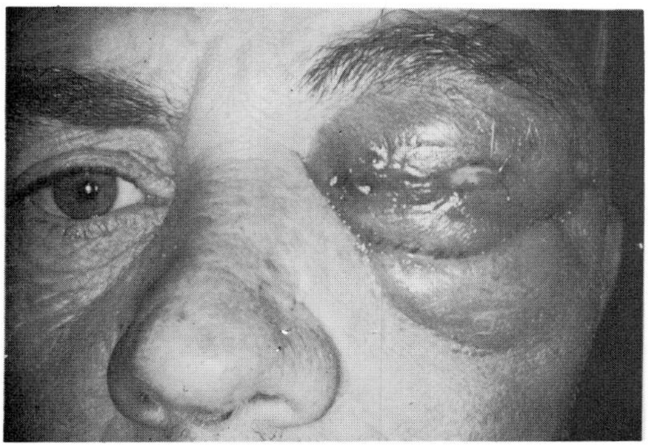

Fig 12-5. Orbital cellulitis. Abscess draining through upper eyelid.

Almost all cases respond well to large doses of penicillin. Hot compresses are useful to localize the inflammatory reaction. Unless the condition is growing steadily worse, surgical drainage should be delayed until absolutely necessary.

If penicillin or other antibiotics fail to bring the condition under control after a vigorous trial of 2-3 days, surgical drainage must be employed. The safest method is to make an incision into the area of greatest fluctuation—avoiding, if possible, the areas of the trochlea of the superior oblique muscle and the lacrimal gland recess. Antibiotics should be continued until the infection clears.

The response to penicillin is generally good. If not, the infection may localize anteriorly and rupture or require drainage; or may extend posteriorly, causing cavernous sinus thrombosis, meningitis, or brain abscess. Optic neuritis with secondary atrophy may follow severe inflammatory reactions. The visual prognosis is excellent in the absence of complications.

ORBITAL PERIOSTITIS

Chronic infection of the periorbita may occur as a result of tuberculous or, less commonly, syphilitic invasion of the bones and tissues of the orbit. Both occur rarely since the antibiotics came into use. Tuberculous periostitis tends to involve the bones and tissues of the lateral orbital rim; syphilitic periostitis, the superior orbital rim. Symptoms consist of painless red swelling with "cold" abscess in tuberculous periostitis; painful swelling in syphilitic.

Treatment is with systemic antisyphilitic or antituberculosis drugs. Tuberculous lesions should be drained.

CAVERNOUS SINUS THROMBOSIS

Orbital signs and symptoms are usually associated with thrombosis of the cavernous sinus within the skull. Exophthalmos with edema of the orbit and eyelids, diminished or absent pupillary reflexes, impaired visual acuity, and papilledema are usually present. Since the 3rd, 4th, and 6th cranial nerves and the ophthalmic division of the 5th cranial nerve traverse the cavernous sinus, involvement of these nerves leads to paresis of the respective muscles and limitations of ocular movement. Fever is of the septic type.

Thrombosis of the cavernous sinus is usually due to infection spreading along the venous channels which drain the orbit, central face, throat, and nasal cavities.

Differentiation from orbital cellulitis is sometimes necessary. Cavernous sinus thrombosis may be bilateral, whereas orbital cellulitis is almost always unilateral. In cellulitis the pupillary reflexes remain normal, there is no papilledema, and pain and tenderness are more severe.

Massive doses of systemic antibiotics are necessary. Prophylactic chemotherapy and avoidance of manipulation of pyogenic infections which may drain into the cavernous sinus is of the greatest importance.

Since the pyogenic bacteria are usually responsible, most patients can be saved with good visual recovery. Before the antibiotics became available, all patients died.

PSEUDOTUMOR OF ORBIT

Pseudotumor of the orbit is an uncommon inflammatory reaction, usually unilateral, which clinically resembles a neoplasm. Exophthalmos is a prominent clinical finding. Many bacteria, viruses, parasites, and other possible causes have been investigated, but the cause has not been determined.

Inflammatory pseudotumor is characterized by restriction of ocular movement, exophthalmos with occasional lateral displacement, swelling of the lids, and resistance to retrodisplacement of the eye with finger pressure. Pain and diplopia are present in about one-half of cases. The onset is usually gradual, and other signs of inflammation such as are seen with the more acute orbital cellulitis are not present.

The resemblance of pseudotumor to neoplasm may lead to exploratory orbital surgery; biopsy of the tissue reveals only signs of chronic inflammation.

Treatment is often difficult. Anti-infective chemotherapeutic and antibiotic drugs and x-ray radiation have been tried without effect. Systemic steroids in high doses have proved to be effective in many cases. Therapy may have to be continued for weeks or months to prevent serious relapse. If the swollen, chronically inflamed tissues impinge upon the optic nerve, there may be permanent damage to the optic nerve. Corticosteroid therapy decreases the chances of optic atrophy.

•   •   •

Bibliography

Beisner, D. H.: Orbital radiography: Orbitography, orbital phlebography and angiography. Survey Ophth **13**:187-99, 1969.

Benedict, W. L.: Diseases of the orbit. Am J Ophth **33**:1-10, 1950.

Haddad, H. M.: Endocrine exophthalmos: Humoral and orbital factors. JAMA **199**: 559-62, 1967.

Howard, G. M.: The orbit. Annual review. Arch Ophth **84**:839-54, 1970.

Lerman, S.: Blowout fracture of the orbit. Brit J Ophth **54**:90-8, 1970.

Long, J. C., & G. D. Ellis: Temporal decompression of the orbit for thyroid exophthalmos. Am J Ophth **62**:1089-97, 1966.

Miller, G. R., & J. S. Glaser: The retraction syndrome and trauma. Arch Ophth **76**: 662-3, 1966.

Zizmor, J., & others: Roentgenographic diagnosis of unilateral exophthalmos. JAMA **197**:343-6, 1966.

13 . . .

Neuro-ophthalmology

The eyes are intimately related to the brain and frequently give important diagnostic clues to CNS disorders. Indeed, the optic nerve is a part of the CNS. Intracranial disease frequently causes visual disturbances because of destruction of or pressure upon some portion of the optic pathways. Cranial nerves III, IV, and VI, which control ocular movements, are also frequently involved, and nerves V and VII are also intimately associated with ocular function.

Anatomy of the Optic Nerve (Fig 13-1)

The optic nerve is a trunk consisting of about 1 million axons arising from the ganglion cells of the retina. These axons comprise the nerve fiber layer of the retina and converge to form the optic nerve. The nerve emerges from the back of the globe through a short, circular opening (0.7 mm long, 1.5 mm in diameter) in the sclera situated 1 mm below and 3 mm nasal to the posterior pole of the eye. The orbital portion of the nerve is 25-30 mm long and travels within the muscle cone to enter the bony optic foramen to gain access to the cranial cavity. The intraosseous portion measures 4-9 mm. After a 10 mm intracranial course, the nerve joins the opposite optic nerve to form the optic chiasm and continues posteriorly to the lateral geniculate bodies. Here synapse occurs on neurons whose axons terminate in the primary visual cortex of the occipital lobes. The nerve fibers become myelinated upon leaving the eye and are supported by neuroglia; this increases the diameter from 1.5 mm (within the sclera) to 3 mm (within the orbit). Eighty percent of the nerve is made up of visual fibers en route to synapse in the lateral geniculate body. Twenty percent are pupillary; these bypass the lateral geniculate body en route to the pretectal area. Since the ganglion cells of the retina and their axons which make up the optic nerve are actually extensions of the CNS, they have no capacity to regenerate if severed.

Sensory impulses are received by the rods and cones of the retina, which may be considered the special end organ. The nuclei of the rods and cones are situated in the outer nuclear layer. The dendrites synapse with the second neuron of this pathway, the bipolar cells. The bipolar cells synapse with the ganglion cells of the retina whose axons form the nerve fiber layer, which collects to form the optic nerve.

Sheaths of the Optic Nerve

The fibrous wrappings which ensheath the optic nerve are continuous with the meninges. The pia mater is loosely attached about the nerve near the chiasm and only for a short distance within the cranium, but it is closely attached around most of the intracranial and all of the intraorbital portions. The pia consists of some fibrous tissue with numerous small blood vessels. It divides the nerve fibers into bundles by sending numerous septa into the nerve substance. The pia continues to the sclera, with a few fibers running into the choroid and lamina cribrosa.

The arachnoid comes in contact with the optic nerve at the intracranial end of the optic foramen and accompanies the nerve to the globe, where it ends in the sclera and overlying dura. This membrane is a diaphanous connective tissue membrane with many septate connections with the pia mater, which it closely resembles. It is more intimately associated with pia than with dura.

The dura mater lining the inner surface of the cranial vault comes in contact with the optic nerve as it leaves the optic foramen. As the nerve enters the orbit from the optic foramen, the dura splits, one layer (the periorbita) lining the orbital cavity and the other forming the outer dural covering of the optic nerve. The dura becomes continuous with the outer two-thirds of the sclera. The dura consists of tough, fibrous, relatively avascular tissue lined by endothelium on the inner surface.

The subdural space is between the dura and arachnoid; the subarachnoid space is between the pia and arachnoid. Both are more potential than actual spaces under normal conditions, but are direct continuations of their corresponding intracranial spaces. Subarachnoid or subdural fluid under sufficient pressure

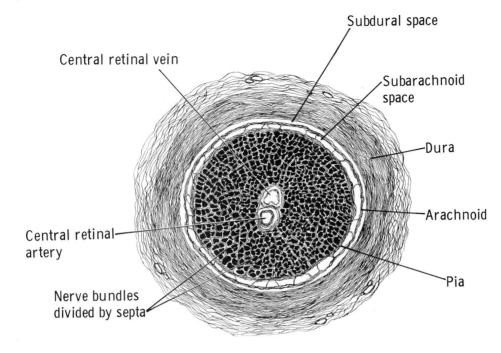

Fig 13-1. Cross section of the optic nerve. (Redrawn and reproduced, with permission, from Wolff: Anatomy of the Eye and Orbit, 5th ed. Blakiston-McGraw, 1961.)

will fill these potential spaces about the optic nerve. The meningeal layers are adherent to each other and to the optic nerve and the surrounding bone within the optic foramen, making the optic nerve resistant to traction from either end.

DISEASES OF THE OPTIC NERVE

OPTIC NEURITIS

Optic neuritis (papillitis) is a broad term denoting inflammation, degeneration, or demyelinization of the optic nerve. A wide variety of diseases can cause optic neuritis (see below). Loss of vision is the cardinal symptom and serves to differentiate optic neuritis from papilledema, which it may simulate ophthalmoscopically.

The term "optic neuritis" also includes retrobulbar neuritis, a form in which the nerve is affected posteriorly so that there are no visible ophthalmoscopic changes of the nerve head unless optic atrophy appears.

Etiologic Classification

A. Demyelinating Diseases:
1. Multiple sclerosis.
2. Post-infectious encephalomyelitis.
3. Other rare demyelinating syndromes, neuromyelitis optica (Devic's disease), diffuse periaxial encephalitis (Schilder's disease).

B. Systemic Infections:
1. Viral - Poliomyelitis, influenza, mumps, measles.
2. Bacterial - Pneumonia and, rarely, other bacterial infections.

C. Nutritional and Metabolic:
1. Diabetes mellitus.
2. Pernicious anemia.
3. Other vitamin deficiencies.
4. Malignant disease.
5. Hyperthyroidism.

D. Leber's disease (hereditary atrophy of the optic nerve; see p 142).

E. Local Extension of Inflammatory Disease:
1. Sinusitis.
2. Meningitis (purulent, tuberculous, syphilitic).

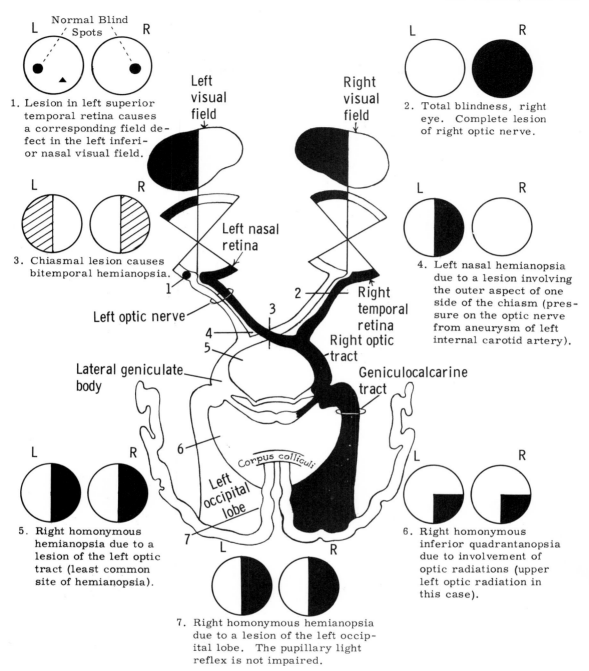

Normal Blind Spots

L R

1. Lesion in left superior temporal retina causes a corresponding field defect in the left inferior nasal visual field.

L R

3. Chiasmal lesion causes bitemporal hemianopsia.

Left visual field

Right visual field

Left nasal retina

Left optic nerve

Right temporal retina

Right optic tract

Lateral geniculate body

Geniculocalcarine tract

Left occipital lobe

Corpus colliculi

L R

2. Total blindness, right eye. Complete lesion of right optic nerve.

L R

4. Left nasal hemianopsia due to a lesion involving the outer aspect of one side of the chiasm (pressure on the optic nerve from aneurysm of left internal carotid artery).

L R

5. Right homonymous hemianopsia due to a lesion of the left optic tract (least common site of hemianopsia).

L R

6. Right homonymous inferior quadrantanopsia due to involvement of optic radiations (upper left optic radiation in this case).

L R

7. Right homonymous hemianopsia due to a lesion of the left occipital lobe. The pupillary light reflex is not impaired.

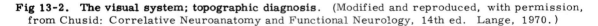

Fig 13-2. The visual system; topographic diagnosis. (Modified and reproduced, with permission, from Chusid: Correlative Neuroanatomy and Functional Neurology, 14th ed. Lange, 1970.)

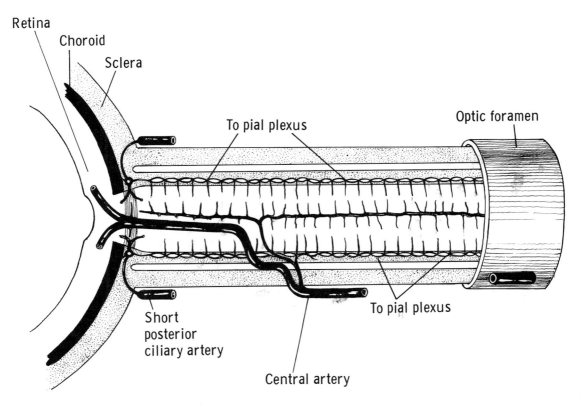

Fig 13-3. Schematic drawing showing optic nerve and central retinal artery. Note sharp bends. (Redrawn and reproduced, with permission, from Wolff: ibid.)

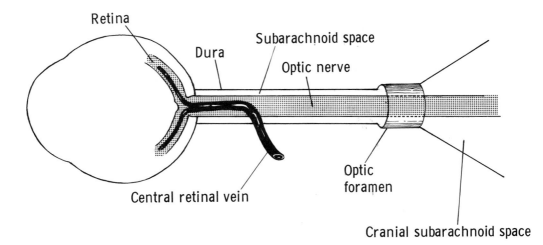

Fig 13-4. Schematic drawing showing optic nerve and central retinal vein. (Redrawn and reproduced, with permission, from Wolff: ibid.)

3. Orbital inflammation.
4. Intraocular (chorioretinitis).
5. Syphilis.

F. Toxic Amblyopias: Tobacco, methanol, quinine, arsenic, salicylates, lead.

G. Blood dyscrasias.

H. Trauma.

Pathology

In the early stages of optic neuritis there is an outpouring of white blood cells, predominantly neutrophils, in the affected area. The nerve fibers are swollen and fragmented. Fat-bearing macrophages soon appear, carrying away degenerated myelin material. As the process becomes more chronic, lymphocytes and plasma cells predominate. In mild attacks, the nerve fibers may be preserved with a minimum amount of scar tissue formation. When nerve tissue is permanently destroyed, fibrous gliosis replaces the nerve elements.

Clinical Findings

There is usually a temporary but severe loss of vision. There may be pain in the region of the eye, especially upon movement of the globe. Vision characteristically improves dramatically within 2-3 weeks.

Central scotomas are the most common visual field defect. They are usually circular, varying widely in size and density. Almost any unilateral field change is possible. The pupil reacts sluggishly to light.

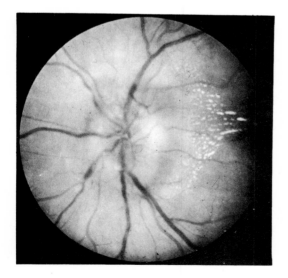

Fig 13-5. Optic neuritis. Note retinal edema on temporal side of optic disk.

Ophthalmoscopically, hyperemia of the optic disk and distention of large veins are early signs. Blurred disk margins and filling of the physiologic cup are common. The process may advance to marked edema of the nerve head, but elevations of more than 3 diopters (1 mm) are unusual. Extensive surrounding retinal edema may be present. Hemorrhages may occur in the nerve fiber layer near the optic disk, and are usually flame-shaped.

Differential Diagnosis

Papilledema is the most common differential diagnostic problem. In papilledema there is often greater elevation of the optic nerve head, nearly normal visual acuity, normal pupillary response to light, associated increased intracranial pressure, and no visual field defect except an enlarged blind spot unless the visual pathway has been interrupted intracranially. Despite these obvious differences, differential diagnosis continues to be a problem because of the similarity of the ophthalmoscopic findings.

Treatment

Ideally, treatment is directed toward the underlying cause. If the cause cannot be effectively treated or is not known, treatment is often unsatisfactory. Systemic corticosteroids have been reported to be helpful in persistent optic neuritis due to any cause, but many patients fail to respond. Since the tendency is in the direction of improvement, many drugs have been reported to be "successful" in the treatment of this disorder.

Course and Prognosis

Loss of vision occurs within the first few hours after onset and is maximal within several days. Visual acuity usually begins to improve 2-3 weeks after onset, and sometimes returns to normal in a few days. Improvement may continue slowly over a period of several months. The appearance of optic atrophy indicates some permanent destruction of nerve fibers with permanent loss of function. Optic neuritis associated with systemic or local inflammatory disease or of unknown etiology does not usually recur. Optic neuritis in demyelinating disease has a favorable prognosis without treatment for an individual attack, but over a period of years significant visual loss is the rule since permanent damage results from recurrent attacks.

RETROBULBAR NEURITIS

Retrobulbar neuritis is optic neuritis which occurs far enough behind the optic disk so that no early changes of the optic disk are visible ophthalmoscopically. Visual acuity is markedly reduced. ("The patient sees nothing and the doctor sees nothing.")

The most frequent cause of retrobulbar neuritis is multiple sclerosis. A diagnosis of multiple sclerosis is eventually made in about half of patients between 20 and 45 years of age who have an attack of retrobulbar neuritis. Other causes are late neurosyphilis, toxic amblyopias, other demyelinating diseases, Leber's optic atrophy, diabetes mellitus, and vitamin deficiency. If the process is sufficiently destructive, a retrograde optic atrophy results. The disk loses its normal pink color and becomes pale. In extreme cases a chalky-white disk with sharp outlines in a blind eye results.

DEMYELINATING DISEASES

MULTIPLE SCLEROSIS

Multiple sclerosis is a chronic, relapsing disorder of the CNS with a tendency to involve the optic nerves and chiasm, brain stem, cerebellar peduncles, and spinal cord, although no part of the CNS is invulnerable. Pathologically, multiple areas of irregular patches of demyelinization are present in the white matter. Early, there is degeneration of the myelin sheaths and a relative sparing of the axons. Glial tissue overgrowth and complete nerve fiber destruction with some round cell infiltration are seen later. The disease has a predilection for the optic nerve and chiasm. Vestibular nystagmus is a common early sign and, unlike most manifestations of the disease (which tend toward remission), it is often permanent (70%).

Optic neuritis (especially retrobulbar neuritis), characterized by acute unilateral loss of vision with a tendency toward recovery, is a frequent initial symptom of multiple sclerosis. The other eye is often involved eventually. With each attack there may be some residual permanent damage (eg, loss of visual acuity or defective color vision). Abnormal electro-retinogram (ERG) findings often parallel the optic nerve damage.

Because of the tendency toward selective involvement of the papillomacular bundle within the optic nerve, central scotoma is by far the most common visual field defect during the acute stage.

Diplopia is a frequent early symptom of extraocular muscle involvement, due most frequently to internuclear ophthalmoplegia. This condition, caused by a lesion of the medial longitudinal fasciculus, is characterized by paresis of one rectus muscle on conjugate lateral gaze to the opposite side while medial rectus function is normal for convergence. Weakness of one medial rectus muscle or ptosis may also occur; less commonly, weakness of the lateral rectus or other muscles, singly or together, also occurs.

NEUROMYELITIS OPTICA
(Devic's Disease)

This rare demyelinating disease of the CNS (considered by many to be a form of multiple sclerosis) is characterized by bilateral optic neuritis and paraplegia. The cause is not known. There is usually a sudden onset of blindness in one eye, followed soon by blindness in the other eye and paraplegia. There is only a moderate tendency to recovery of both elements of the disease. The mortality rate is 50% in some series.

There is no treatment.

DIFFUSE PERIAXIAL ENCEPHALITIS
(Schilder's Disease)

This rare disease of young children is characterized pathologically by widespread demyelinization of the white matter in the brain. Clinically there is an acute onset of rapidly developing cortical blindness,* mental deterioration, convulsions, bilateral spastic weakness, and paralysis progressing to coma and death.

---

*Cortical blindness is due to bilateral widespread destruction of the visual cortex. A striking feature of cortical blindness is the patient's subjective unawareness of his disability (Anton's syndrome). Despite being totally blind, the patient believes that he can see.

PAPILLEDEMA AND OPTIC ATROPHY

PAPILLEDEMA
(Choked Disk)

Papilledema is a noninflammatory congestion of the optic disk associated with increased intracranial pressure. Papilledema will occur in any condition causing persistent increased intracranial pressure; the most com-

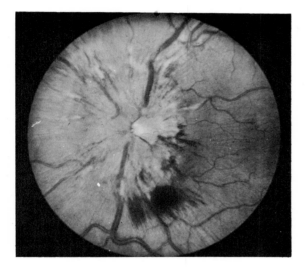

Fig 13-6. Papilledema. Note obliteration of disk margins, edema of nerve head and adjacent retina, and flame-shaped peripapillary hemorrhages.

mon causes are cerebral tumors, abscesses, subdural hematoma, hydrocephalus, and malignant hypertension. An important factor in the mechanism of papilledema is obstruction to the venous flow caused by pressure on the central retinal vein where it leaves the optic nerve and passes through the subarachnoid and subdural spaces.

Edema of the optic nerve is the principal pathologic finding. Edema may be present in the adjacent nerve fiber layer of the retina. Subhyaloid hemorrhages and hemorrhages in the nerve fiber layers are common. Inflammatory signs are minimal, and leukocytes are seen histologically only in the later stages. Degeneration of nerve fibers may eventually occur.

Clinical Findings
The blind spot is enlarged. Visual acuity and visual fields are otherwise normal. Early ophthalmoscopic findings include hyperemia of the disk, blurring of the disk margins, and distention of retinal veins. It is difficult to be sure about early papilledema. One helpful sign is the absence of pulsation of the central retinal vein or failure to produce a pulsation with light digital pressure on the globe. Frank (measurable) swelling of the disk, peripapillary retinal edema, and hemorrhages radially about the disk in the nerve fiber layers appear later. Papilledema may elevate the disk to 6 or 10 diopters, and hemorrhages in severe cases are subhyaloid, occasionally breaking into the vitreous and markedly affecting vision.

Differential Diagnosis
The common differential diagnostic problem of papilledema and optic neuritis is discussed above (p 139).

A condition known as pseudopapilledema is sometimes noted in normal optic disks, particularly in farsighted persons, that have a "blurred" disk-margin that suggests papilledema. A normal blind spot and normal intracranial pressure rule out true papilledema.

Myelinated nerve fibers of the retina adjacent to the nerve head may be confused with papilledema (Fig 13-8).

Complications
Papilledema may persist for a long time without permanently affecting vision, or secondary optic atrophy may occur as a complication. Following reduction of increased intracranial pressure, papilledema improves rapidly. Hemorrhages, exudates, and retinal edema usually clear promptly. If optic atrophy does follow, slight to total permanent loss of vision results.

Treatment
Treatment depends upon the underlying cause. Papilledema associated with hypertensive retinopathy is an indication for vigorous treatment with potent hypotensive drugs.

Caution: Although it is at times undertaken as a calculated risk with proper precautions, lumbar puncture is usually contraindicated in patients with papilledema because of the danger of herniation of the brain into the tentorial incisure or into the foramen magnum. Such herniation causes pressure particularly on the medulla and can cause sudden death.

Course and Prognosis
In general, the more rapid the onset, the greater the danger of permanent visual loss.

Papilledema of more than 5 diopters, extensive retinal hemorrhages and exudates, and macular stars imply a poor visual prognosis. Early pallor of the disk, once the edema of the nerve head clears, indicates that some optic atrophy will follow.

OPTIC NERVE ATROPHY

Etiologic Classification

A. Vascular: Occlusion of the central retinal vein or artery; arteriosclerotic changes within the optic nerve itself, disturbing its normal nutrition; or post-hemorrhagic, due to sudden massive blood loss (eg, bleeding peptic ulcer, traumatic amputation).

B. Degeneration: Consecutive atrophy secondary to retinal disease, with destruction of ganglion cells (eg, retinitis); or as part of a systemic degenerative disease (eg, cerebromacular degeneration).

C. Secondary to Papilledema: See p 141.

D. Secondary to Optic Neuritis (Including Retrobulbar Neuritis): See pp 136 and 139.

E. Pressure Against the Optic Nerve: Aneurysm of the anterior circle of Willis, bony pressure at the optic foramen (eg, osteitis deformans), intraorbital or intracranial tumors, adhesive constricting basal arachnoiditis.

F. Toxic: End result of toxic amblyopia. See pp 163-165.

G. Metabolic Diseases: Eg, diabetes mellitus.

H. Traumatic: Direct injury to a nerve (ie, severing, avulsion).

I. Glaucomatous: See Chapter 15.

Clinical Findings

Loss of vision is the only symptom. Pallor of the optic disk and loss of pupillary reaction are usually proportionate to visual loss.

Treatment, Course, and Prognosis

It is rarely possible to treat the underlying cause effectively. Changes in visual function occur very slowly over weeks or months. It is difficult to assess prognosis on the basis of ophthalmoscopic findings alone. Atrophic cupping, attenuation and reduced number of vessels on the disk, and pallor with papilledema are unfavorable prognostic signs. Optic atrophy secondary to vascular, traumatic, degenerative, and some toxic causes usually has a very bad prognosis. Visual loss due to optic atrophy secondary to pressure against the optic nerve may be restored, particularly if the cause is relieved early.

GENETICALLY DETERMINED OPTIC ATROPHY

Leber's Disease

This rare disease, characterized by bilateral progressive optic atrophy, occurs in young men age 20-30 (very rarely in women). It has classically been considered to be due to a sex-linked recessive gene, but its real mode of inheritance must still be considered in doubt. Vision is not totally lost, but there is no known treatment.

Congenital or Infantile Hereditary Optic Atrophy

This occurs in a severe autosomal recessive form and a milder autosomal dominant form. The recessive form is present at birth or within 2 years, and is accompanied by nystagmus. The more common dominant form has an insidious onset in childhood, with little progression thereafter. There is characteristically a centrocecal scotoma with variable loss of central visual acuity.

Behr's Hereditary Optic Atrophy

This rare autosomal recessive disease is characterized by (1) bilateral optic atrophy, rarely complete; and (2) associated neurologic findings such as mild ataxia, a positive Babinski sign, clubfoot, mental deficiency, nystagmus, and other findings, at times with generalized slow progression to a static condition by late adolescence. There is no known treatment.

DISEASES OF THE OPTIC CHIASM

Anatomy (Fig 13-9)

The optic chiasm is variably situated near the top of the diaphragm of the sella turcica (most often posteriorly, projecting over the dorsum sellae) and usually separated from it by several mm of subarachnoid space. Above, the lamina terminalis forms the anterior wall of the third ventricle. The internal carotid arteries lie just laterally, adjacent to the cavernous sinuses. The chiasm is made up of the junction of the 2 optic nerves and provides for crossing of the nasal fibers to the opposite optic tract and the passage of temporal fibers to the ipsilateral optic tract. The macular fibers are arranged similarly to the rest of the fibers

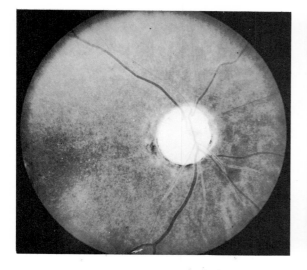

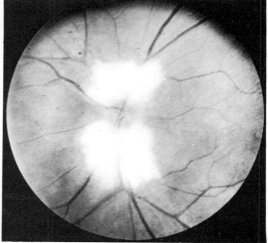

Fig 13-7. Optic atrophy due to syphilitic optic neuritis. Note pallor of optic disk and lack of small vessels coursing over disk edges.

Fig 13-8. Myelinated nerve fibers adjacent to optic nerve head. Depending upon the size and distribution, they may be mistaken for retinal exudates, papilledema, or optic neuritis.

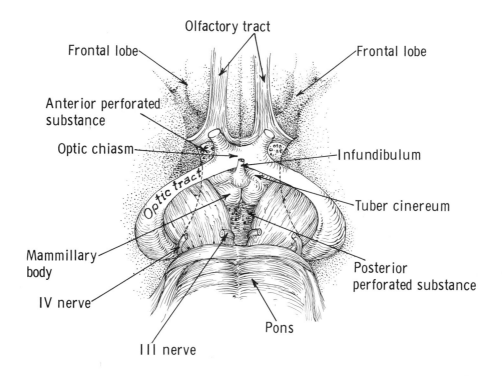

Fig 13-9. Relationship of optic chiasm from inferior aspect. (Redrawn and reproduced, with permission, from Duke-Elder: System of Ophthalmology, Vol. II. Mosby, 1961.)

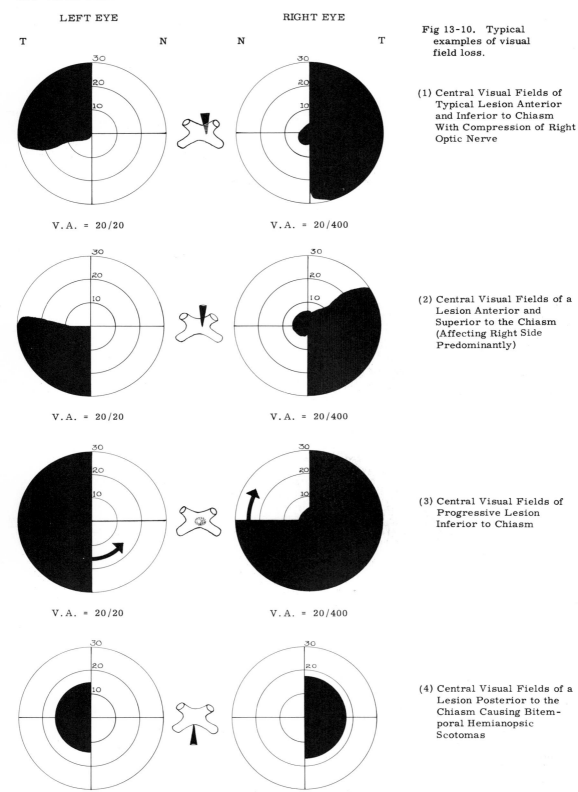

LEFT EYE   RIGHT EYE

T   N   N   T

Fig 13-10. Typical examples of visual field loss.

(1) Central Visual Fields of Typical Lesion Anterior and Inferior to Chiasm With Compression of Right Optic Nerve

V.A. = 20/20   V.A. = 20/400

(2) Central Visual Fields of a Lesion Anterior and Superior to the Chiasm (Affecting Right Side Predominantly)

V.A. = 20/20   V.A. = 20/400

(3) Central Visual Fields of Progressive Lesion Inferior to Chiasm

V.A. = 20/20   V.A. = 20/400

(4) Central Visual Fields of a Lesion Posterior to the Chiasm Causing Bitemporal Hemianopsic Scotomas

V.A. = 20/20   V.A. = 20/20

except that their decussation is farther posteriorly. In general, lesions of the chiasm cause bitemporal hemianopsic defects.

LESIONS AFFECTING THE OPTIC CHIASM

Lesions Posterior and Inferior to the Chiasm
Intrasellar tumors such as pituitary tumors (see below) are the most common causes. Papilledema is rare, and destruction and enlargement of the sella turcica is seen by x-ray. Visual fields reveal superior bitemporal field involvement with or without macular loss. Progression of such a lesion will then cause loss of the inferior temporal field, inferior nasal field, and finally the superior nasal field.

Lesions Anterior and Inferior to the Chiasm (Common)
Pituitary tumors, meningitis, and arachnoiditis are most commonly responsible. Superior bitemporal quadrants are affected with one or both optic nerves involved, causing central scotoma due to involvement of the papillomacular bundle (the most susceptible fibers).

Lesions Posterior to the Chiasm (Uncommon)
These are due to suprasellar tumors, Rathke pouch tumors, and tumors of the third ventricle. Increased intracranial pressure may be present, and x-rays often reveal suprasellar calcification and destruction of the sella. The visual fields show bitemporal central scotomas due to compression of the posteriorly placed crossing macular fibers. Since the nasal field (uncrossed) macular fibers are preserved, good visual acuity remains.

Lesions Anterior and Superior to the Chiasm (Rare)
Aneurysms of the circle of Willis, particularly of the anterior cerebral artery, cause a descending optic atrophy. Angiography is often diagnostic in these cases. Inferior temporal quadrant visual field defects with a central scotoma on the side of the optic atrophy are usually found.

Lesions Posterior and Superior to the Chiasm (Rare)
These are caused by internal hydrocephalus resulting from tumors of the wall of the third ventricle, such as hypothalamic tumor. Signs of increased intracranial pressure are present, and ventriculograms reveal the hydrocephalus. The visual fields will show inferior bitemporal loss. (Same as the second diagram in Fig 13-10, illustrating anterior and superior

lesions, except that good central vision is usually retained longer.)

Lesions Lateral to the Chiasm
Aneurysm of the internal carotid artery is the most common cause, but tumors such as meningiomas or intrasellar or extrasellar tumors occasionally cause lateral pressure upon the optic chiasm. The visual field change is a unilateral nasal hemianopsia. Binasal hemianopsia is a rare defect which occurs if there is lateral pressure on both sides of the chiasm. Lesions causing lateral pressure on the chiasm include meningioma of the lesser wing of the sphenoid, arachnoiditis, aneurysm of the internal carotid artery, and arteriosclerosis of the carotid artery.

INTRASELLAR PITUITARY TUMORS

The anterior lobe of the pituitary gland is the site of origin of pituitary tumors. Three types of cells are normally present (basophils, eosinophils, and neutrophils), and any one type can predominate in a tumor. Symptoms and signs include loss of vision and field changes (90%), x-ray evidence of bony erosion of the sella (80%), pituitary dysfunction (60%), extraocular nerve palsies (10%), and papilledema (rarely).

Surgical removal is the usual method of treatment. Irradiation has been equally effective in many instances. Visual loss or endocrine dysfunction is an indication for treatment. Visual acuity and visual fields may improve dramatically after pressure has been removed from the chiasm. X-ray evidence of erosion of the sella is frequently seen as an incidental finding on skull films in patients over 50 with benign asymptomatic tumors. No treatment is indicated in such cases.

Chromophobe Adenoma (Neutrophilic)
This is by far the most common pituitary tumor. The onset is gradual, and the incidence increases with age; these tumors are most commonly seen in the 50's and 60's. Headache and visual loss are the most common presenting complaints. Later, bitemporal field defects and eventually optic atrophy appear along with symptoms of hypopituitarism.

Chromophile Adenoma (Eosinophilic)
Eosinophilic adenoma causes marked endocrine disturbance: gigantism before the epiphyses of long bones are closed and acromegaly thereafter. The visual field changes appear later, after the tumor has eroded

through the sella or pushed against the chiasm. Acromegaly may progress slowly for years.

CRANIOPHARYNGIOMA
(Rathke Pouch Tumor)

Craniopharyngiomas are a group of rare tumors arising from epithelial remnants of Rathke's pouch (80% of the population normally have such remnants) and characteristically are first seen between the ages of 10 and 25 years. They are usually suprasellar, occasionally intrasellar. The signs and symptoms vary tremendously with the age of the patient and the exact location of the tumor as well as its rate of growth. When a suprasellar tumor occurs, chiasmal syndrome field defects are prominent. Pituitary deficiency may result, and posterior pressure may cause hypothalamic disturbances such as diabetes insipidus. With the passage of years, calcification and ossification of parts of the tumor give a characteristic radiographic appearance. Treatment consists of surgical removal, if possible, but evacuation of the cystic contents and removal of cyst wall is often all that can be done.

SUPRASELLAR MENINGIOMAS

Suprasellar meningiomas arise from the dura covering the circle of venous sinuses around the chiasm and sella. The tumor is usually anterior and superior to the chiasm, and the visual field changes are characteristic. The optic nerves are often involved early (but asymmetrically) in the slowly progressive damage to the visual pathway. Skull x-rays may reveal stippled calcification within the tumor, but the sella turcica is normal. Carotid anteriograms usually show displacement of the normal vessels and often filling of abnormal tumor vessels as well. Treatment consists of surgical removal.

GLIOMA OF THE OPTIC CHIASM

Optic chiasm glioma is a rare disorder of childhood that sometimes occurs as part of the clinical picture of neurofibromatosis. Onset is sudden, with rapid loss of vision. Optic atrophy occurs, and visual field defects reveal a chiasmal syndrome. Orbital x-rays may reveal enlargement of the optic foramen; air

contrast studies may reveal displacement of the third ventricle. Treatment is by irradiation, since surgical removal results in blindness.

THE OPTIC PATHWAY

Anatomy (Fig 13-11)
The second cranial nerve is the pathway for the special sense of vision. It is made up of visual fibers (80%) and afferent pupillary fibers (20%). The nerve has been described in detail on p 135. At the chiasm, more than half of the fibers (those from the nasal retinas) decussate and join the uncrossed temporal fibers of the opposite side to form the optic tracts. All of the fibers receiving impulses from the right visual field are thus projected to the left cerebral hemisphere; those from the left field to the right cerebrum.

Each optic tract sweeps around the hypothalamus and cerebral peduncle to end in the lateral geniculate body, with a smaller portion carrying pupillary impulses continuing to the pretectal area and superior colliculi. (The pupillary pathway is diagrammed in Fig 13-12.) The visual fibers synapse in the lateral geniculate body. The cell bodies of this structure give rise to the geniculocalcarine tract, the final neuron of the visual pathway. The geniculocalcarine tract passes through the posterior limb of the internal capsule and then fans into the optic radiation, which traverses parts of the temporal and parietal lobes en route to the occipital cortex.

Detection of Lesions of the Optic Pathways
The primary method of localizing lesions of the optic pathways is by central and peripheral visual field examination, the technic of which is discussed on p 21. Fig 13-2 shows the types of field defects caused by lesions in various locations of the pathway. Lesions anterior to the chiasm (of the retina or optic nerve) cause unilateral field defects; lesions anywhere in the visual pathway posterior to the chiasm cause contralateral homonymous defects. Chiasmal lesions cause bitemporal defects and are discussed separately.

Multiple isopters (field tests with several objects of different sizes) should be used in order to evaluate the defects thoroughly. A field defect shows evidence of actively spreading disease when there are areas of "relative scotoma" (ie, a larger field defect for a smaller test object). Such visual field defects are said to be "sloping." This is in contrast to

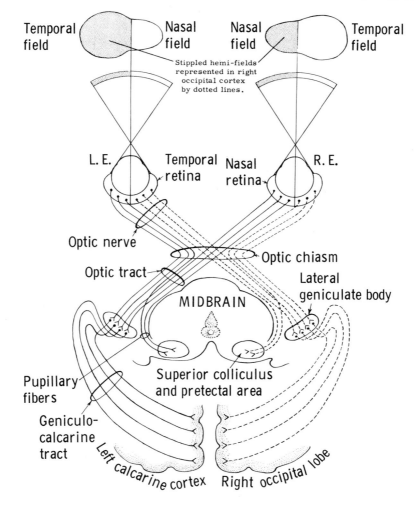

Fig 13-11. The optic pathway. The dotted lines represent nerve fibers from the retina to the occipital cortex that carry visual and pupillary afferent impulses from the left half of the visual field.

old inactive lesions with steep borders (ie, the defect is the same size no matter what size test object is used).

Another important generalization is that the more congruous (ie, the more similar the 2 fields) the homonymous field defects, the farther posterior the lesion is in the visual pathway. A lesion in the occipital region causes identical defects in each field, whereas optic tract lesions cause incongruous (dissimilar) homonymous field defects. Also, the more posterior the lesion, the more likely that there will be macular sparing and, therefore, maintenance of good visual acuity.

The Normal Pupil

The size of the normal pupil varies at different ages and from person to person. The normal pupillary diameter is usually about 3-4 mm, tending to be larger in childhood and progressively smaller with advancing age. Many normal persons have a slight difference in pupil size (physiologic anisocoria). Occasionally there is a marked difference in normal pupil size. Mydriatic and cycloplegic drugs work more effectively on blue eyes than on brown eyes. The function of the pupil is to control the amount of light entering the eye to give best visual function under the varieties of light intensity normally encountered. The pathways controlling this purely reflex function are described below and are diagrammed in Fig 13-11.

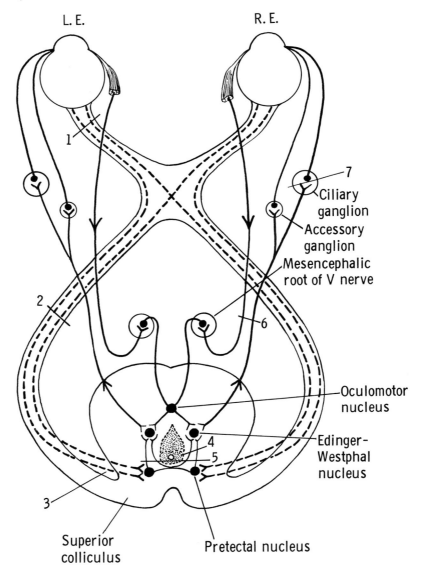

(1) Lesion at optic nerve. Loss of direct and opposite consensual reaction. Retention of near reflex.

(2) Lesion at optic tract. Contralateral hemianopsic loss of reaction (Wernicke's).

(3) Lesion at optic tract beyond the exit of the pupillary fibers. No pupillary reaction loss (right homonymous hemianopsia present).

(4) Lesion between decussation and Edinger-Westphal nucleus. Loss of ipsilateral direct and consensual reaction. Near reflex intact (unilateral Argyll Robertson pupil).

(5) Lesion of all fibers from pretectal nucleus to Edinger-Westphal nucleus. Loss of all light response. Retention of near reflex (complete Argyll Robertson pupil).

(6) Lesion of cranial nerve III. Absolute ipsilateral pupillary paralysis.

(7) Lesion of ciliary ganglion. Ipsilateral loss of light reflex with retention of near reflex (unilateral Argyll Robertson pupil).

Fig 13-12. Pupillary pathways for light reflex and miosis of accommodation. Solid lines = efferent pathway. Dotted lines = afferent pathway. (Redrawn and reproduced, with permission, from Duke-Elder: Text-book of Ophthalmology, Vol. IV. Mosby, 1949.)

THE PUPILLARY PATHWAYS

The evaluation of the pupillary reactions is important in localizing lesions involving the optic pathways. A knowledge of the neuroanatomy of the pathway for reaction of the pupil to light and the miosis associated with accommodation is very important.

Neuroanatomy of the Pupillary Pathways

A. Light Reflex: The pathway for the light reflex is entirely subcortical. The afferent pupillary fibers are included within the optic nerve and pathway until they leave the optic tract just before the visual fibers synapse in the lateral geniculate body. They go to the pretectal area of the midbrain and synapse. Impulses are then relayed by crossed fibers through the posterior commissure to the opposite Edinger-Westphal nucleus. Some fibers also go directly ventral to the ipsilateral Edinger-Westphal nucleus. The efferent pathway is via the third nerve to the ciliary ganglion within the retrobulbar extraocular muscle cone. The postganglionic fiber goes via the short ciliary nerves to innervate the sphincter muscle of the iris.

B. The Near Reflex: When the eyes look at a near object, 3 reactions occur: **accommodation, convergence,** and **constriction of the pupil,** bringing a sharp image into focus on corresponding retinal points. There is convincing evidence that the final common pathway is mediated through the oculomotor nerve with a synapse in the ciliary ganglion. The afferent pathway has not been worked out, but there is evidence that it enters the midbrain ventral to the Edinger-Westphal nucleus and sends fibers to both sides of the cortex. Although the 3 components are closely associated, it cannot be considered a pure reflex as each component can be neutralized while leaving the other two intact—ie, by prism (neutralizing convergence), by lenses (neutralizing accommodation), and by weak mydriatic drugs (neutralizing miosis).

ARGYLL ROBERTSON PUPIL

A typical Argyll Robertson pupil is very suggestive of CNS syphilis associated with tabes dorsalis or general paresis. The pupil is less than 3 mm in diameter (miotic) and does not respond to light stimulation. The pupil does constrict with accommodation. The finding is nearly always bilateral. The pupils are commonly irregular and eccentric and dilate poorly with mydriatics. Less commonly, the sign is incomplete (slow response to light) or unilateral. Some degree of Argyll Robertson pupil is present in over 50% of patients with CNS syphilis. A wide variety of other CNS diseases infrequently cause incomplete Argyll Robertson pupil. These include diabetes, chronic alcoholism, encephalitis, multiple sclerosis, CNS degenerative disease, and tumors of the midbrain. The site or sites of the CNS lesion are not definitely known, but Fig 13-12 shows the most likely locations.

TONIC PUPIL

This not uncommon entity is characterized by a delayed or diminished direct and consensual reaction to light (80% unilateral) in a pupil larger than normal. It may be associated with loss of tendon reflexes (Adie's syndrome). The cause is obscure but definitely is not syphilis, and it is important that tonic pupil be differentiated from Argyll Robertson pupil. It is most frequently seen in young adult women. It may come on abruptly and be noticeable to the patient because of increased sensitivity to light. A weak (2.5%) solution of methacholine (Mecholyl®) instilled into the conjunctival sac causes a tonic pupil to constrict; normal pupils are not affected. The tonic pupil dilates slowly in the dark and reacts promptly to mydriatics.

HORNER'S SYNDROME

Horner's syndrome is caused by a lesion of the sympathetic pathway in the brain stem, upper spinal cord, or cervical sympathetic chain. Unilateral miosis, ptosis, mild enophthalmos, and absence of sweating on the ipsilateral face and neck make up the complete syndrome. Causes of Horner's syndrome include cervical vertebral fractures, tabes dorsalis, syringomyelia, cervical cord tumor, apical tuberculosis, goiter, enlarged cervical lymph glands, apical bronchogenic carcinoma, mediastinal tumor, and aneurysm of the carotid or subclavian artery.

EXTRAOCULAR MOVEMENTS

This section deals with the neural apparatus that controls the movements of the eyes and causes them to move simultaneously in tandem up or down and side to side as well as in convergence or divergence.

1. SUPRANUCLEAR PATHWAYS

The supranuclear neural pathways of the extraocular muscles innervate conjugate lateral and vertical gaze as well as the disjunctive movements of convergence and divergence. They consist of CNS connections to the nuclei of cranial nerves III, IV, and VI located in the midbrain. The highest centers for these functions are located in the frontal lobe (voluntary or command movement) and the occipital lobe (involuntary or fixation movement).

Anatomy of Voluntary Conjugate Movements

A. Horizontal: The cortical center that controls horizontal conjugate movements of the eyes is situated posteriorly in the second convolution of the frontal lobe. The pathway descends with the pyramidal tract in the internal capsule through the basal ganglia and into the brain stem. The fibers leave the pyramidal tract in the midbrain, cross, and probably go to the vestibular nucleus. Impulses then go to a hypothetical nucleus for conjugate lateral gaze which may be identical with the abducens nucleus. The ipsilateral lateral rectus and the contralateral medial rectus muscles are stimulated to produce conjugate movement via the medial longitudinal fasciculus. (See Fig 13-13.)

B. Vertical: The centers and pathways are probably the same as for horizontal move-

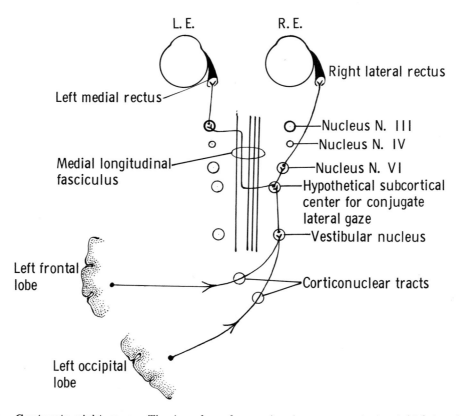

Fig 13-13. Conjugate right gaze. The impulses for conjugate movements in right lateral gaze are initiated in the left frontal lobe (voluntary) and the left occipital lobe (involuntary). (After Spiegel and Sommer. Redrawn with modifications and reproduced, with permission, from Adler: Physiology of the Eye, 5th ed. Mosby, 1970.)

ment except that the subcortical pathway leaves the pyramidal tract somewhat higher and synapses in the pretectal area. The impulses then go to the medial longitudinal fasciculus and are distributed to the appropriate oculomotor nuclei to effect vertical gaze. The vestibular nuclei undoubtedly affect this pathway also.

C. Convergence: It is probable that the supranuclear impulses for convergence travel much the same pathway as do those for conjugate horizontal and vertical gaze, arriving at a midbrain synapse near or in the oculomotor nucleus. From this synapse stimulating impulses go to each medial rectus and inhibitory inpulses go to each lateral rectus via the medial longitudinal fasciculus.

D. Divergence: Electromyography has established divergence as an active process (not a relaxation of convergence, as was once thought). The supranuclear pathway is probably more or less the same as for convergence, arriving at a midbrain center near the 6th nerve nuclei. Stimulating impulses go to each lateral rectus and inhibitory impulses to each medial rectus via the medial longitudinal fasciculus as the eyes undergo divergence.

Anatomy of Involuntary Conjugate Movements
A. Horizontal and Vertical: The cortical center is a large ill-defined area of the occipital lobe. The descending pathway is not definitely known, but in general it follows a route similar to the voluntary pathway into the internal capsule, midbrain, vestibular nuclei, and medial longitudinal fasciculus. This pathway carries the impulses of the "following movement" as demonstrated by optokinetic nystagmus. The eyes will "follow" a slowly moving object even when the voluntary pathway is non-functioning. When both pathways are intact, the voluntary influence dominates the involuntary.

B. Convergence and Divergence: Convergence has a strong involuntary component which dominates the voluntary. This is in contrast to the conjugate movements, where the voluntary component predominates. The pathway is not definitely known but probably follows that of the conjugate pathways, finally arriving at its subcortical center in the midbrain.

Divergence must be innervated by a similar supranuclear pathway which sends impulses to the midbrain center, probably located in or near the 6th nerve nuclei.

LESIONS OF SUPRANUCLEAR PATHWAYS

Frontal Lobe
Irritative lesions of the frontal lobe involving the supranuclear ocular pathways may cause involuntary turning of the eyes to the side opposite the lesion. Destructive lesions cause deviation to the same side, and the eyes cannot be turned to the opposite side. This is termed a gaze palsy. The "following reflex" is retained since the involuntary pathway is unaffected. There is no diplopia. An exaggerated end point nystagmus is often the first sign of a gaze palsy or may occur as a residuum of a clearing gaze palsy.

Occipital Lobe
The "following reflex" may be lost with lesions of the visual cortex. The patient is unable to follow a slowly moving object in the direction of the gaze palsy. The command movement is not lost.

PARINAUD'S SYNDROME

This syndrome is characterized by loss of voluntary upward gaze and (frequently) loss of the pupillary light response with retention miosis response in the near reflex. Nystagmus retractorius, which consists of retraction movements of the globe on attempted upward gaze or convergence, is also frequently present. There may also be accommodative spasm, a loss of conjugate voluntary downward gaze associated with loss of convergence and accommodation, ptosis or lid retraction, papilledema, or third nerve palsy. Surrounding structures may also be involved depending upon the size and location of the lesion. Conjugate horizontal ocular movements are usually not affected. The syndrome results from tectal or pretectal lesions affecting the periaqueductal area. Pinealomas, infiltrating gliomas, vascular lesions, and trauma may also produce this picture.

LESIONS OF THE BRAIN STEM

Lesions of the brain stem are common causes of gaze palsies. The lesions most frequently encountered (in order of frequency) are vascular accidents, multiple sclerosis, tumors, and encephalitis.

Table 13-1. Differentiation of cortical and brain stem lesions causing gaze palsies.

Lesion Above Brain Stem	Lesion in Brain Stem
1. Conjugate deviation is usually present early and is usually of large magnitude.	1. Conjugate deviation is rarely present is of small magnitude.
2. Conjugate deviation is toward the side of the lesion.	2. Gaze palsy is away from the side of the lesion.
3. Gaze palsy is of short duration.	3. Gaze palsy is present as long as the lesion remains.
4. Lesion is frequently irritative.	4. Lesion is rarely irritative.
5. Head is turned in direction of deviation.	5. Head is straight or turned in direction opposite the ocular deviation.
6. Individual infranuclear muscle palsy not present; diplopis is never present.	6. Infranuclear muscle palsy is often present; diplopia is common.

OCULOGYRIC CRISIS

Oculogyric crisis is a tonic, conjugate, spastic upward movement of the eyes; it is frequently associated with a backward head tilt. It occurs most commonly in parkinsonism, epidemic encephalitis, and as a consequence of phenothiazine toxicity. Tabes dorsalis, multiple sclerosis, cerebral tumors, and hysteria are rarer causes. Generalized painful sensations, opened mouth, and protruding tongue are other characteristic signs of an attack which may last from a few seconds to several hours. Attacks occur sporadically or frequently, at times even daily, and are often followed by sleep. The specific cause is not known, but this disorder is generally considered to be due to malfunction of the extrapyramidal system.

Oculogyric crisis is a poor prognostic sign in parkinsonism, often just preceding invalidism or death. Recent neurosurgical procedures have relieved or reduced oculogyric crisis. Mild cycloplegics such as hyoscine given topically may shorten or abort an individual attack.

SUPRANUCLEAR SYNDROMES INVOLVING DISJUNCTIVE OCULAR MOVEMENTS

Spasm of the Near Reflex
The near reflex consists of 3 components: convergence, accommodation, and constriction of the pupil. Spasm of the near reflex is usually caused by hysteria, although encephalitis, tabes dorsalis, and meningitis may cause spasm by irritation of the supranuclear pathway. It is characterized by convergent strabismus with diplopia, miotic pupils, and spasm of accommodation.

If hysteria is the cause, atropine, 1%, 2 drops in each eye twice daily, or minus (concave) lenses may give temporary relief. Psychiatric consultation is indicated for treatment of an underlying mental cause.

Convergence Paralysis
Convergence paralysis is characterized by a sudden onset of diplopia for near vision, with absence of any individual extraocular muscle palsy. It is caused by hysteria or destructive lesions of the supranuclear pathway for convergence. Multiple sclerosis, encephalitis, tabes dorsalis, tumors, aneurysms, minor cerebrovascular accidents, and Parkinson's disease are the most common organic causes.

SUPRANUCLEAR LESIONS AND STRABISMUS

Strabismus is dealt with in Chapter 14, but it should be mentioned here that idiopathic esotropias and exotropias with onset early in life may result from abnormalities of the supranuclear pathways regulating divergence and convergence.

2. NUCLEAR AND INFRANUCLEAR CONNECTIONS

Peripheral and Intermediate Connections of the Nuclei of Cranial Nerves III, IV, and VI
A. Oculomotor (III): The motor fibers arise from a group of nuclei in the central gray matter ventral to the cerebral aqueduct at the level of the superior colliculus. Mainly uncrossed fibers course through the red nucleus

and the inner side of the substantia nigra to emerge on the medial side of the cerebral peduncles. The nerve runs alongside the sella turcica, in the outer wall of the cavernous sinus, and through the superior orbital fissure to supply the internal, superior, and inferior rectus muscles and the inferior oblique and levator palpebrae muscles.

The parasympathetics arise from the Edinger-Westphal nucleus just rostrad to the motor nucleus of the third nerve and pass via the nasociliary branch of the third nerve to the ciliary ganglion. From there the short ciliary nerves are distributed to the sphincter muscle of the iris. The upper portion of the medial nucleus of the third nerve passes via the ciliary ganglion and short ciliary nerves to the ciliary muscle, which controls the shape of the lens during accommodation.

B. Trochlear (IV): Motor (entirely crossed) fibers arise from the trochlear nucleus just caudad to the third nerve at the level of the inferior colliculus, run posteriorly, decussate in the anterior medullary velum, and wind around the cerebral peduncles. From here the 4th nerve follows the third nerve along the cavernous sinus to the orbit, where it supplies the superior oblique muscle.

C. Abducens (VI): Motor (entirely uncrossed) fibers arise from the nucleus in the floor of the 4th ventricle in the lower portion of the pons near the internal genu of the facial nerve. Piercing the pons, the fibers emerge anteriorly, the nerve running a long course over the tip of the petrous portion of the temporal bone to the outer wall of the cavernous sinus. It enters the orbit with the 3rd and 4th nerves to supply the lateral rectus muscle.

Central Reflex Connections of the Nuclei of Cranial Nerves III, IV, and VI

The central reflex connections of these nuclei originate in 5 areas: (1) From the pretectal region via the posterior commissure to the Edinger-Westphal nuclei for mediation of ipsilateral and consensual light reflexes. Interruption of this pathway may cause an Argyll Robertson pupil. (2) From the superior colliculi via the tectobulbar tract to the nuclei of cranial nerves III, IV, and VI for the mediation of miosis associated with accommodation. (3) From the inferior colliculi via the tectobulbar tract to the eye muscle nuclei for reflexes correlated with hearing. (4) From the vestibular nuclei via the medial longitudinal fasciculus for reflex gaze movement correlated with equilibrium. (5) From the cortex through the corticobulbar tract for mediation of voluntary and involuntary conjugate movements of the eyes.

SUMMARY OF DISORDERS OF CRANIAL NERVES III, IV, AND VI

Oculomotor Paralysis (Cranial Nerve III)

A. Complete Oculomotor Paralysis: The lesion involves the third nerve anywhere from the nucleus (midbrain) to the peripheral branches in the orbit. It causes divergent strabismus since the eye is turned out by the intact lateral rectus muscle and slightly depressed by the intact superior oblique muscle. There is a dilated fixed pupil, absent accommodation, and ptosis of the upper lid, often severe enough to cover the pupil. The eye may only be moved laterally. Trauma, carotid aneurysm, and diabetes are the most common causes. In diabetes, the normal pupillary responses are usually intact; in carotid aneurysm, they almost never are spared.

B. Complete Internal Ophthalmoplegia: This consists of a dilated and fixed pupil and paralysis of accommodation. The lesion is nearly always peripheral in the ciliary ganglion.

Trochlear Paralysis (Cranial Nerve IV)

There may be esotropia (convergent strabismus) in the primary position, with diplopia relieved by tilting the head to the side opposite the affected superior oblique muscle— a valuable diagnostic clue. There is difficulty in turning the eye downward, which may cause difficulty in reading or in descending stairs. This is the least common oculomotor palsy; it occurs most often due to trauma, pressure on the nerve by an aneurysm, or with any disorder that causes third nerve palsy.

Abducens Paralysis (Cranial Nerve VI)

This is the most common single muscle palsy, since one nerve with a long intracranial course supplies one extraocular muscle. Abduction of the eye is absent; esotropia is present in the primary position and increases upon gaze to the affected side. Movement of the eye to the opposite side is normal. Cerebrovascular accidents are the most common cause; basilar artery disease, increased intracranial pressure, tumors at the base of the skull, meningitis, diabetes, and trauma are other frequent causes.

Symptoms and Signs of Extraocular Muscle Palsies

Diplopia occurs when the visual axes are not aligned. This is especially true when the onset of strabismus is after age 6 (suppression and abnormal retinal correspondence cannot develop). Dizziness is often associated. Head tilt occurs, especially in paresis of the superior oblique or superior rectus muscle, when the head tilt is to the opposite side to avoid diplopia by moving the eye out of the field of action of the paralyzed muscle.

Ptosis is caused by weakness or paralysis of the levator muscle.

SYNDROMES AFFECTING CRANIAL NERVES III, IV, AND VI

Peripheral Involvement of Cranial Nerves III, IV, and VI

A. Gradenigo's Syndrome: This is characterized by pain in the face (from irritation of the trigeminal nerve) and abducens palsy. The syndrome is produced by meningitis at the tip of the petrous bone and most often occurs as a complication of otitis media.

B. Cavernous Sinus Syndrome: See p 133.

C. Orbital Fissure Syndrome: All extraocular peripheral nerves pass through the orbital fissure and can be involved by a traumatic bone fracture in this area or by tumor encroaching on the fissure from the orbital or cranial side.

D. Orbital Apex Syndrome: This is similar to the orbital fissure syndrome with the addition of optic nerve signs. It is caused by an orbital tumor or trauma which damages the optic and extraocular nerves.

Brain Stem Syndromes

A. Chronic Progressive External Ophthalmoplegia:* This rather rare disease involves all 3 extraocular nerves. It is characterized by a slowly progressive inability to move the eyes and, quite often, ptosis, with normal pupillary reactions and accommodation. It may begin at any age and progresses over a period of 5-15 years to complete external ophthalmoplegia. Generalized muscular dystrophy occasionally ensues. Most authorities believe that this disease is a variant of a type of hereditary muscular dystrophy primarily affecting extraocular muscles. There is no effective treatment, although cosmetic surgery for strabismus or ptosis is often necessary. Myasthenia gravis is the major differential problem.

---

*"External ophthalmoplegia" is a general term that denotes inability to move the eyes normally as a result of any nuclear or infranuclear involvement of cranial nerves III, IV, or VI; the pupillary reaction and accommodation are normal.

B. Benedikt's Syndrome: Ipsilateral oculomotor paralysis, which may be partial, and a contralateral hyperkinesis from involvement of the red nucleus are caused by a lesion of the red nucleus in the midbrain which involves oculomotor fibers (cranial nerve III) passing through it. A cerebrovascular accident is the most frequent cause.

C. Weber's Syndrome: Crossed hemiplegia (including the lower face) and ipsilateral oculomotor paresis are caused by a lesion in the upper portion of the midbrain (see below) involving the peduncle and cranial nerve III. Cerebrovascular accidents and tumors are the most frequent causes.

D. Foville's Syndrome: Ipsilateral paralysis of the muscles of facial expression, with abducens palsy and loss of conjugate lateral gaze to the same side, is caused by a lesion in the pons involving the abducens nucleus and facial fibers which arch around it before making their central exit. It may also include Horner's syndrome, loss of taste, deafness, and facial analgesia on the same side.

E. Millard-Gubler Syndrome: This is essentially the same as Foville's syndrome except that the lesion is lower in the pons and misses the supranuclear pathway for conjugate lateral gaze. The pyramidal tract is affected along with fibers of cranial nerves VI and VII as they leave the pons. There is therefore a crossed hemiplegia and ipsilateral facial and abducens palsy without a horizontal gaze palsy.

F. Wernicke's Syndrome: This syndrome consists of bilateral external ophthalmoplegia,* nystagmus, ataxia, and Korsakoff's psychosis. Ptosis is present in 50% of cases; internal ophthalmoplegia is less frequently present. Other cranial nerves are commonly affected, and polyneuritis may occur elsewhere. Although severe chronic alcoholism is the most frequent clinical setting in which this disorder occurs, hyperemesis gravidarum and other malnutritional states may be causative. The metabolic defect has been clearly shown to be thiamine deficiency. Treatment consists of immediate parenteral thiamine and should also include alcohol withdrawal and proper diet with other vitamin supplementation. This will effect a complete cure if the disease is not too far advanced. Without treatment the course is rapidly downhill to stupor, delirium, and death within several weeks.

NYSTAGMUS

Nystagmus is defined as involuntary, rhythmically repeated oscillations of one or both eyes in any or all fields of gaze. The movements are either pendular, with undulatory movements of equal speed, amplitude, and duration in each direction; or jerky, with slower movements in one direction (slow component) followed by a rapid return to the original position (fast component). The full mechanism remains unknown, and the location of the defect can usually not be specified.

Nystagmus is classified as grade I, present only with the eyes directed toward the fast component; grade II, present also with the eyes in primary position; or grade III, present even with the eyes directed toward the slow component. The movements may be horizontal, vertical, oblique, rotatory, circular, or a combination of these. The direction may change depending upon the direction of gaze. Amplitude refers to the extent of the movement; rate refers to the frequency of oscillation. Generally, the faster the rate, the smaller the amplitude and vice versa.

Known factors relating to ocular movements, malfunction of which can cause nystagmus, are as follows: The labyrinth exerts influence on eye movements by 2 mechanisms: (1) The otolith apparatus influences torsional eye movements in response to head position; (2) the semicircular canals influence eye movements in response to acceleration and deceleration. The gaze mechanism influences the supraconnections of extraocular muscle function (see 152-3). These complicated pathways are known in a general way, but many details are far from established. The fixation mechanism also is not completely understood but undoubtedly involves the retina, the visual pathways, the brain stem, and the cerebellum.

Physiology of Symptoms

Reduced visual acuity is caused by inability to maintain steady fixation. False projection is evident in vestibular nystagmus, where past-pointing is present. Head tilting is usually involuntary, to decrease the nystagmus. The head is turned toward the fast components in jerky nystagmus, or set so that the eyes are in a position which minimizes ocular movement in pendular nystagmus. The patient sometimes complains of illusory movements of objects (oscillopsia). This is more apt to be present in nystagmus due to lesions of lower centers, such as the labyrinth, or associated with the sudden arrest of nystagmus in an adult. The apparent movement of the environment occurs during the slow component and causes an extremely distressing vertigo, so that the patient is unable to stand. Head nodding is most apt to accompany congenital nystagmus, spasmus nutans, and miner's nystagmus. Nystagmus is noticeable and cosmetically disturbing except when excursions of the eye are very small.

Classification of Nystagmus
A. Physiologic Nystagmus:
1. End point.
2. Optokinetic.
3. Stimulation of semicircular canals.

B. Pathologic Nystagmus:
1. Congenital -
   a. Sensory defect type.
   b. Motor defect type.
   c. Latent.
2. Nystagmus due to poor illumination -
   a. Spasmus nutans.
   b. Miner's nystagmus.
3. Nystagmus due to neurologic fixation mechanisms -
   a. Acquired pendular or jerky nystagmus.
   b. Ocular flutter.
   c. See-saw nystagmus.
   d. Nystagmus retractorius.
4. Vestibular nystagmus.
5. Gaze nystagmus.
6. Voluntary and hysterical nystagmus.

1. PHYSIOLOGIC NYSTAGMUS

The following 3 types of nystagmus can be elicited in the normal person. Alteration of normal response may be helpful diagnostically.

End Point Nystagmus
A jerky type of nystagmus of small amplitude with the fast component in the direction of gaze commonly occurs in extreme lateral gaze after a latent period of not more than 30 seconds. The nystagmus appears earlier and is of larger amplitude in general fatigue states.

Optokinetic Nystagmus
This is a jerky type of nystagmus which may be elicited in all normal individuals, most easily by means of a rotating drum with alternating black and white lines. The slow component follows the object and the fast component moves rapidly counterwise to fixate each succeeding object. Unilateral or asymmetrical horizontal response usually indicates a parietal lobe tumor. Anterior cerebral (ie, frontal lobe) lesions may inhibit this response only

temporarily, which suggests the presence of a compensatory mechanism which is much greater than for lesions situated farther posteriorly. Asymmetry of response in the vertical plane suggests a brain stem lesion.

Nystagmus Elicited by Stimulation of Semicircular Canals

A. Bárány Rotating Chair: The horizontal canals are horizontal with the floor when the chair is depressed 30° on the chest. Rotation of the subject causes a jerky nystagmus in the direction of the turning. The slow component is in the opposite direction, the same as the flow of endolymph in the semicircular canals.

B. Caloric Stimulation: With the subject supine and the head flexed on the chest, cold water ear irrigation produces nystagmus with the slow component toward the side of irrigation while warm water produces nystagmus with the slow component away from the side of irrigation.

2. PATHOLOGIC NYSTAGMUS

CONGENITAL NYSTAGMUS

Sensory Defect Type

Congenital impairment of vision in any part of the eye or optic nerve can result in pendular nystagmus. Causes include corneal opacity, cataract, albinism, posterior polar chorioretinitis, aniridia, and optic atrophy. Oscillations of the head which are synchronous with the nystagmus but in the opposite direction often accompany sensory defect congenital nystagmus.

Motor Defect Nystagmus

This is manifested as a jerky nystagmus on gaze to either side with the fast component in the direction of gaze. The eyes are otherwise normal except when strabismus is associated (20%). There is always a position of relative rest. If this position is with the eyes deviated to one side, the head will be turned toward the opposite side to obtain the best possible vision. This condition shows some spontaneous improvement up to about age 10. The cause is not known, but a lesion of the brain stem is probably responsible. About 20% of cases are inherited as an autosomal recessive trait.

Latent Nystagmus

Latent nystagmus occurs upon occlusion of either eye. The nystagmus is conjugate and jerky, with the fast component toward the side of the covered eye. The condition has no known neurologic significance and is only of consequence when the affected individual loses one eye.

NYSTAGMUS DUE TO POOR ILLUMINATION

Spasmus Nutans

This uncommon condition occurs in infants 4-12 months of age who are kept in poorly illuminated surroundings. The nystagmus is of the dissociated vertical or asymmetrical horizontal pendular type and is often associated with nonsynchronous head nodding. The cause is not known. The prognosis is good; recovery occurs within a few months to 2 years.

Miner's Nystagmus

A fine, rapid, pendular nystagmus commonly occurs in persons working in poorly lighted surroundings for long periods of time. The prognosis is excellent with return to adequate lighting.

NYSTAGMUS DUE TO NEUROLOGIC FIXATION MECHANISMS

Pendular or Jerky Nystagmus

Acquired pendular or jerky nystagmus is usually horizontal (occasionally vertical) and causes oscillopsia. It is frequently seen in demyelinating disease (occasionally in vascular disease) and is due to a lesion of the brain stem.

Ocular Flutter

Ocular flutter is a sign of cerebellar disease. It consists of a series of pendular horizontal movements while fixating an object.

See-Saw Nystagmus

This rare type of nystagmus consists of regular reciprocating oscillations in which one eye rises while the other falls. Tumors in the region of the optic chiasm and diencephalon are the most frequent cause.

Nystagmus Retractorius

With convergence or on upward gaze, nystagmus associated with retraction of the eyes is present. It is diagnostic of a lesion of the upper brain stem and may be associated with signs of lid retraction, loss of upward gaze (Parinaud's syndrome), and abnormal pupillary reactions.

VESTIBULAR NYSTAGMUS

Vestibular nystagmus is always of the jerky type. The slow component is considered to be a response to impulses originating in the semicircular canals; the fast component is a corrective movement. Vestibular nystagmus is not dependent upon visual stimuli, ie, it is present with the lids closed as well as open and can be elicited in blind individuals also. Rotatory movements are especially characteristic of vestibular nystagmus, but horizontal or vertical vestibular nystagmus also occurs.

Physiologic nystagmus elicited by stimulation of the semicircular canals by means of the Bárány chair or caloric stimulation depends upon normal vestibular function.

The following characteristics of vestibular nystagmus demonstrate its origin in labyrinthine and vestibular nerve disease: (1) Vertigo, tinnitus, and deafness are apt to be associated. (2) Nystagmus is maximal early in the disease, and tends to improve or disappear in 2-3 weeks (unless the vestibular nuclei are affected directly, in which case nystagmus may be permanent). (3) The lesion is always destructive, and its direction (fast component) is away from the side the lesion is on.

Specific Lesions Causing Vestibular Nystagmus

Vestibular nystagmus may be due to labyrinthitis, Ménière's disease, traumatic (including surgical) destruction of one labyrinth; vascular, inflammatory, or neoplastic lesions of the vestibular nerves; lesions of the vestibular nuclei (encephalitis, multiple sclerosis, syringobulbia, poliomyelitis, thrombosis of the posteroinferior cerebellar artery), or cerebellar tumors and abscesses (probably as a result of pressure on the vestibular pathways). (**Note:** There is some dispute about whether a cerebellar lesion per se can cause nystagmus. Evidence suggests that nystagmus in such cases results from pressure on the vestibular structures. An alternative explanation is that the cerebellar hemispheres exert an inhibitory influence on nystagmus on its own side through the cerebellobulbar tract. Thus a lesion on one side causes nystagmus toward the side of the lesion.)

GAZE NYSTAGMUS

Gaze nystagmus is probably the most common nystagmus and often represents the first sign or the residuum of a gaze palsy. These patients have no nystagmus on forward gaze but develop nystagmus in one or more fields of gaze with the fast component in the direction of gaze.

The causes are variable and include drug toxicity (especially diphenylhydantoin, but barbiturates also) and demyelinating, degenerative, neoplastic, or vascular disease. Gaze nystagmus is of no specific localizing value except that it is suggestive of lesions of the posterior fossa.

VOLUNTARY AND HYSTERICAL NYSTAGMUS

Voluntary nystagmus is an uncommon "parlor trick." The individual "wills" a rapid horizontal nystagmus of high frequency and low amplitude which can be maintained only a few seconds.

Hysterical nystagmus is similar to voluntary nystagmus. It may be even more rapid, and is particularly common in anxiety neuroses.

CENTRAL NERVOUS SYSTEM TUMORS OF NEURO-OPHTHALMOLOGIC IMPORTANCE

CEREBRAL TUMORS

Frontal Lobe Tumors

Mental changes (depression, euphoria, or mental deficiency) and contralateral hemiparesis are the most frequent signs of frontal lobe tumors. Pressure upon the olfactory tracts may cause anosmia. Ophthalmologic signs include the following:

A. Papilledema (50%): Due to increased intracranial pressure.

B. Visual Field Changes (30%): These are not characteristic. Almost any defect is possible as a result of pressure upon the optic pathway.

C. Irregular Nystagmus (5-10%): This is of no localizing value.

D. Gaze Palsies: Irritative lesions cause the eyes to deviate to the opposite side. Destructive lesions cause deviation to the same side. These gaze palsies are usually incomplete and last only a few weeks, or may be manifested by an end point nystagmus only.

Temporal Lobe Tumors

Gliomas are the most common type. Meningiomas are next most common and angiomas are rare.

Temporal lobe tumors may cause psychomotor convulsions and uncinate fits, sometimes preceded by an aura of abnormal smell. Visual hallucinations may occur. A generalized or localized convulsion (chewing, sucking, or smacking movements) follows. Auditory disturbances are not common. Aphasia (involvement of the left side in right-handed people) is commonly present. Ophthalmologic signs include papilledema (often) and incongruous visual field changes (usually). The typical visual field change is an incongruous contralateral homonymous hemianopsia of the upper quadrants. Aphasia, alexia, acalculia, and agnosia may also be present if the dominant side is involved.

Occipital Lobe Tumors

The occipital lobe is only rarely involved by tumor. Gliomas, meningiomas, and metastatic tumors may occur. Epileptic attacks (grand or petit mal) as well as mild mental abnormalities may be present. Papilledema can be extreme (up to 6 or 8 diopters). Contralateral homonymous hemianopsia occurs in 85% of cases. It tends to be congruous with sparing of the macula. Loss of involuntary conjugate eye movements is due to a lesion of the supranuclear pathway. Visual agnosia occurs as a result of involvement of the visual association areas.

CEREBELLAR TUMORS

Cerebellar tumors are the most common brain tumors before age 15. Gliomas are common, and about one-fourth of these are the very malignant medulloblastomas of the roof of the 4th ventricle. Astrocytomas of the cerebellar hemisphere also occur, mainly in children. Papilledema due to increased intracranial pressure and abducens palsy due to pressure on the 6th nerve at the base of the brain are common findings. Vestibular nystagmus also occurs. Systemic cerebellar signs include ataxia, hypotonia, and tremor.

BRAIN STEM TUMORS

Tumors of the Midbrain

Lesions of the upper part of the midbrain (near the quadrigeminal bodies) cause Parinaud's syndrome, sometimes associated with retraction of the lids or ptosis. Lesions of the lower midbrain produce paralysis of downward gaze, paralysis of convergence, loss of pupillary reaction to light or accommodation (or both), and unequal pupil size. Increased intracranial pressure is often present as a result of obstruction of the cerebral aqueduct. Papilledema may be an early or a late sign. Gliomas and pinealomas are the most common tumors, especially in children.

Lesions involving the red nucleus produce Benedikt's syndrome and Weber's syndrome. Cerebellar signs (ataxia, hypotonia, and nystagmus) due to pressure on or direct involvement of the cerebellum may also be present.

Tumors of the Pons

Gliomas are the most common pontine tumors. Multiple nuclear palsies (particularly in childhood) involve principally the 5th, 6th, 7th, and 8th cranial nerves in combination with motor and sensory long tract signs in the limbs. Increased intracranial pressure develops late. Foville's syndrome is sometimes present. The course is usually chronic and progressive.

Tumors of the Medulla

Early manifestations include vertigo, cardiac irregularities, swallowing difficulties, and hoarseness. Paralysis of the tongue and papilledema develop later. Eye signs are not prominent. Death usually occurs early.

OTHER INTRACRANIAL TUMORS OF NEURO-OPHTHALMOLOGIC IMPORTANCE

Meningioma of Sphenoidal Ridge

The tumor arises from the small wing of the sphenoid bone. Ipsilateral slight (occasionally severe) progressive exophthalmos is present in about 40% of cases and is often the presenting sign. Visual field changes are at first unilateral and later bilateral, and are not characteristic. Headache is common. All changes occur gradually over many years, since the tumor grows quite slowly.

Tumors of the Cerebellopontine Angle

Neurofibroma (or neurinoma) of the acoustic nerve sometimes occurs as part of Recklinghausen's disease. More often, the tumor occurs alone. A cerebellopontine angle tumor may also be a meningioma. Cerebellar signs include hypotonia, ataxia, and unsteady gait. Vestibular nystagmus is common as a result of pressure on the brain stem. Increased intracranial pressure causes papilledema. Cranial nerve palsies include facial paresis (7th nerve), tinnitus, deafness, vertigo (8th nerve), loss of corneal sensation and sneeze reflex (5th nerve), and dysphagia (10th nerve). Motor involvement produces contralateral hemiplegia (pyramidal).

Complete or partial excision of the tumor is usually possible.

Pineal Tumor

This rare tumor (2% of all gliomas) may occur at any age. Papilledema occurs early as a result of blockage of the cerebral aqueduct. Parinaud's syndrome develops later. Argyll Robertson pupil is common. Pressure on adjacent structures commonly occurs, causing cerebellar signs, extraocular muscle palsies, and deafness.

Surgical removal, sometimes followed by irradiation, continues to be the only treatment. The mortality and morbidity rate continues to be very high despite advances in neurosurgical and radiation technics.

CEREBROVASCULAR LESIONS OF OPHTHALMOLOGIC IMPORTANCE

Vascular Insufficiency of the Vertebral-Basilar Arterial System

Brief episodes of transient bilateral blurring of vision commonly precede a basilar artery stroke. An attack seldom leaves any residual visual impairment, and the episode may be so minimal that the patient or doctor does not heed the warning. The blurring is described as a graying of vision just as if the house lights were being turned down at a theater. The change seldom lasts more than 5 minutes (often only a few seconds) and may be associated with other transient symptoms of vertebral-basilar insufficiency. Such episodes of visual loss are termed amaurosis fugax.

Thrombosis of the Basilar Artery

Complete or extensive thrombosis of the basilar artery nearly always causes death. With partial occlusion or basilar "insufficiency" due to arteriosclerosis, a wide variety of brain stem and cerebellar signs may be present. These include nystagmus, supranuclear oculomotor signs; and involvement of cranial nerves III, IV, VI, and VII. Abnormal pupillary responses are nearly always present; the pupils are usually small and unresponsive to light.

Prolonged anticoagulant therapy has become the accepted treatment of partial basilar artery occlusion or "insufficiency."

Thrombosis of the Middle Cerebral Artery

This disorder may produce severe contralateral hemiplegia, hemianesthesia, and homonymous hemianopsia. The lower quadrants of the visual fields (upper radiations) are most apt to be involved. Aphasia may be present.

Vascular Insufficiency and Thrombosis of the Internal Carotid Artery

Episodes of amaurosis fugax frequently occur as a result of atherosclerotic lesions of the ipsilateral internal carotid artery. Cerebral and retinal disturbances occur as a result of small emboli breaking loose from the sclerotic plaque and lodging in cerebral or retinal arterioles (occlusion of the central retinal artery or a major branch can occur). Reduced ophthalmic artery pressure as determined by ophthalmodynamometry, bruits over the internal carotid artery, and angiography all help confirm the diagnosis.

Removal of the plaque by carotid endarterectomy is frequently indicated, and may prevent a major stroke or a central retinal artery occlusion.

Thrombosis of the Posterior Cerebral Artery

Occlusion of the posterior cerebral artery seldom causes death. Occlusion of the cortical branches (most common) causes homonymous hemianopsia, usually superior quadrantic (the artery supplies primarily the visual cortex). Lesions on the left in right-handed persons can cause aphasia and dyslexia. Occlusion of the proximal branches may produce the thalamic syndrome (thalamic pain, hemiparesis, hemianesthesia, choreo-athetoid movements), and cerebellar ataxia. Weber's, Benedikt's, or Parinaud's syndrome may result.

Cavernous Sinus Thrombosis

See p 133.

HEAD TRAUMA

SUBDURAL HEMORRHAGE

Subdural hemorrhage results from tearing or shearing of the veins bridging the subdural space from the pia mater to the dural sinus. It leads to an encapsulated accumulation of blood in the subdural space, usually over one cerebral hemisphere. It is nearly always caused by trauma to the head. The trauma may be minimal and may precede the onset of neurologic signs by weeks or even months.

In infants, subdural hemorrhage produces progressive enlargement of the head with bulging fontanels. The diagnosis is established by finding bloody spinal fluid on tapping the subdural space and by enlarged head measurements. Ocular signs include strabismus, pupillary changes, papilledema, and retinal hemorrhages.

In adults the symptoms of chronic subdural hematoma are severe headache, drowsiness, and mental confusion, usually appearing hours to weeks (or even months) after trauma. Symptomatology is similar to that of cerebral tumors. Papilledema is present in 30-50% of cases. Retinal hemorrhages occur in association with papilledema. Ipsilateral dilatation of the pupil is the most common and most serious pupillary sign and is an urgent indication for immediate surgical evacuation of blood. Unequal, miotic, or mydriatic pupils can occur, or there may be no pupillary signs. Other signs, including vestibular nystagmus and cranial nerve palsies, also occur. Many of these signs result from herniation and compression of the brain stem, and hence often appear late with stupor and coma.

Skull films may show a shift of a calcified pineal gland. Carotid arteriography frequently confirms the diagnosis.

Treatment consists of surgical evacuation of the blood. Without treatment, the course is progressively downhill to coma and death. With early and adequate treatment, the prognosis is good except for infants, in whom repeated subdural taps may be only temporarily life-saving or may result in residual damage (convulsions, low mentality, motor and sensory defects).

SUBARACHNOID HEMORRHAGE

Subarachnoid hemorrhage most commonly results from ruptured congenital berry aneurysms of the circle of Willis in the subarachnoid space. It may also result from trauma, birth injuries, intracranial hemorrhage, hemorrhage associated with tumors, arteriovenous malformations, or systemic bleeding disorders.

The most prominent symptom of subarachnoid hemorrhage is sudden, severe headache, usually occipital and often associated with signs of meningeal irritation (eg, stiff neck). Drowsiness, loss of consciousness, coma, and death may occur rapidly. Ocular symptoms are not always present. Extraocular muscle palsies are the most common single ocular sign. An oculomotor palsy with associated numbness and pain in the distribution of the ipsilateral trigeminal nerve is pathognomonic of a supraclinoid, internal carotid, or posterior communicating artery aneurysm. Papilledema appears late when it does occur. Various types of retinal hemorrhage occur infrequently (preretinal hemorrhages are the most common). Exophthalmos may occur as a result of extravasation of blood into orbital tissues. Pressure of an aneurysm on the optic nerve may cause blindness in one eye.

Arteriography following injection of radiopaque substances may help to demonstrate and localize the aneurysms. Blood is present in the CSF.

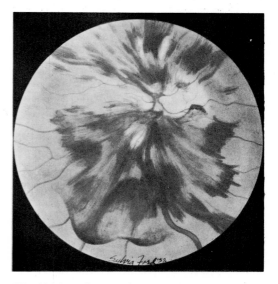

Fig 13-14. Subhyaloid hemorrhage around optic disk associated with subarachnoid hemorrhage. (Drawing.)

Ligation of aneurysmal vessels or of parent arterial trunks may be advisable. Supportive treatment, including control of blood pressure, is at times all that can be done.

INTRACRANIAL INFECTIONS OF OPHTHALMOLOGIC IMPORTANCE

MENINGITIS

Acute Bacterial Meningitis

Acute meningitis may be due to Neisseria meningitidis, Diplococcus pneumoniae, Hemophilus influenzae, Staphylococcus aureus, or Streptococcus viridans. There are many ocular manifestations of general meningeal irritation, depending upon the main area of associated inflammation. Basal meningitis causes oculomotor palsies (abducens palsy is the most common). Ptosis and pupillary changes, including sluggish light reaction and anisocoria, are also frequent. Papilledema indicative of increased intracranial pressure may be prominent. Locally the disease may be complicated by chemosis of the conjunctiva and edema of the lids, with photophobia a common symptom. Metastatic uveitis with resulting endophthalmitis and loss of all function occurs at times, especially in children. Treatment consists of massive systemic administration of sulfonamides and antibiotics (and intrathecal antiinfectives administered by lumbar puncture). Culture of the spinal fluid nearly always establishes the etiologic diagnosis.

Tuberculous Meningitis

Tuberculous meningitis is a more chronic form of bacterial meningitis. It occurs rarely, and usually in children. The general symptomatology is the same as outlined above for acute bacterial meningitis. When miliary lesions can be seen ophthalmoscopically as small oval yellowish lesions in the choroid, the prognosis for life is very bad. In the past, tuberculous meningitis was uniformly fatal. Long-term systemic administration of isoniazid (INH) combined with aminosalicylic acid (PAS) and at times with streptomycin has reduced the mortality rate significantly.

Syphilitic Meningitis

Acute syphilitic meningitis may be quite similar to acute infectious meningitis. The cranial nerves—particularly the oculomotor nerves—are very often involved, causing diplopia. Papilledema and visual field changes,

indicating chiasmal arachnoiditis (bitemporal hemianopsia), are also common. All manifestations of meningitis clear well on antisyphilitic therapy.

Encephalomyelitides Associated With Infectious Diseases

Measles, mumps, vaccinia, chickenpox, and smallpox are the most common viral diseases having neurologic complications. Complications may be due to activation of a neurotropic virus, a toxin, or an allergic phenomenon. There is no treatment.

Neurologic signs result from cerebral, cerebellar, or cord involvement as well as optic neuritis. Most patients recover completely, but permanent sequelae and deaths do occur, especially in smallpox and vaccinia.

BRAIN ABSCESS

Abscesses form in the brain by direct extension of infection from the nasal sinuses (frontal lobe) and middle ear (temporal lobe or cerebellum). Penetrating head wounds and septicemia may also produce brain abscesses. Symptoms include persistent headache, fever, and vomiting. Increased intracranial pressure may develop rapidly. Papilledema is present, usually on the side of the lesion. Localizing cerebral signs of cerebral abscess are the same as for cerebral tumors. Diagnosis is more difficult today because of the masking effect of inadequate antibiotic therapy. Treatment consists of systemic antibiotics and surgical drainage of the abscess.

•   •   •

THE PHAKOMATOSES

These 4 disease entities are logically grouped together because they are characterized by combination skin and CNS lesions with frequent ocular involvement. All are genetically determined as autosomal dominants.

Neurofibromatosis (Recklinghausen's Disease)

Neurofibromatosis is a generalized hereditary disease characterized by multiple tumors of the skin, CNS, peripheral nerves, and nerve sheaths. Other developmental anomalies, particularly of the bones, may be associated. Inheritance is autosomal dominant with incomplete penetrance. Thus the disease can be quite mild in one generation and appear as a full-blown debilitating disease in the next.

Neurofibromas are made up of randomly oriented or palisaded cells of either fibroplastic or Schwann cell origin. Nerve fibers often course through or over the tumor. The tumors are discrete and benign but may undergo sarcomatous degeneration.

Tumors may occur anywhere in the body, including the eye. Café au lait spots (small pigmented areas of skin) tend to enlarge and darken with age. Tumors of the lids are often present. Tumors of the orbital portion of the optic nerve are particularly common, causing papilledema and retrobulbar neuritis early and optic atrophy later in the disease. There may be iris nodules and corneal nerve changes.

Neurofibromatosis of the lid is associated rarely with unilateral infantile glaucoma.

Intracranial gliomas may be associated with neurofibromatosis. Spinal cord neurofibromas frequently occur. The acoustic nerve is the cranial nerve most commonly involved and produces the syndrome of the cerebellopontine angle.

Bone development is affected when the tumor involves periosteum. Pulsating exophthalmos occasionally occurs when an osseous defect of the posterior orbit is present.

Orbital or intracranial surgery may be needed to remove tumors for functional or cosmetic reasons.

When lesions are confined to the skin, the prognosis is good. Intracranial and intraspinal lesions are usually multiple and have a bad prognosis. The disease tends to be fairly stationary, with only slow progression over long periods of time.

Angiomatosis Retinae (Lindau-Von Hippel Disease)

This rare disease occurs most commonly in men in the third decade, but can appear at any age up to 60. The earliest signs are dilatation and tortuosity of the retinal vessels, which later develop into an angiomatous formation with hemorrhages and exudates. A stage of massive exudation, retinal detachment, and absolute glaucoma occurs later, and usually destroys the eye within 5-15 years after onset. The disease is unilateral in 65% of cases. In 25% of cases the retinal angiomatosis is associated with a similar generalized process, most often affecting the cerebellum and less commonly the pancreas, kidney, adrenal gland, and other organs. The evidence at present suggests that this is all one genetically determined disease showing autosomal dominant inheritance with variable expression. Several reports of abnormal chromosomal patterns have been reported.

Early treatment of retinal lesions with photocoagulation has been effective in some cases. Cerebral and cerebellar tumors have been successfully removed, but if the CNS is involved the prognosis for life is poor. A downhill course and death, usually by middle age, is the rule.

Sturge-Weber Syndrome

This uncommon disease is recognizable at birth by a characteristic nevus flammeus (port wine stain type of angioma) on one side of the face following the distribution of one or more branches of the 5th cranial nerve. Unilateral infantile glaucoma on the affected side frequently develops if there is extensive involvement of the eye with uveal hemangioma. Lid and conjunctival involvement nearly always implies ultimate intraocular involvement and glaucoma. Extensive venous aneurysms in the meningeal sheaths extending into the brain substance account for the high incidence of CNS disturbances, of which jacksonian convulsive seizures are the most common. These cranial lesions are on the same side as the skin lesions and usually become manifest within the first decade. Radiographically, calcification in the cerebral cortex is usually present. The disease follows an autosomal dominant hereditary pattern with variable expression. There is at least one study reporting a 22 trisomy on cytogenic study.

There is no effective treatment of Sturge-Weber syndrome, although the glaucoma can be controlled in rare cases by cyclodiathermy. Other glaucoma operations have been unsuccessful.

The prognosis for life as well as for sight is poor, with death before age 30 the rule.

Tuberous Sclerosis (Bourneville's Disease)

This is a generalized disease whose manifestations include adenoma sebaceum (85%), CNS tumors, retinal tumors (50%), renal tumors (50%), and multiple lung cysts. The signs may be present at birth or may develop within the first few years of life. Onset is with convulsive seizures and mental retardation. The large papular skin lesions have the appearance of overgrown "blackheads," and are often the earliest sign of the disease. The retinal tumors appear as oval or circular white areas in the peripheral fundus, and characteristically have a mulberry-like appearance (see Fig 16-12). Histologically, the retinal tumors are composed of hyaline material with areas of calcification.

The disease is inherited as an autosomal dominant with high penetrance. No treatment is available. The prognosis is very poor, with a progressive downhill course and death in adolescence the rule.

CEREBROMACULAR DEGENERATION

Genetically determined (autosomal recessive) neuronal lipid storage diseases of the brain may affect the neural elements of the retina as well. The clinical forms are classified mainly by the age of onset. The pathologic changes are present at birth, with clinical manifestations occurring as a critical level of intraneuronal lipidosis is reached. A definite diagnosis can be established readily by rectal biopsy or appendectomy showing ganglioside accumulation even before clinical signs are present. Five forms of cerebromacular degeneration (ganglioside lipidosis) are recognized: Congenital, infantile (Tay-Sachs), late infantile, juvenile (Spielmeyer-Vogt), and adult.

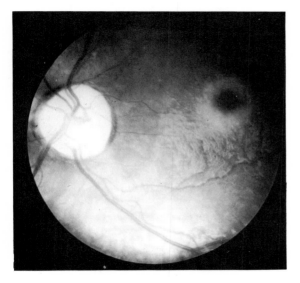

Fig 13-15. Cherry-red spot of Tay-Sachs disease in an 18-month-old child.

Severe mental and physical deterioration occurs, usually causing death within a few years. The later the onset, the milder the disease. The liver and spleen show increased gangliosides. The striking ocular finding of a cherry-red spot in the macula is seen in congenital and infantile cases. Optic atrophy and retinal pigmentary changes are frequently present in the juvenile and adult forms. Extraocular muscle dysfunction is a less frequent finding in all forms.

The exact enzyme abnormality is still not known, but a deficiency of serum fructose-1-phosphate aldolase is present in carriers as well as affected persons.

NIEMANN-PICK DISEASE
(Sphingomyelin-Sterol Lipidosis)

This entity is quite similar to the ganglioside lipidosis. There is a deposition of glycolipid in the ganglion cells of the brain and retina. The spleen, liver, and other reticuloendothelial organs are massively infiltrated with glycolipid. Inheritance is autosomal recessive, and 2 clinical forms are recognized. The infantile form is the most common and most severe, with death usually occurring in 2 or 3 years. A cherry-red spot in the macula may be present. The juvenile or adult form is much more benign and usually without eye findings.

MISCELLANEOUS DISEASES OF NEURO-OPHTHALMOLOGIC IMPORTANCE

AMBLYOPIA DUE TO METHANOL (METHYL ALCOHOL) POISONING

Methyl alcohol (wood alcohol) has long been used as an intoxicating drink, either by mistake or because ethyl alcohol was not available. It may be mixed either accidentally or purposely with ethyl alcohol, and its breakdown product, formaldehyde, can cause severe poisoning marked by gastroenteritis, pulmonary edema, cerebral edema, and extensive retinal damage. There are great individual variations in tolerance; small amounts (1 oz) may cause profound effects in some persons while much larger amounts cause no poisonous effects in others. Significant systemic absorption has been reported from inhaled fumes and, very rarely, through the skin.

There is a marked destruction of the ganglion cells of the retina as well as degeneration of nerve fibers in the optic nerve, occasionally extending well past the optic chiasm in severe cases.

Clinical Findings

A. Symptoms and Signs: Acute symptoms appear within 18 hours of ingestion. Weakness, anorexia, nausea, vomiting, headache, dizziness, Kussmaul respiration, and pain in the back, extremities, and abdomen may occur in succession or almost simultaneously. Extensive exposure will lead to delirium, convulsions, coma, and death.

Visual disturbances range from "spots before the eyes" to complete blindness. The

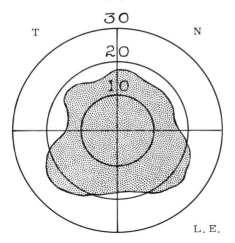

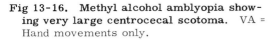

Fig 13-16. Methyl alcohol amblyopia showing very large centrocecal scotoma. VA =
Hand movements only.

field defects are quite extensive and nearly
always include the centrocecal area (Fig 13-16).
    Hyperemia of the disk is the first ophthal-
moscopic finding. Within the first 2 days a
whitish, striated edema of the disk margins
and nearby retina appears. Papilledema can
last up to 2 months, and is followed by optic
atrophy of mild to severe degree.
    Decreased pupillary response to light oc-
curs in proportion to the amount of visual loss.
In severe cases the pupils become dilated and
fixed. Extraocular muscle palsies and ptosis
may also occur.

    B. Laboratory Findings: The most im-
portant laboratory determination is the blood
CO_2 combining power. A reduced CO_2 combining power (below 25 mEq/liter) indicates
acidosis, which requires alkali therapy; a level below 10 mEq/liter is critical.

Treatment
    If ethanol and methanol are ingested or
inhaled simultaneously, the effects of methanol
will not become evident until most of the ethanol
is excreted. If the patient is seen soon after
exposure, gastric lavage should be performed.
Acidosis should be controlled with large and
repeated doses of bicarbonate. Ethanol inhibits the metabolic oxidation of methanol;
therefore, a blood ethanol concentration of
100 mg/100 ml blood should be maintained until all methanol has been excreted.

Course and Prognosis
    Patients with dilated, fixed pupils during
the acute attack usually die. If they survive,
they have severe visual loss. Patients with

retinal edema usually have moderate to marked
permanent visual loss. The initial loss of
vision shows an early improvement that may be
only transitory. Visual improvement occurs
only during the first week; if little or no immediate improvement occurs, eventual optic atrophy with very low visual acuity is the rule.
Only in mild cases is normal visual function re-
gained.

NUTRITIONAL AMBLYOPIA
(Tobacco-Alcohol Amblyopia)

    Nutritional amblyopia is the preferred
term for the entity sometimes referred to as
tobacco-alcohol amblyopia, tobacco amblyopia,
or alcohol amblyopia since they are all the
same entity. Persons with poor dietary hab-
its, particularly if the diet is deficient in vitamin B complex, may develop centrocecal scotomas that are usually of constant density.
When density of the scotoma varies, the most
dense portion usually lies between fixation and
the blind spot.

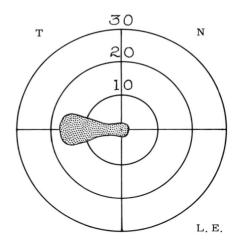

Fig 13-17. Nutritional amblyopia showing
centrocecal scotoma. VA = 20/200.

    Heavy drinking with or without heavy smok-
ing is most often associated with the poor nutritional state. Occasionally, heavy smoking
without drinking is present.
    Bilateral loss of central vision is present
in over 50% of patients, reducing visual acuity
below 20/200. Most of the others have severe
central loss in one eye with some deficit, often
about 20/50 visual acuity, in the better eye.

Central visual fields reveal scotomas which nearly always include both fixation and the blind spot (centrocecal scotoma). Pallor of the optic disks may be present. Loss of the ganglion cells of the macula, destruction of myelinated fibers of the optic nerve, and sometimes of the chiasma as well are the main histologic changes.

Chiasmal lesions can cause similar visual field changes, but the scotomas generally stop at the mid-line allowing differentiation. Rarely, multiple sclerosis, pernicious anemia, methanol poisoning, retrobulbar neuritis, or macular degeneration may cause diagnostic confusion.

Adequate diet plus vitamin B supplementation is nearly always effective in completely curing the disease. Withdrawal of tobacco and alcohol is advisable and may hasten the cure, but innumerable cases are known in which adequate nutrition alone effected the cure despite continued excessive intake of alcohol or tobacco or both. Improvement usually begins within 1-2 months, although occasionally significant improvement may not occur for a year. In nearly all cases, visual function returns to normal or nearly normal sooner or later; permanent optic atrophy occurs in a low percentage of cases with long-standing nutritional deficiency.

AMBLYOPIA DUE TO QUININE AND RELATED COMPOUNDS

Quinine and quinacrine (Atabrine®), used primarily in the treatment and prevention of malaria, occasionally cause visual disturbances on an idiosyncratic basis. The onset is acute, most often following a single dose. Other symptoms are a feeling of fullness in the head, ringing in the ears, and deafness. There is constriction of the visual field (Fig 13-18) and, rarely, total blindness. The tendency is toward partial recovery, with permanent peripheral field defects the rule. The ganglion cells of the retina are affected first, presumably as a result of marked vasoconstriction of the retinal arterioles, easily visible with an ophthalmoscope. Varying degrees of retinal edema early, and optic atrophy later, occur bilaterally.

The most important treatment is drug withdrawal, after which there may be some improvement, no change, or gradual continued deterioration of visual function. Vasodilators such as amyl nitrate, acetylcholine, and sodium nitrite may favorably influence some cases in the acute phase.

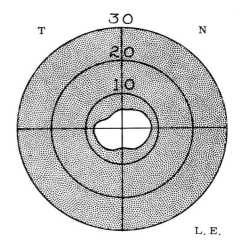

Fig 13-18. Quinine amblyopia showing only a central cone of field remaining. VA = 20/25.

AMBLYOPIA DUE TO ORGANIC ARSENIC COMPOUNDS

Sudden permanent visual loss sometimes resulted from organic arsenic compounds used in the treatment of syphilis. Peripheral field contraction and general field depression were followed by optic atrophy with no tendency toward recovery. In some cases, despite stopping the medication, complete blindness occurred.

AMBLYOPIA DUE TO SALICYLATES

Salicylic acid derivatives in very large doses cause a clinical picture of toxicity which is quite similar to that caused by quinine. Constriction of the visual field like that seen in quinine amblyopia (Fig 13-18), dilated pupils, tinnitus, and deafness may all be present. Upon withdrawal of the drug, visual function usually improves, but complete recovery is rare.

HERPES ZOSTER
(Shingles)

Infection with herpes zoster virus is characterized by the appearance of vesicles upon the skin along the course of a nerve. The virus has a predilection for the gasserian ganglion and the first 2 divisions of the 5th cranial nerve. Severe pain over one side of the face may precede by several days the eruption of vesicles on the forehead and eyelids on one side. The vesicles contain clear fluid which rapidly becomes purulent. These rupture, leaving ulcers which usually become secondarily infected and form crusts. Some permanent scarring always results. The eyelids become red and edematous, and there is tearing with scanty discharge. The conjunctiva is red and the cornea shows discrete white subepithelial opacities (involvement of the nasociliary branch of the first division of the 5th cranial nerve). Corneal sensitivity is markedly decreased, favoring exposure and secondary infection. The keratopathy lasts several months and may clear with minimal scarring. Complications of keratitis include secondary glaucoma, iritis, and scleritis. Corneal opacity may persist and markedly reduce vision. Severe, persistent neuralgia may be a late manifestation.

Complete internal and external ophthalmoplegia occurs rarely. Incomplete palsy of the third nerve is the most common type of involvement. Optic neuritis is rare but is quite serious if it does occur since recovery of function is minimal. Gaze palsies and encephalitis seldom occur.

There is no specific therapy for shingles. Eye treatment is directed toward protecting the exposed cornea and combating secondary infection. Antibiotic ointments are used locally. Dilatation of the pupil with homatropine, 2-5%, puts the eye at rest and is particularly useful if iritis is present. Local corticosteroids have been used with some success in shortening the course of the keratitis. Systemic corticosteroids do not help, and there are several reports of death following their administration.

The prognosis is good, and recurrences are almost unknown.

NEUROPARALYTIC KERATITIS

Loss of function of the sensory nerve to the cornea (nasociliary branch of the ophthalmic division of the 5th cranial nerve) can lead to trophic changes in the cornea. Punctate epithelial lesions appear first, usually as small vesicles which lead to irritation, photophobia, and ciliary injection. If the process continues, epithelium is lost and a corneal ulcer may develop with secondary infection. Iritis, hypopyon, and, at times, an overwhelming endophthalmitis with loss of the eye can occur.

Neuroparalytic keratitis usually occurs as a complication of section of the sensory 5th nerve root in the treatment of tic douloureux, and it also occurs following herpes zoster keratitis, posterior fossa tumor extirpations, and other rarer conditions.

Protection of the cornea and treatment of secondary infection are the only available measures. Antibiotic ointments should be applied locally, particularly at night. Protective eye shields may be necessary. In well established cases, suturing the lids together temporarily may be the best way to control keratitis.

MARCUS GUNN PHENOMENON
(Jaw Winking)

This rare congenital condition consists of elevation of a ptotic eyelid upon movement of the jaw. Acquired cases occur after damage to the oculomotor nerve with subsequent abnormal regeneration of nerve fibers. Muscular palsies may be present.

Treatment is surgical. The best results have been obtained by severing the levator muscle completely and then doing a ptosis operation later, utilizing the frontalis muscle.

DUANE'S SYNDROME

This uncommon congenital, stationary, nearly always unilateral condition consists of deficient horizontal ocular motility originally thought to be due to fibrous rectus muscles. Recent evidence based on electromyographic studies of extraocular muscles suggests that Duane's syndrome may be partly a disorder of innervation. It is genetically determined, usually as an autosomal recessive. The lateral rectus muscle is usually more involved than the medial rectus, and attempted adduction movements result in retraction of the globe and narrowing of the lid fissure. The visual handicap is seldom severe. Visual acuity is normal, and the eye is otherwise normal. Unless the deviation is very large, strabismus surgery is best avoided.

MIGRAINE

Migraine is a common episodic illness of unknown etiology and varied symptomatology characterized by severe unilateral headache, visual disturbances, nausea, and vomiting. It is associated with dilatation of the external carotid artery and its branches. Autosomal dominant inheritance is nearly always present. The disease usually becomes manifest between ages 15 and 30. It is equally common in the 2 sexes but is often more severe in women, perhaps because of endocrine factors. Prodromal symptoms are common and include drowsiness, paresthesias, "scintillating" scotomas, blurred vision, and other symptoms. In some patients, homonymous hemianopsia can be accurately recorded on the tangent screen during attacks. The visual symptoms usually last no longer than 15-30 minutes. Many factors, particularly emotional ones, may predispose or contribute to attacks.

Ergotamine tartrate, when given early in an attack, is often effective. Once the attack is well under way, treatment is of little value. The headaches last from several hours to several days. Bed rest is often helpful if not essential.

CRANIOSYNOSTOSIS
(Oxycephaly)

Under this general heading are grouped a number of rare dysostoses causing distortion of the face and head and having recessive or irregular dominant inheritance. In oxycephaly the sutures of the bones of the face and head close before the brain growth is complete. Continued growth of frontal bone allows for brain expansion, leading to tower skull or other abnormal shapes of the skull. At times the sphenoid bone does not develop properly, leaving an inadequate optic canal and constricting the optic nerve and causing optic atrophy. Increased intracranial pressure may result from the inadequate cranial vault volume. One variant of particular note is gargoylism (Hurler's disease), a form of dwarfism with oxycephaly and hypertelorism (widely spaced eyes). Gargoylism is an autosomal recessive disease due to overproduction of mucopolysaccharides. Acid mucopolysaccharides and glycoproteins are deposited in the cornea, abdominal organs, and CNS, causing death before age 20.

MANDIBULOFACIAL DYSOSTOSIS
(Franceschetti's Syndrome)

Patients with this rare disorder have a characteristic antimongoloid facies with a temporally placed notch in the lower lids, hypoplasia of some facial bones, high palate, and other less striking facial changes. The disease is genetically determined as an irregular dominant.

WAARDENBURG'S SYNDROME

This rare entity is distinguished by wide separation of the inner canthi, broad nasal root, heavy eyebrows, heterochromia of the iris, white forelock, and congenital deafness. It is inherited as an irregular dominant.

MYASTHENIA GRAVIS

This disease, characterized by ease of fatigability of the striated muscles, often is first manifested by weakness of extraocular muscles. Unilateral ptosis is a frequent first sign, with subsequent bilateral involvement of extraocular muscles so that diplopia is often an early symptom. Generalized weakness of the arms and legs, difficulty in swallowing, weakness of jaw muscles, and difficulty in breathing may follow rapidly in untreated cases. There are no sensory changes. The disease is not rare, and usually affects young adults age 20-40 though it may occur at any age.

The onset may follow an upper respiratory infection or an injury, and has been noted as a transitory condition in newborn infants of myasthenic mothers. The disease has been associated with hyperthyroidism, collagen disease and diffuse metastatic carcinoma. Accumulating evidence suggests that an autoimmune mechanism is a significant factor.

The differential diagnosis includes progressive nuclear ophthalmoplegia, brain stem lesions, epidemic encephalitis, bulbar and pseudobulbar palsy, and postdiphtheritic paralysis.

Although substantial neurophysiologic evidence indicates that the site of the disorder is the neuromuscular junction, convincing evidence of morphologic changes has not been presented. It is known that there is insufficient utilization of acetylcholine at the motor end plate. Thymomas have been reported in 25% of myasthenic persons over age 35. About half of patients with thymomas have myasthenia gravis. The 2 diseases must be related, but the mechanism remains obscure.

Cholinesterase destroys acetylcholine at the myoneural junction, and cholinesterase-inhibiting drugs (neostigmine) markedly improve the condition. The edrophonium chloride (Tensilon®) test is used in addition to the neostigmine-atropine diagnostic test. Edrophonium, 2 mg (0.2 ml), is given IV over 15 seconds. Relief of ptosis constitutes a positive response and confirms the diagnosis of myasthenia gravis. If no response occurs in 30 seconds, an additional 8 mg (0.8 ml) are given. The test is most critical when marked ptosis is present. It is best performed with the patient looking upward, as this most effectively demonstrates improvement in levator action (30-60 seconds after injection).

Neostigmine bromide (Prostigmin®) remains the drug of choice in most cases. A typical dose is 15 mg 4 times daily. Pyridostigmine (Mestinon®) is also widely used. Topical anticholinesterase drops, especially demecarium bromide (Humorsol®), sometimes help with ocular signs, which are often particularly resistant to systemic therapy. Ptosis usually does respond to treatment, but extraocular muscle weakness often does not respond. Thymectomy, once widely used, is now reserved for severe cases. Its benefit still remains to be substantiated.

The course of this chronic disease is not steady, and remissions are frequent. During severe exacerbations the patient may die from paralysis of respiration.

The prognosis depends to a great extent upon the patient's response to medication and his ability to regulate his medication. An intelligent patient, well oriented to his disease, can live a normal life span.

CENTRAL NERVOUS SYSTEM COMPLICATIONS OF USE OF ORAL CONTRACEPTIVES

Since 1964, a number of reports have appeared of cerebrovascular accidents in younger women taking birth control pills of all types. The sudden onset of homonymous hemianopsia, hemiplegia, convulsions, and other signs and symptoms has occurred in persons in good health receiving no other medication. Warnings against the use of such drugs in persons with a history of thrombophlebitis or other vascular problems were issued by the drug industry prior to issuing oral contraceptives. Migraine has also been noted to develop in persons taking oral contraceptives, and migraine sufferers should be advised against using such drugs. The CNS effects have cleared in some cases and have resulted in permanent neurologic deficits in others. While the percentage of complications reported so far is very low and the relationship to oral contraceptives is not always clear-cut, it is important for physicians to be aware of the possibility of the complications that can occur with such a widely used group of drugs.

•   •   •

Bibliography

Adler, F. H. : Physiology of the Eye, 5th ed. Mosby, 1970.

Benton, C. D. , & F. P. Calhoun, Jr. : The ocular effects of methyl alcohol poisoning. Tr Am Acad Ophth 56:875-85, 1952.

Birge, H. L. : Ophthalmic diagnosis and management of impending cerebrovascular lesions. JAMA 172:1998-2005, 1960.

Carr, R. E. : Optics and visual physiology. Annual review. Arch Ophth 84:238-51, 1970.

Carroll, F. D. : Nutritional amblyopia. Arch Ophth 76:406-11, 1966.

Chizek, J. , & A. T. Franceschetti: Oral contraceptives: Their side effects and ophthalmological manifestations. Survey Ophth 14:90-105, 1969.

Chusid, J. G. : Correlative Neuroanatomy and Functional Neurology, 14th ed. Lange, 1970.

Cogan, D. G. : Congenital nystagmus. Canad J Ophth 2:4-10, 1967.

Cogan, D. G. : Neurology of the Ocular Muscles, 3rd ed. Thomas, 1963.

Cogan, D. G. : Ocular correlates of inborn metabolic defects. Canad MAJ 95:1055-65, 1966.

Duke-Elder, W. S. : Textbook of Ophthalmology, Vol. IV. Mosby, 1949.

Dunphy, E. B. : Alcohol and tobacco amblyopia: a historical survey. Am J Ophth 68:569-78, 1969.

Ehrenfeld, W. K. , Hoyt, W. F. , & E. J. Wylie: Embolization and transient blindness from carotid atheroma: surgical considerations. Arch Surg 93:787-94, 1966.

Fahmy, J. A. , Knudsen, V. , & S. Y. Andersen: Intraocular hemorrhage following subarachnoid hemorrhage. Acta Ophth 47:550, 1969.

Harrington, D. O. : The Visual Fields, 2nd ed. Mosby, 1964.

Hollenhorst, R. W. : Ocular manifestations of insufficiency or thrombosis of the internal carotid artery. Am J Ophth 47:753-66, 1959.

Hollenhorst, R. W. : Vascular status of patients who have cholesterol emboli in the retina. Am J Ophth 61:1159-65, 1966.

Hoyt, W. F. : Transient bilateral blurring of vision. Arch Ophth 70:746-51, 1963.

Kimi, M. M. , King, D. W. , & J. R. Cooper: Biochemistry of methanol poisoning. J Neurochem 9:119-24, 1962.

Knox, D. L. : Neuro-ophthalmology. Annual review. Arch Ophth 85:111-26, 1971.

Lowenfeld, I. E. : The Argyll Robertson pupil, 1869-1969. A critical survey of the literature. Survey Ophth 14:199-299, 1969.

Reed, H. : The Essentials of Perimetry. Oxford, 1960.

Retzlaff, J. A. , & others: Lancaster red-green test in evaluation of edrophonium effect in myasthenia gravis. Am J Ophth 67:13-20, 1969.

Rucker, C. W. : The causes of paralysis of the third, fourth and sixth cranial nerves. Am J Ophth 61:1293-8, 1966.

Walsh, F. B. , & W. F. Hoyt: Clinical Neuro-ophthalmology, 3rd ed. (3 Vols.) Williams & Wilkins, 1969.

Wolf, S. M. : The relationship between thymoma and myasthenia gravis. Bull Los Angeles Neurol Soc 31:107-13, 1966.

14 . . .

Strabismus

Under normal conditions the image of the object of regard falls on the fovea of each eye. When the eyes are positioned so that the image falls upon the fovea of one eye but not the other, the second eye is deviating (squinting) and strabismus is present. The deviation may be inward, outward, up, or down. The amount of deviation is a measurement of the angle formed by the visual axes of the 2 eyes.

Strabismus is present in about 5% of children. Treatment should begin as soon as the diagnosis is definite in order to ensure the development of the best possible visual acuity and a good cosmetic result and increase the chance for normal binocular visual function. The idea that "the child may outgrow his crossed eyes" should be discouraged.

ANATOMY

Muscles

Six extraocular muscles control the movement of each eye: 4 rectus and 2 oblique muscles.

A. Rectus Muscles: The 4 rectus muscles originate at a common ring tendon (annulus of Zinn) surrounding the optic nerve at the posterior apex of the orbit. They are named according to their insertion into the sclera on the medial, lateral, inferior, and superior surfaces of the eye. The muscles are about 40 mm long, becoming tendons 4-6 mm from insertion, and are about 10 mm wide at the point of insertion. The approximate distances of insertion from the corneal limbus are as follows: medial rectus, 5 mm; inferior rectus, 6 mm; lateral rectus, 7 mm; and superior rectus, 8 mm (Fig 14-1).

B. Oblique Muscles: The 2 oblique muscles control primarily torsional movement and, to a lesser extent, upward and downward movement. The inferior oblique muscle arises from the nasal orbital wall several mm behind the orbital rim; it passes under the inferior rectus and curves around the eyeball, making a large arc of scleral contact, and inserts in the posterior lateral quadrant of the eye just under the lateral rectus muscle. The main muscle body of the superior oblique muscle originates from the annulus of Zinn just above the origin

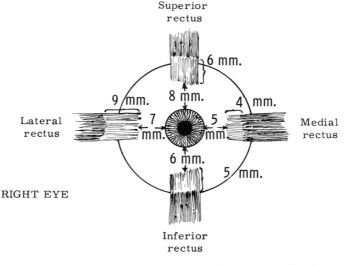

Fig 14-1. Approximate distances of the rectus muscles from the limbus, and the approximate lengths of tendons.

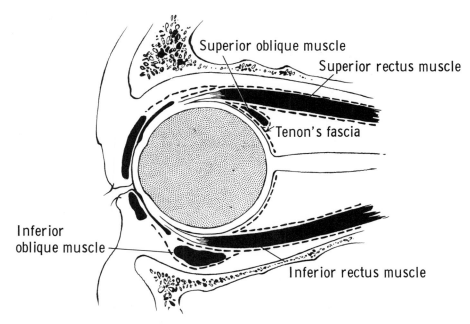

Fig 14-2. Fascia about muscles and eyeball (Tenon's capsule).

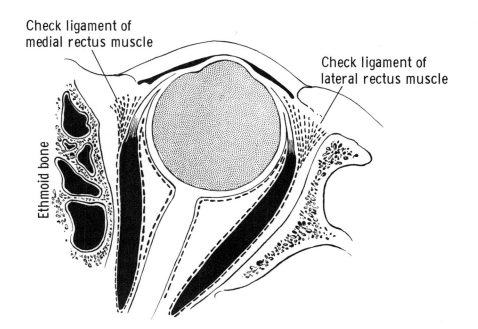

Fig 14-3. Check ligaments of medial and lateral rectus muscles, right eye (diagrammatic).

of the superior rectus muscle and passes to the cartilaginous pulley (trochlea) attached to the nasal side of the superior orbital rim. At the pulley it is reflected downward, outward, and posteriorly at a 55° angle, passing under the tendon of the superior rectus muscle to insert into the sclera.

Innervation

The abducens nerve innervates the lateral rectus muscle; the trochlear nerve innervates the superior oblique muscle; and the oculomotor nerve innervates the other 3 rectus muscles and the inferior oblique muscle.

Fascia

The rectus and oblique muscles are ensheathed by fascia. Near the points of insertion of these muscles the fascia is continuous with Tenon's capsule, which is between the sclera and conjunctiva. Fascial condensations to adjacent orbital bony structures serve as check ligaments for the extraocular muscles and limit ocular rotation.

DEFINITIONS

Angle kappa: The angle between the visual axis and the central pupillary line. When fixing a light, if the corneal reflection is centered on the pupil, the visual axis and the central pupillary line coincide and the angle kappa is zero. Ordinarily, the light reflex is 2-4° nasal to the pupillary center, giving the appearance of slight exotropia (positive angle kappa). A negative angle kappa gives the false impression of esotropia.

Ductions: Monocular rotations (other eye covered).
  Adduction: Inward rotation.
  Abduction: Outward rotation.
  Supraduction: Upward movement.
  Infraduction: Downward movement.

Fusion: The cortical integration of the images received simultaneously by the 2 eyes.

Heterophoria (or phoria): A deviation of the eyes corrected by the fusion mechanism.
  Esophoria: Tendency for one eye to turn inward.
  Exophoria: Tendency for one eye to turn outward.
  Hyperphoria: Tendency for one eye to deviate upward.
  Hypophoria: Tendency for one eye to deviate downward.

Heterotropia (or tropia): Strabismus, or "squint"; deviation of the eyes not corrected by the fusion mechanism.

Esotropia: "Crossed eyes"; convergent strabismus.

Exotropia: "Wall eyes"; divergent strabismus.

Hypertropia: Deviation of one eye upward.

Hypotropia: Deviation of one eye downward. By common usage one usually refers to a vertical deviation in terms of hypertropia rather than hypotropia.

Orthophoria: The absence of any tendency of either eye to deviate when fusion is suspended. This state is rarely seen clinically. A small degree of phoria is "normal."

Primary deviation: The deviation measured with the normal eye fixing and the eye with the paretic muscle deviating.

Prism diopter (Δ): A unit to measure deviations. One Δ is that strength of prism that will deflect a ray of light 1 cm at a distance of 1 meter. The deflection is toward the base of the prism. Another commonly used unit, a degree (°), equals about 2 Δ. (For technic of measurement, see p 176.)

Secondary deviation: The deviation measured with the paretic eye fixing and the normal eye deviating.

Torsions: Wheel-like motion of the eye on its anteroposterior axis.
  Intorsion (incycloduction): Torsion of superior limbus toward the nose.
  Extorsion (excycloduction): Torsion of superior limbus away from the nose.

Vergences (disjunctive movements): Movement of the 2 eyes in opposite directions.
  Convergence: The eyes turn inward
  Divergence: The eyes turn outward.

Versions: Binocular voluntary movement of the eyes in conjugate gaze.
  Dextroversion (levoversion): Movement of the eyes to right (or left).
  Supraversion (infraversion): Movement of the eyes up (or down).
  Dextrocycloversion: Torsional movement of both eyes to the right (clockwise).
  Levocycloversion: Torsional movement of both eyes to the left (counterclockwise).

PHYSIOLOGY: MOTOR ASPECTS

Individual Muscle Functions

The lateral rectus muscle has the lone function of abducting the eye; the medial rectus muscle, that of adducting the eye; the other muscles have both primary and secondary actions which vary according to the position of the eye.

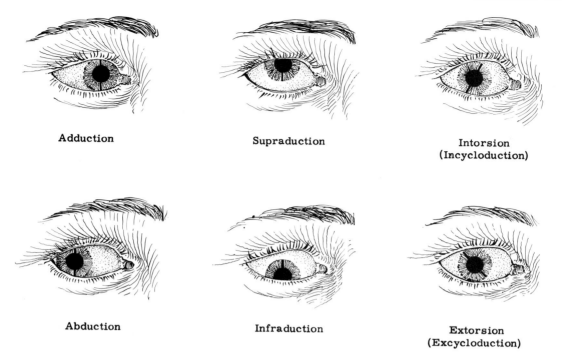

Adduction

Supraduction

Intorsion (Incycloduction)

Abduction

Infraduction

Extorsion (Excycloduction)

Fig 14-4. Ductions (monocular rotations), right eye.

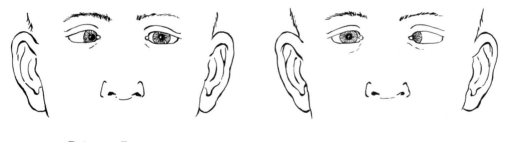

Primary Deviation (Left Eye Fixing)

Secondary Deviation (Right Eye Fixing; "inshoot" of sound left eye)

Fig 14-5. Paresis of horizontal muscle (right lateral rectus). Secondary deviation is greater than primary deviation because of Hering's law. With the left eye fixing, the right eye is deviated inward because of the paretic right lateral rectus. For the right eye to fix, the paretic right lateral rectus muscle must receive excessive stimulation. The yoke muscle, the left medial rectus, also receives the same excessive stimulation (Hering's law), which causes "inshoot" shown above.

Table 14-1. Functions of the ocular muscles.

Muscle	Primary Action	Secondary Action
Lateral rectus	Abduction	None
Medial rectus	Adduction	None
Superior rectus	Elevation	Adduction, intorsion
Inferior rectus	Depression	Adduction, extorsion
Superior oblique	Depression	Intorsion, abduction
Inferior oblique	Elevation	Extorsion, abduction

The elevation-depression actions of the superior and inferior rectus muscles increase as the eye is abducted; the elevation-depression actions of the superior and inferior oblique muscles increase as the eye is adducted.

Field of Action

The field of action of a muscle is that direction in which its primary action is greatest. Every movement of the eye involves the cooperation of all the muscles (each contracting or relaxing as its antagonist relaxes or contracts), but in each of the 6 cardinal directions of gaze there is always one muscle of each eye whose pull predominates.

Synergistic and Antagonistic Muscles (Sherrington's Law)

Two or 3 muscles of the same eye work together to produce a certain movement. In elevation, for example, the superior rectus and inferior oblique muscles are synergistic. Synergistic muscles for one function may be antagonists for another, eg, the superior rectus and inferior oblique are synergists for elevation but antagonists for torsional movement since the superior rectus causes intorsion and the inferior oblique extorsion. In normal ocular movement, neural inhibition of the antagonist of the directly acting muscle allows smooth ocular movement (Sherrington's law of reciprocal innervation). Thus, in dextroversion (eyes turning to the right), the right medial and left lateral rectus muscles receive inhibitory impulses that cause them to relax.

Yoke Muscles (Hering's Law)

In coordinated eye movements, a muscle of one eye is paired with a muscle of the opposite eye to produce movement in the 6 cardinal directions of gaze. (Eyes straight up and eyes down are not considered primary directions of gaze since no single pair of yoke muscles is primarily responsible for this action.) These paired primary movers are termed yoke muscles. In any conjugate movement, the yoke muscles receive equal innervation (Hering's law). Table 14-2 lists the yoke muscle combinations.

The Evolution of Binocular Movement

The movements of the eyes at birth are irregular and uncoordinated. By 5-6 weeks of age, the conjugate fixation reflexes are sufficiently developed so that the infant's eyes follow a slowly moving light. By 3 months of age the eyes will follow any moving object, but occasional deviations or "wandering" eye movements are seen until age 6 months. If a deviation is still present after 6 months, the child has strabismus and should be under the care of an ophthalmologist.

PHYSIOLOGY: SENSORY ASPECTS

Binocular Vision

In normal binocular vision, the image of the object of regard falls on the 2 foveas. The impulses travel along the optic pathways to the occipital cortex, where a single image is perceived. This is known as **fusion**. With normal use of the eye, the fovea looking at an object in space has a visual direction of "straight ahead." The foveas have a common visual direction and are the principal corresponding points. An extrafoveal point (or area) of one

Table 14-2. Yoke muscle combinations.

Cardinal Direction of Gaze	Yoke Muscles
Eyes up, right	Right superior rectus and left inferior oblique
Eyes right	Right lateral rectus and left medial rectus
Eyes down, right	Right inferior rectus and left superior oblique
Eyes down, left	Right superior oblique and left inferior rectus
Eyes left	Right medial rectus and left lateral rectus
Eyes up, left	Right inferior oblique and left superior rectus

eye having the same visual direction as an extrafoveal point of the other eye is called a corresponding point. Fusion is a relative process regardless of the alignment of the eyes, and therefore is classified into 3 grades or degrees (see p 179).

Sensory Changes in Strabismus

Up to the age of 6 or 7, the sensory pattern of the eyes is not entirely fixed and the eye is capable of adjusting to new mechanical alignments. If one eye deviates, the image of an object observed by the nondeviating eye falls on an extrafoveal area of the deviating eye. If the sensory conditions are normal, **diplopia** will result. The fovea of the deviating eye will also be directed toward another object in space, and this second object will be perceived as if it were superimposed upon the object seen by the nondeviating eye. This causes confusion of images. Under these conditions, **suppression** rapidly occurs. Suppression consists of the development of a scotoma which involves the macula as well as the point on which the image of regard falls (the image of the object being fixed by the dominant eye). Suppression exists only under binocular conditions, and is a method of obtaining relief from the diplopia and confusion caused by the deviating eye. With the nondeviating eye covered, there is no discernible loss of vision or demonstrable scotoma. Under binocular conditions using suitable testing apparatus, a "suppression scotoma" can be elicited.

If monocular strabismus persists untreated, suppression will usually deepen into **amblyopia** of the deviating eye. In this case the visual acuity may be reduced to finger counting only or perception of hand movements.

Abnormal (Anomalous) Retinal Correspondence

An extrafoveal area of the deviating eye may adapt to give a new sense of "straight ahead." The fovea of the fixing eye and the extrafoveal area of the deviating eye will then experience a common visual direction. This is called anomalous retinal correspondence and represents a crude attempt at binocular vision in the presence of strabismus. In alternating strabismus the sensory pattern changes, depending upon which eye is fixing, so that when the right eye is being used for fixation the left eye is suppressed (and vice versa).

Eccentric Fixation

In eyes with amblyopia, an extrafoveal area is usually employed for fixation even when the dominant eye is covered (monocular conditions). This is termed eccentric fixation. It may be a retinal area near the fovea and detectable only with special pleoptic instruments (see p 182), or it may be an area dis-tant from the fovea depending upon such variables as angle of deviation, duration of strabismus, age, and other poorly understood factors. Gross eccentric fixation can be readily identified clinically by occluding the dominant eye and directing the patient's attention to a light source held directly in front of him. An eye with gross eccentric fixation will not point toward the light source but will appear to be looking in a different direction.

EXAMINATION:
STRABISMUS EVALUATION

History

A careful history is of great aid in the diagnosis, prognosis, and treatment of strabismus.

A. Family History: Strabismus is frequently present; autosomal dominant inheritance is common.

B. Age at Onset: The single most important factor in prognosis. The earlier the onset, the worse the prognosis for fusion.

C. Type of Onset: May be gradual, sudden, or associated with systemic disease.

D. Type of Deviation: Under what conditions does the patient notice strabismus? When viewing near objects? When tired? Is the amount of deviation constant? It is most important to know if the eyes are straight at any time.

E. Fixation: Is it always the same eye that deviates? Alternating strabismus?

Visual Acuity

Visual acuity must be evaluated even if only a rough approximation or comparison of the 2 eyes is possible. The illiterate "E" chart can be used with children as young as $3^{1}/2$ years of age.

Determination of Refractive Error

It is important to determine the full cycloplegic refractive error by retinoscopy (see p 276). Up to 6 years of age, atropine, 0.5 or 1%, is used. Homatropine, 5%, or cyclopentolate (Cyclogyl®), 1%, is adequate for older children.

Inspection

Inspection alone will show whether the strabismus is constant or intermittent, alternating or monocular, and variable or constant.

Associated ptosis and abnormal position of the head may also be noted. The quality of fixation of each eye separately and both eyes together is important. Nystagmoid movements indicate poor fixation and reduced visual acuity.

Prominent epicanthal folds commonly confuse laymen as well as some physicians. The folds obscure a portion of the nasal sclera and may give the child the appearance of esotropia ("pseudoesotropia"). This pitfall can be avoided if the positions of the corneal reflec-

tions are noted. When the child is observing a light source, the corneal reflection of this light should be centered in the 2 pupillary areas. Prominent epicanthal folds usually disappear by 4 or 5 years of age.

Determination of Angle of Strabismus (Angle of Deviation)

A. Cover-Uncover Test: (See Fig 14-6.) In addition to determining the presence of a heterophoria or heterotropia, its degree can be measured by placing the appropriate prism

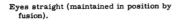

Eyes straight (maintained in position by fusion).

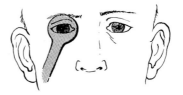

Position of eye under cover in orthophoria (fusion-free position). The right eye under cover has not moved.

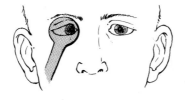

Position of eye under cover in esophoria (fusion-free position). Under cover, the right eye has deviated inward. Upon removal of cover, the right eye will immediately resume its straight-ahead position.

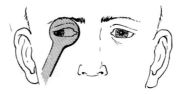

Position of eye under cover in exophoria (fusion-free position). Under cover the right eye has deviated outward. Upon removal of the cover, the right eye will immediately resume its straight-ahead position.

Fig 14-6. Cover-uncover test. The patient is directed to look at a small light source at eye level 20 feet away. **Note:** In the presence of heterotropia, the deviation will remain when the cover is removed.

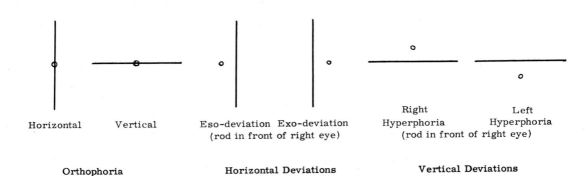
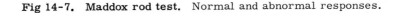

Horizontal	Vertical	Eso-deviation Exo-deviation (rod in front of right eye)	Right Hyperphoria	Left Hyperphoria (rod in front of right eye)

Orthophoria   Horizontal Deviations   Vertical Deviations

Fig 14-7. Maddox rod test. Normal and abnormal responses.

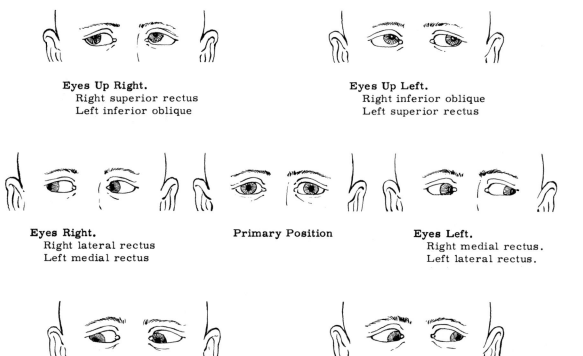

Eyes Up Right.
Right superior rectus
Left inferior oblique

Eyes Up Left.
Right inferior oblique
Left superior rectus

Eyes Right.
Right lateral rectus
Left medial rectus

Primary Position

Eyes Left.
Right medial rectus.
Left lateral rectus.

Eyes Down Right.
Right inferior rectus
Left superior oblique

Eyes Down Left.
Right superior oblique
Left inferior rectus

Fig 14-8. Normal version movement (binocular rotations). Yoke muscles primarily concerned with ocular movement in the cardinal directions are shown.

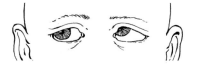

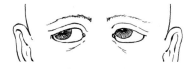

Eyes Up Right (Right Eye Fixing). Shows upshoot of left eye, indicating overaction of left inferior oblique. Excessive stimulation is needed to move right eye into position due to paretic right superior rectus muscle. The yoke muscle (left inferior oblique) receives the same excessive stimulation and "overacts." Secondary deviation; eye with paretic muscle is fixing.

Eyes Up Right (Left Eye Fixing). Shows underaction of right superior rectus. The left eye moves up and to the right with normal stimulation of the left inferior oblique muscle. The same normal impulse (Hering's law) to the right superior rectus muscle is insufficient to move the right eye up normally. Primary deviation; eye with nonparetic muscle is fixing.

Fig 14-9. Testing versions. Example of paretic right superior rectus muscle.

in front of one eye. For eso-deviations, the prism is placed base-out in such strength that, when the cover is moved from one eye to the other, the eye being uncovered no longer moves to obtain fixation upon the target light.

B. Maddox Rod Test: This test is an accurate method of measuring a deviation if normal retinal correspondence is present. It is particularly useful for measurement of heterophoria, but can also be used in heterotropia. A Maddox rod consists of a series of thin red glass cylinders placed side by side, usually mounted in a circular holder that can be held before the eye. When a target light is seen through the Maddox rod, its image is a red focal line perpendicular to the axes of the cylinders. Thus, one eye sees the light directly while the other views its image through the Maddox rod. In orthophoria the red line appears to run through the light. When the Maddox rod is held so that the cylinders are horizontal, a vertical red line is seen which in cases of horizontal deviation is displaced laterally. A prism can be held in front of one eye so that the red line appears to "run through the light." The strength of such a prism reflects the angle of deviation. By rotating the Maddox rod 90°, a horizontal line is produced (cylinders of the rod are vertical). Its displacement can also be measured by prisms as described above for horizontal deviations.

C. Objective Tests: If the patient is uncooperative or has eccentric fixation, some purely objective method of testing must be used to measure the deviation. Two methods are available. Results by both methods or any objective method must be modified by allowing for the angle kappa.

1. Hirschberg method - The patient fixes a light at a distance of about 13 inches. The decentering of the light reflection is noted in the deviating eye. By allowing 15Δ for each mm of decentration, an estimate of the angle of deviation can be made.

2. Prism reflex method (modified Krimsky test) - The patient fixes a light at any distance. The strength of a prism placed before the fixing eye required to center the corneal reflection of the deviating eye measures the angle of deviation.

Ductions (Monocular Rotations)

With one eye covered, the other eye follows a moving light in all directions of gaze so that any weakness of rotation can be noted. Such a weakness can be due to a muscle paralysis or to a mechanical anatomic anomaly.

Versions (Conjugate Ocular Movements)

According to Hering's law, yoke muscles receive equal stimulation during any conjugate ocular movement. The versions are tested by having the eyes follow a light at 13 inches in the cardinal directions of gaze and evaluating any "overaction" or "underaction" noted. First one eye and then the other is made to fix the light. "Overaction" of a muscle results when the eye with the paretic muscle is fixing the light placed in the cardinal directions of gaze controlled primarily by the set of yoke muscles in question (eg, eyes up and to the right for the right superior rectus and left inferior oblique muscles). The paretic muscle receives excessive innervation. Its yoke muscle receives the same excessive stimulation and therefore "overacts."

The evaluation of versions is most important in diagnosing paretic muscles, particularly those acting vertically. They are more important than monocular rotations (ductions), which can appear normal in testing mildly paretic muscles.

Disjunctive Movements

A. Convergence: As the eyes follow an object approaching, they must turn inward in order to maintain alignment of the visual axes with the object of regard. The medial rectus muscles are contracting and the lateral rectus muscles are relaxing under the influence of neural stimulation and inhibition. (Neural pathways of supranuclear control are discussed in Chapter 1.)

Convergence is an active process with a strong voluntary as well as involuntary component. An important consideration of extraocular movements in evaluating strabismus is the function of convergence.

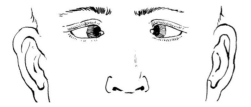

Fig 14-10. Convergence. The normal position of the eyes at the near point of convergence (NPC) is shown at left. The break point is within 50 mm of the bridge of the nose.

To test convergence, a small object or light source is slowly brought toward the bridge of the nose. The patient's attention is directed to the object by saying, "Keep the light from going double as long as possible." Convergence can normally be maintained until the object is nearly to the bridge of the nose. An actual numerical value is placed on convergence by measuring the distance from the bridge of the nose (in mm) at which the eyes "break" (ie, when the nondominant eye swings laterally so that convergence is no longer maintained). This point is termed the near point of convergence (NPC), and a value of up to 50 mm is considered within normal limits.

B. Divergence: Electromyography has established that divergence is an active process, not merely a relaxation of convergence as previously believed by some authorities. Clinically, this function is seldom tested except in considering the amplitude of fusion (see below).

The Major Amblyoscope (Grades of fusion, amplitude, suppression, retinal correspondence.)

This is the most important testing device for evaluation of the sensory status of the eyes. Other devices are used, some of which are smaller and simpler, but the major amblyoscope is the best instrument. It consists essentially of 2 adjustable tubes which present an illuminated image to each eye separately, using a mirror system. The tubes can be moved horizontally or vertically, and are calibrated. The light source illuminates the images separately, alternately, or together. Pairs of slides, one for each eye, are placed in the end of each tube. With appropriate slide pairs and a cooperative child (at least age 3), the sensory status can be evaluated. Orthoptic therapy can also be carried out with the aid of the amblyoscope.

A. Grades of Fusion: Grades of fusion as measured with the amblyoscope are as follows:

1. Grade I: (Simultaneous macular perception.) Dissimilar test targets (bird on one side, cage on the other side) are presented to the maculas. If the person sees both objects (can see the bird in the cage), grade I fusion is present. If one object is not seen, this eye is suppressing.

2. Grade II: (Fusion under stress with some amplitude.) Pairs of test targets are used which individually lack some detail but which when superimposed form a complete image. If these are perceived as a single image and this fusion maintained as the tubes are moved for 5 to 10 diopters, grade II fusion exists.

3. Grade III: (Stereopsis.) The test targets are so devised that an impression of depth is given if the observer has normal binocular vision.

B. Amplitude of Fusion: If grade II or III fusion exists, it is important to evaluate the stability of fusion. This is done by measuring the amplitude of fusion. Starting at the zero point, the arms are gradually converged until diplopia occurs. Normally, this is at least 25 or 30 diopters. The same test is performed for divergence, with 5 diopters being a minimal normal value. Vertical dissociation is also tested, and a normal person should overcome at least 5 diopters.

C. Suppression: Although grade I targets may disclose suppression (as above), foveal suppression can only be tested by using targets with very small central check marks.

D. Retinal Correspondence: Normal retinal correspondence has been defined as being present when anatomically corresponding retinal areas have the same subjective visual direction in space. To test retinal correspondence, the amblyoscope is set at the patient's objective angle of strabismus (angle measured by cover test; see p 176). If the grade II test targets are superimposed, normal retinal correspondence exists. If the images are double, abnormal retinal correspondence exists. Conversely, as a check, the patient is asked to place the tubes so that the images are together or as close together as possible. If this coincides with the angle of strabismus, normal retinal correspondence exists.

After-Image Test

This is a good simple test for determining whether a constant deviation in one eye has caused an extrafoveal area to take on the rudimentary function of the fovea in binocular vision (abnormal retinal correspondence).

The room is darkened and the patient instructed to cover his right eye. His left eye is then exposed to a horizontal beam of light for 10 seconds. This procedure is then repeated, covering the left eye and exposing the right eye to a vertical beam of light for 10 seconds. The patient is then asked to describe what he "sees." If the after-images of the 2 lines cross at the center, the patient has normal retinal correspondence. If not, abnormal retinal correspondence is present.

ORTHOPTIC THERAPY
WITH THE AMBLYOSCOPE

Before or after strabismus surgery, orthoptic therapy may materially aid in the treatment of strabismus by improving the quality of fusion. An attempt can be made to eliminate suppression by stimulating the fovea of the suppressing eye, or to break down abnormal retinal correspondence by presenting the maculas simultaneously with grade II test targets (see above). If grade II fusion is present or is developed, the amplitude of fusion can be improved by using grade II targets and varying the angle while maintaining fusion. In association with glasses or, at times, as an aid in reducing the strength of glasses required or eliminating them altogether, orthoptic exercises are useful in accommodative esotropia.

In special instances heterophorias of significant degree in adults may be aided by various orthoptic exercises.

PRINCIPLES OF
THERAPY OF STRABISMUS

There are 3 main objectives in the treatment of strabismus:

(1) Good visual acuity in each eye, achieved by occluding the good eye to force the child to use the deviating eye or, in some cases, by means of pleoptics (see p 182).

(2) A good cosmetic appearance. The eyes can be "straightened" by surgery or spectacles, or by a combination of both.

(3) Binocular vision (fusion, stereopsis). This also depends upon surgery, orthoptics, and refractive lenses.

Poor visual acuity and cosmetic defects are easier to correct if the child is seen early; the ideal age at which to begin therapy is 6 months. Normal fusion is difficult to obtain unless the child has already developed his powers of binocular vision before the onset of strabismus; it is the ideal objective of therapy, but is attained less than half the time. It is a satisfactory result in strabismus therapy to obtain 2 straight eyes with good vision but without good fusion. (Absence of fusion is not a serious handicap, affecting depth perception and estimation of distance to a limited degree.)

Occlusive therapy ("patching") may be required for variable periods depending upon the age at which strabismus is discovered.and the presence of amblyopia. It is essential to secure (and maintain, if necessary by frequent urging) the complete cooperation of the child

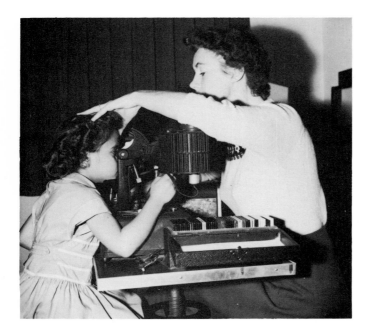

Fig 14-11. Giving eye exercises with the major amblyoscope.

and his parents; it must be carefully explained to them that this simple procedure will prevent the loss of vision in one eye. Patching is effective up to age 7. In older children, pleoptics may be effective.

Surgical correction of muscle imbalance should not be undertaken until maximal visual acuity has been restored by means of patching or pleoptics. (It is important to emphasize that strabismus surgery does not correct the visual disturbance nor the underlying cause of ocular deviation, but merely the cosmetic deformity.) Two or more operations may be required before the eyes are straightened, as there is no mathematically precise relationship between the number of mm the surgeon will recess or resect and the number of degrees of deviation corrected. However, in each case the surgeon can usually make a good estimate of how many mm he should recess or resect; these clinical estimates are based on the degree of deviation and the size of the muscle as observed at surgery.

In most cases it does not greatly matter whether surgery is performed on the straight eye or the deviating eye, but the deviating eye is usually chosen since this is easier to explain to parents.

In general, strabismus surgery can be regarded as a type of calculated "trial and error" surgery which creates an artificial defect in one or more extraocular muscles in an effort to compensate for an existing defect of unknown cause (probably, in most cases, neural).

CLASSIFICATION OF STRABISMUS

A. Esotropia:
  1. Nonparalytic (comitant) - The angle of deviation is constant in all directions of gaze.
    a. Nonaccommodative
    b. Accommodative
    c. Combined accommodative and nonaccommodative
  2. Paretic (noncomitant) - The angle of deviation varies in different directions of gaze.
B. Exotropia:
  1. Intermittent
  2. Constant
C. Hypertropia:
  1. Paralytic
  2. Nonparalytic

ESOTROPIA
(Convergent Strabismus, "Crossed Eyes")

Esotropia is by far the most common type of strabismus, comprising about 75% of cases. It is divided into paralytic (due to paresis or paralysis of one or more extraocular muscles) and nonparalytic (comitant). Comitant esotropia is the most common type in infants and children; it may be accommodative, nonaccommodative, or a combination of both. Paralytic strabismus comprises nearly all cases of adult and a minority of childhood strabismus.

NONPARALYTIC ESOTROPIA

1. NONACCOMMODATIVE ESOTROPIA

More than half of all cases of esotropia fall into this group. In most cases the cause is obscure. Characteristically, the convergent deviation is manifest early in life, usually by the first year and often at birth. By definition, the deviation is comitant, ie, the angle of deviation is approximately the same in all directions of gaze and is not affected very much by accommodation. The cause, therefore, is not related to the refractive error nor dependent upon a paretic extraocular muscle. It is probable that some cases are due to anomalous insertions of the horizontally acting muscles, abnormal check ligaments, or various other fascial abnormalities. It is also quite likely that many cases are due to faulty innervational development, especially of the supranuclear pathways for controlling convergence and divergence.

There is also good evidence that "idiopathic" strabismus may occur on a genetically determined basis. Esophoria and esotropia are frequently passed on as an autosomal dominant trait. Siblings often have similar ocular deviations. At other times, when there is no apparent family history, the parents of an esotropic child may be found to have significant esophoria, and have passed on the defect in a more severe form. An accommodative element is often superimposed upon comitant esotropia, ie, a correction of the hyperopic refractive error corrects some but not all of the deviation.

Clinical Findings

Aside from the cosmetic defect and the personality problems it may create in older children, there are usually no symptoms due to strabismus.

The deviation may be monocular (ie, the same eye always deviates) or alternating (either eye may deviate). The refractive error in alternating esotropia is approximately the same in each eye; in monocular esotropia the refractive error is frequently more marked in one eye (anisometropia). Adduction is commonly increased and abduction decreased in one or both eyes. Convergence may be unaffected. Visual acuity is not affected in alternating esotropia, but it usually becomes reduced in the deviating eye in monocular esotropia. The deviation usually varies only slightly when the eyes are focused on near and distant objects, and correction of the refractive error does not appreciably affect the deviation.

If the strabismus has been present for several months, alternating esotropia will usually result in alternate suppression and often abnormal retinal correspondence (but not amblyopia). Monocular strabismus is most likely to cause amblyopia. Retinal correspondence is often abnormal.

Treatment

A. Occlusive Therapy: The objective of occlusive therapy is to equalize the visual acuity in both eyes. Early diagnosis followed by patching the good eye is the best means of preventing amblyopia. However, even with patching and successful surgical correction, many patients (especially those who have strabismus at birth) do not develop normal fusion. In general, the earlier the deviation is discovered and the fixing eye patched, the sooner will the deviating eye develop useful visual acuity. Even a few days of patching may be sufficient prior to age 1, whereas several months may be necessary by age 5. After age 7, only pleoptics can help develop or restore visual function, and this is a very time consuming procedure in which there is no assurance of success.

Occlusion has a favorable effect upon abnormal sensory patterns but rarely on the degree of deviation. When nothing further can be accomplished by occlusion, surgical realignment of the eyes is indicated.

Occlusive therapy may be combined with orthoptics (see p 180), utilizing the amblyoscope in an effort to develop better binocular function. The sensory abnormalities of suppression and abnormal retinal correspondence are also broken down, if possible, by orthoptic means.

B. Pleoptics: The value of pleoptics as a practical therapeutic tool has not lived up to early expectations. It is more widely used in Europe than in the USA. A wide variety of technics have been utilized, all designed to disrupt eccentric fixation and establish foveal fixation. One frequently used technic is based on stimulating the dormant fovea while discouraging the eccentric fixation point by dazzling and blocking out appropriate retinal areas. The entire parafoveal area out to 30 degrees is dazzled with an ophthalmoscope light source which has a central dark shield to protect the macula from the dazzle. After the light is removed, the macula stands out as a positive after-image. Shortly thereafter, a negative after-image becomes apparent to the patient. The patient is then taught that the after-image is in the straight-ahead position, and in this way foveal vision can be gradually reoriented to the straight-ahead position. Many concentrated hours of pleoptic work are required to attain proper macular and foveal orientation so that improved visual acuity can occur. Some patients respond fairly quickly, but others require months or years of treatment. For ideal results, hospitalization is necessary—an almost prohibitive financial factor in the USA. The average visual improvement is from 20/200 to 20/70, but some exceptional cases have improved from hand movement visual acuity to 20/25. Even many of these apparently successfully treated patients have reverted to previous visual levels shortly after cessation of treatment.

The best age group for treatment is from age 7 to 14, but a few remarkable results have been reported on amblyopic eyes of elderly patients who have lost the vision of the dominant eye from some organic cause.

C. Surgical Treatment: There are basically 2 surgical approaches to the correction of strabismus: strengthening a muscle or weakening a muscle. In the case of the horizontal muscles, the strengthening operation is usually resection and the weakening operation is usually recession. Other rarely used procedures include tucking and advancement, for strengthening; and various types of tenotomy for weakening.

1. Recession of the medial rectus muscle - A conjunctival incision is made over the insertion of the medial rectus muscle and carried down through Tenon's capsule. The muscle is then isolated and exposed for a short distance away from its insertion. The immediate check ligaments are severed. The muscle is then severed at the insertion and resutured into the sclera 4-5 mm behind this point, depending upon the amount of adjustment desired. The overlying conjunctiva is then reapproximated.

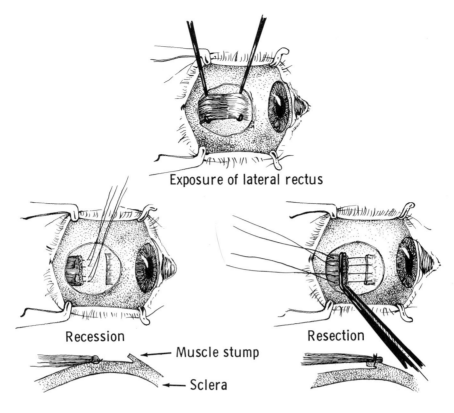

Exposure of lateral rectus

Recession

Resection

← Muscle stump

← Sclera

Fig 14-12. Surgical correction of strabismus (right eye).

This operation is usually done under general anesthesia, and the patient may be ambulatory within hours after surgery. The eye is patched for a few days postoperatively. Conjunctival injection is present immediately postoperatively, but gradually disappears within 2-3 weeks.

2. Resection of the lateral rectus muscle - A conjunctival incision is made over the insertion of the lateral rectus muscle and carried through Tenon's capsule. The insertion of the lateral rectus is isolated and the muscle clamped and detached from the sclera. One or 2 sutures are then placed through the sclera at the original point of insertion. The sutures are then passed through the muscle 6-10 mm from its detached end and tied. The excess muscle tissue is dissected off, and the conjunctival incision reapproximated.

3. Discussion of surgery - There is no precise rule for the amount of recession or resection needed to correct a given amount of deviation. There are many variables, including the technic of the surgeon, which determine how much correction will be achieved by a given amount of surgery. In general, the surgeon first decides how many muscles are

to be operated on and then varies the amount of surgery within rather narrow limits. In the case of esotropia, deviations of less than 20 Δ can usually be corrected by surgery on one muscle (eg, 4-5 mm recession of one medial rectus muscle). For deviations of 20-35 Δ it is usually necessary to operate on 2 muscles. Some surgeons prefer to operate upon 2 muscles of one eye, doing a recession of the medial rectus and a resection of the lateral rectus; others prefer so-called symmetrical surgery, eg, bilateral recession of both medial rectus muscles.

To some extent the type of strabismus influences the type of surgery. In the case of monocular strabismus with an amblyopic eye, most surgeons prefer to operate upon the deviating eye. In the case of alternating esotropia, recession of both medial rectus muscles is preferable. In deviations above 45 Δ it may be necessary to operate on 3 or even 4 muscles.

Prognosis

Strabismus surgery is empirical, and consistent results cannot be predicted. The patient and his parents should be warned that

2 or more operations may be necessary before a good result is obtained. One of the best opportunities to improve fusion occurs just before and just after strabismus surgery since the sensory status is made temporarily more flexible by strabismus surgery.

2. ACCOMMODATIVE ESOTROPIA

About a third of cases of esotropia fall into this group; another 15-20% have some accommodative factor. These patients are hyperopic, usually 2 Δ or more. For this reason they must accommodate for clear distance vision. Accommodation is associated with a certain amount of convergence; if the amount of convergence is too great to be overcome by the available fusional amplitude, convergent strabismus results. Accommodative esotropia sometimes takes the form of esophoria for distance and esotropia for near. In these cases there is an over-response of convergence in association with accommodation.

Clinical Findings
The onset of this type of esotropia is characteristically between 18 months and 4 years of age (because the faculty of accommodation is not well developed until then). The deviation is most often monocular, but may be alternating. The hyperopic refractive error is usually from +2 to +5 Δ. Sensory findings reveal that suppression develops rapidly in the deviating eye, but normal retinal correspondence is usually retained.

Treatment
Pure accommodative esotropia responds satisfactorily to correction of hyperopia with eyeglasses if treatment is instituted within a fairly short time, usually not more than 6 months after onset. If treatment is delayed beyond this time, the abnormal sensory pattern is apt to have become so well established that glasses alone will not correct the strabismus. In this event, treatment is generally as outlined above for nonaccommodative esotropia. If amblyopia has developed in one eye, occlusion is indicated, and this may so reverse the abnormal sensory pattern that nonsurgical cure is possible. More frequently, however, surgical treatment will be necessary in long-standing cases. In cases which have a partial accommodative factor, a prescription for hyperopic eyeglasses will reduce the amount of deviation and the residual deviation must be corrected surgically. Bifocals may be prescribed if the deviation is much greater for near than for distance.

Long-acting miotics in weak strengths (echothiophate [Phospholine®] iodide, 0.06 or 0.12% solution; or isoflurophate [Floropryl®] ointment, 0.025%) applied once daily have been used with success in treating accommodative esotropia. In younger children (age 2-4), these drugs can be used instead of glasses if the hyperopia is less than 4 diopters and there is little astigmatism. Miotics are particularly useful in cases where hyperopic eyeglasses align the eyes for distance vision but esotropia remains at near vision. These drugs act by altering the accommodative convergence relationship in a favorable way so that fusion is maintained despite accommodation. In addition, the miotic effect allows clear vision with less accommodation both for near and distance.

PARETIC (NONCOMITANT) ESOTROPIA
(Abducens Palsy)

In noncomitant strabismus there are always one or more paretic extraocular muscles. In the case of noncomitant esotropia, the paresis is always of one of the lateral rectus muscles, usually as a result of palsy of the abducens nerve. These cases are most often seen in adults who have had cerebrovascular accidents, but abducens palsy may occasionally be the first sign of a tumor or of inflammatory disease involving the CNS. Head trauma can also produce abducens palsy.

Noncomitant esotropia is also seen in infants and children, but much less commonly than comitant esotropia. These cases result from birth injuries or congenital anomalies of a lateral rectus muscle, its nerve supply, or its fascial attachments.

Clinical Findings
If the lateral rectus muscle is totally paralyzed, the eye will not move temporally beyond the midline. Paralysis of a right lateral rectus muscle causes a right monocular esotropia which becomes more marked as the eyes attempt to fix an object moving to the right of the midline. The deviation is absent upon conjugate movement of the eyes to the left.

In children age 6 or younger, suppression will develop under conditions of deviation but entirely normal binocular relationships may remain when the eyes are aligned in the field of gaze opposite the side of the paretic lateral rectus muscle. There may even be a change of retinal correspondence from normal to abnormal as one passes into the field of strabismus. In adults with a sudden onset of paralytic esotropia, the patient experiences diplopia whenever an eye deviates, since the sensory

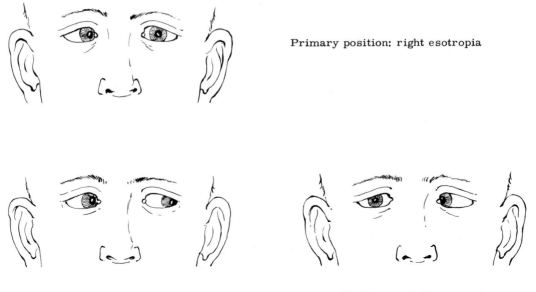

Primary position: right esotropia

Left gaze: no deviation   Right gaze: left esotropia

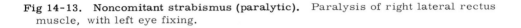

Fig 14-13. **Noncomitant strabismus (paralytic).** Paralysis of right lateral rectus muscle, with left eye fixing.

pattern is fixed and the object of regard falls on noncorresponding retinal areas.

Treatment

The treatment of persistent paralytic esotropia is exclusively surgical. In adults who have a sudden onset of strabismus, a period of at least 6 months is allowed to pass before surgery since the condition may correct itself. During this period, occlusion of the eye with the paretic muscle is necessary to relieve diplopia.

In children, or in adults who have had no improvement after 6 months, surgical treatment is indicated. In paresis of the lateral rectus muscle, an attempt may be made to strengthen this muscle by resection, sometimes combined with advancement of the insertion. In this operation the resection is carried out as described for nonparalytic esotropia. Placement of the sutures anterior to the original insertion effects an advancement. In addition, the medial rectus muscle of the same eye may also be weakened by recession to enhance the effect of the surgery. The type and amount of surgery will depend on the extent of the deviation. In the case of total paralysis of the lateral rectus muscle, strengthening by resection of the muscle will not attain the desired result. The Hümmelsheim operation is preferred, ie, half of the superior rectus and half of the inferior rectus tendons are transplanted to the insertion of the lateral rectus muscle to aid in abduction of the eye. This is combined with recession of the medial rectus muscle. The surgical treatment of noncomitant esotropia is seldom a total success, but some improvement can usually be obtained. Knapp has advocated transplanting the entire superior and inferior rectus muscles to the insertion of the paretic lateral rectus. This not only greatly improves abduction, but does not significantly affect upward or downward movement of the eye.

EXOTROPIA
(Divergent Strabismus)

Exotropia is less common than esotropia, particularly in infancy and childhood. Its incidence increases gradually with age. Not infrequently, a tendency to divergent strabismus beginning as exophoria progresses to intermittent exotropia and finally to constant exotropia if no treatment is given. Other

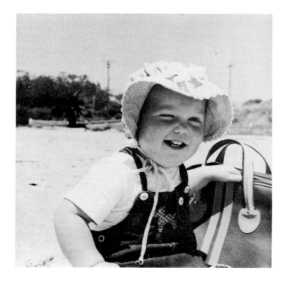

Fig 14-14. Child with
intermittent exotropia
squinting in sunlight.

cases begin as a constant or intermittent exotropia and remain stationary. As in esotropia,
there is a strong hereditary element. Exophoria and exotropia (considered as a single
entity of divergent deviation) is frequently
passed on as an autosomal dominant trait, so
that one or both parents of an exotropic child
may demonstrate exotropia or a high degree
of exophoria.

INTERMITTENT EXOTROPIA
(Divergence Excess)

Intermittent exotropia comprises well over
half of cases of exotropia. The onset of the
deviation may not be noted prior to age 2 or 3.
The history reveals that the condition has become progressively worse. A characteristic
symptom is closing one eye in bright sunlight.
There is usually a manifest exotropia for distance. The patient can fuse for near vision,
overcoming a moderate to large angle exophoria. Convergence is frequently excellent.
There is no correlation with a specific refractive error.

Since the child fuses at least part of the
time, there is usually no gross sensory abnormality. For distance, with one eye deviated, there is suppression but normal retinal
correspondence and no amblyopia. Many patients demonstrate only grade II fusion with
limited amplitude.

Treatment is principally surgical, sometimes enhanced by preoperative orthoptic exercises or optical devices such as base-in
prisms or excessive minus lenses. Fusion exercises may "increase the quality of fusion"
and set the stage for a better functional result
following surgery.

The choice of surgical procedure is based
on a number of considerations, the most important of which is the amount of deviation
and a comparison of near and distance measurements. When the deviation is greater for
distance than for near, recession of each lateral rectus muscle gives the best results.
If the near deviation is approximately equal to
the distance, many surgeons prefer a recession of one lateral rectus and a resection of
the medial rectus of the same eye. As with
other types of strabismus, one operation does
not always result in the desired result and a
second operation may be required.

CONSTANT EXOTROPIA

Constant exotropia is much less common
than intermittent exotropia. It may be present
at birth or may occur when intermittent exotropia progresses to constant exotropia. Some
cases have their onset later in life, particularly following loss of vision in one eye.

As with esotropia, the cause of exotropia
is usually not known. Congenital constant
exotropia may be the result of anomalous insertions of the extraocular muscles, other
defects of the muscles, or faulty innervation.
It has been postulated that in infants and young
children a tendency toward excessive convergence may be present which is controlled by
nuclear and infranuclear pathways and held in
check by supranuclear influences which maintain the proper alignment of the eyes. There
probably also is a divergence center with

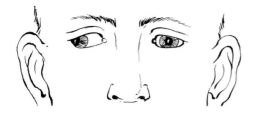

Fig 14-15. Right exotropia.

similar supranuclear influences, and both esotropia and exotropia may well result from abnormalities of the supranuclear influences.
Such common terms as ''convergence excess
and convergence insufficiency'' and ''divergence excess and divergence insufficiency''
are merely descriptive. For example, ''divergence excess'' means an exo-deviation,
either phoria or tropia, which is greater for
distance than for near; ''convergence excess''
means an eso-deviation which is greater for
near than for distance. It is true that the tendency toward divergence becomes greater as
age increases. If there is no fusion, as in the
case of one blind eye, the blind eye usually
deviates inward in a person up to age 6 and
usually deviates outward if the visual loss
occurs after age 6. Many cases of exotropia
develop as a result of loss of vision in one eye,
with subsequent progressive exotropia.

The most important consideration is the
psychic factor resulting from the cosmetic
appearance. The minimal loss of depth perception which occurs is of practical importance only to a person requiring the best depth
perception, such as a pilot. There is a minimal handicap for most athletes.

Constant exotropia is most often monocular
(the same eye always deviating), but may be
alternating. Abduction is frequently increased
and adduction decreased in both eyes, with
little or no convergence. Hypertropia of varying degree is often associated. The deviations
vary from as little as 10 Δ to 80 Δ or more.

In children age 6 or under with alternating
exotropia, alternate suppression characteristically develops. If the squint is monocular,
amblyopia of the deviating eye results. Abnormal retinal correspondence is an infrequent
sensory change. Eccentric fixation of the deviated eye almost never occurs. Exotropia
very seldom has its onset in adulthood unless
there is significant loss of visual acuity in the
deviating eye, and diplopia is therefore not
usually a troublesome symptom.

Surgery is the only treatment available.
A practical goal is a good cosmetic appearance
with maintenance of good vision in each eye.
In general, slight over-correction is attempted
since the resultant small angle esotropia is
less likely to revert to exotropia. If surgery

leaves a residual small angle exotropia, the
eye is apt to deviate outward again.

Even in children with good vision in each
eye, a good fusional result is difficult to obtain.

In monocular exotropia it is usually necessary to operate upon at least the 2 horizontal
muscles of the deviating eye, resecting the
medial rectus and recessing the lateral rectus.
(Technic is described under treatment of nonaccommodative esotropia, p 182.) In large
deviations, 3 or all 4 horizontal muscles may
have to be altered to straighten the eyes.

•   •   •

''A'' AND ''V'' SYNDROMES

Increasing importance has been attached
to 2 types of horizontal strabismus in which
the deviation is significantly different in upward and downward gaze. The terminology is
intended to be descriptive of the position of the
eyes where the deviation is greatest. In ''A''
esotropia, deviation is greater on eyes up than
on eyes down; in ''A'' exotropia, deviation is
greater on eyes down than eyes up. Conversely, in ''V'' esotropia, deviation is greater on
eyes down than eyes up; and in ''V'' exotropia,
deviation is greater on eyes up than eyes down.

When these findings are present in significant degree, most ophthalmic surgeons alter
their surgical approach.

HYPERTROPIA

Vertical deviations are designated according to the eye that is deviated upward. ''Right
hypertropia'' means that the right eye deviates
upward when the left eye is fixating. The same
condition could be called a left hypotropia when
the right eye is fixating, but this terminology
is seldom used. Hypertropia is much less
common than horizontal deviation, and usually
has its onset later in life.

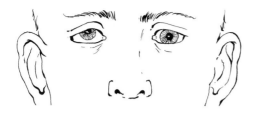

Fig 14-16. Right hypertropia.

There are many causes of hypertropia. Frequent causes are muscle paralysis due to trauma and individual paralyses of the vertically acting muscles. Abnormal insertions, abnormal fascial attachments, and other congenital anomalies may also cause hypertropia.

Complications of systemic disease also account for a great number of cases, eg., myasthenia gravis, multiple sclerosis, thyrotoxicosis, orbital tumor, and brain stem disease. Many of the specific entities are considered in the chapter on neuro-ophthalmology. The discussion here will be limited to "idiopathic cases," ie, those due to paralysis of unknown cause involving one or more of the vertically acting muscles.

Clinical Findings (See also Figs 14-7 and 14-8)

Hypertropia with onset after age 6 causes diplopia if both eyes have good visual acuity. There may be an associated head tilt or abnormal posture of the head.

The deviation may vary from slight (a few prism diopters) to marked. At onset and for a variable period thereafter, the deviation will be greater in one position or direction of gaze than in others. Subsequently, heterotropia tends to become comitant, since secondary contraction of the direct antagonist and other extraocular muscles occurs. It is important to determine which muscle or muscles are at fault. This becomes more difficult if the disorder is of long duration. Many tests are available which are of aid in specific muscle diagnosis. In any one case all tests may not be consistent, but the bulk of evidence will point toward paresis of one or more specific muscles. Treatment is based upon these determinations.

A. Measurement of the Deviation: The deviation must be measured in the 6 cardinal directions of gaze both for near and for distance, and with each eye fixing. Secondary deviation is larger than primary deviation (see p 174); therefore, the deviation measured while the eye containing the paretic muscle is fixing will be larger than that measured while the eye with the nonparetic muscle is fixing. In general, a deviation which is greater for near than for distance implicates an oblique muscle rather than a rectus muscle and vice versa, since in adduction (position of the eyes for near) the eyes depend more upon the oblique muscles than the rectus muscles for elevation and depression. With the eyes in the straight-ahead position (as for distance), the rectus muscles are more prominent as elevators and depressors than are the oblique muscles.

The deviation in the cardinal directions is measured with prisms. In general, if deviation is greater in one of the cardinal directions, this points toward a specific vertical muscle paralysis. For example, in right hypertropia, if the deviation is greater with the eyes up and to the right, this indicates underaction of the left inferior oblique muscle.

B. Head Tilt (Bielschowsky's) Test: (See Fig 14-16.) A person with a paretic oblique muscle may tilt his head toward one shoulder. This is often useful in diagnosing paralysis of an oblique muscle. Normally, when tilting the head toward the right shoulder, the incycloductors of the right eye (superior oblique and superior rectus) and the excycloductors of the left eye (inferior oblique and inferior rectus) tend to cycloduct each eye to neutralize the tilted head position. The oblique muscle predominates in this torsion movement. For example, if the right superior oblique is paretic, the patient will have a right hypertropia and carry his head tilted to the left. This is because the intorsional movement of the right eye is in this instance produced by the right superior rectus; its elevating action is unopposed, since its antagonist in vertical movement is the right superior oblique. With the head tilted to the left, the excycloduction (see p 173) required of the right eye is accomplished by the right inferior oblique and right inferior rectus. The vertical component is balanced, and no hypertropia is present. Thus, in order to avoid vertical diplopia, the patient will usually carry his head tilted to the left.

The head tilt test of Bielschowsky utilizes the above principle to aid in the diagnosis of paretic oblique muscles. The patient fixes a light at 20 feet. The eye to be tested may be placed under cover (still visible to the examiner), but this is not necessary. The head is tilted first toward one shoulder and then the other. An increased hypertropia is diagnostic of oblique paralysis.

Example: The right eye is covered (may be left uncovered) and the head is tilted 45° upon the right shoulder. The eye moves upward. This indicates paralysis of the right superior oblique muscle. This occurs upon tilting the head because the 2 incycloductors (right superior rectus and right superior oblique) receive impulses to contract (as above). In addition to their synergistic function of incycloduction, these muscles are antagonistic in the function of elevation and depression; the normal superior rectus (elevation) will not be balanced by the paretic superior oblique (depression), and the eye will elevate.

C. Sensory Changes in Hypertropia: As in other forms of strabismus, a sensory adaptation will take place if the strabismus has its onset before age 6. The sensory pattern may vary with the position of the eyes, so that suppression or even abnormal retinal correspondence may be present in the direction of gaze of strabismus and normal retinal correspondence without suppression in directions of gaze where strabismus is absent. If the onset is after age 6, there is no sensory adaptation and diplopia is constant.

Treatment

A. Conservative Treatment: In smaller deviations, usually under 10 Δ with relatively comitant strabismus, prisms may neutralize the hypertropia. In the case of a right hypertropia of 8 Δ, a 4 Δ prism base down, right eye, and a 4 Δ prism base up, left eye, may be incorporated into the eyeglasses and fusion reestablished. With larger deviations or in cases where the strabismus is noncomitant even though not of great magnitude, surgery is usually indicated. If there are medical contradications, such as systemic disease, or if there is a good possibility that the strabismus may clear or improve subsequently, temporizing measures are necessary to relieve the diplopia. This frequently consists of patching one eye. When hypertropia is due to a complication of a systemic disease, treatment of the underlying disease will materially affect the hypertropia (eg, myasthenia gravis).

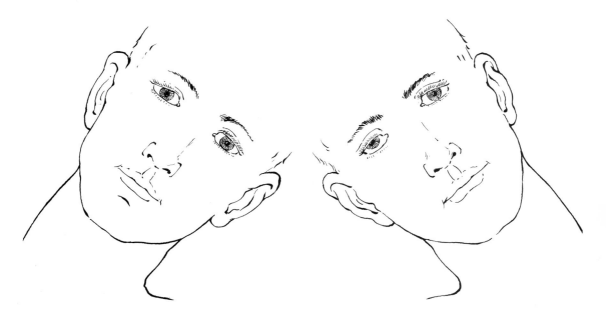

Fig 14-17. Head tilt test (Bielschowsky). Left: Paresis of right superior oblique muscle. Head is carried to shoulder on sound side (left), where fusion is obtained. This is a postural attitude called a ''head tilt.'' **Right:** When the head is tilted to the shoulder on the paretic side, the right hypertropia becomes exaggerated. This is a positive forced head tilt test of Bielschowsky.

B. Surgical Treatment: Many approaches are used in the surgical treatment of hypertropia. The recent tendency has been to strengthen the weakened muscle. At times it may be necessary to weaken the direct antagonist or the yoke muscle, or both. The vertically acting rectus muscles can be recessed or resected in the same manner as the horizontally acting rectus muscles, although within somewhat smaller limits. The superior oblique muscle can be strengthened by tucking the tendon. This effectively shortens the superior oblique tendon by as much as 10 mm and therefore strengthens the muscle. The superior oblique muscle can also be weakened by intrasheath tenotomy, in which the sheath of the superior oblique tendon is opened and a full tenotomy performed. The sheath is then resutured. This gives a fairly predictable amount of correction, usually about 15 Δ. The inferior oblique muscle can be effectively weakened by a recession of 8 to 10 mm, or by myotomy. A number of other operations that both strengthen and weaken the verticle muscles are available but are used less commonly.

HETEROPHORIA

Heterophoria is a deviation of the eyes which is held in check by the fusion mechanism. Almost all individuals have some degree of heterophoria, so that small amounts are considered normal. Larger degrees of heterophoria are a common cause of "eye-strain" (asthenopia), since a strain is placed upon the extraocular muscles to overcome the latent deviation. From an etiologic standpoint, heterophoria and heterotropia differ only in degree. The same etiologic concepts that have been discussed above apply to the 3 types of heterophoria. As with heterotropia, many of the causal factors are unknown. Heterophoria is clinically significant only if it causes symptoms. Symptoms will not always correlate well with the degree of heterophoria, since the personality and occupation of the individual are important in determining the symptomatology.

Asthenopia ("eyestrain") as a symptom of heterophoria takes a wide variety of forms. There may be a feeling of tiredness or discomfort of the eyes varying from a dull ache to deep pain located in or behind the eyes. Headaches of all types occur. Easy fatigability and blurring of vision and occasionally even diplopia, especially after prolonged intense use of the eyes, are less common.

In general, the same diagnostic tests used in evaluating heterotropia are used for heterophoria. The most important test is the cover-uncover test, which allows one to differentiate a heterophoria from heterotropia.

The Maddox rod with prism measurement is especially useful in evaluating measurements in the cardinal directions of gaze when dealing with hyperphoria.

The sensory pattern as determined by the amblyoscope is nearly always normal, including normal retinal correspondence and absence of suppression or amblyopia.

The **prism vergence test** determines whether an individual has the reserve fusional mechanism required to overcome any heterophoria that is present. The test is carried out by asking the patient to fixate on a small light at 20 feet with both eyes uncovered. Prisms of gradually increasing strength or the rotary prism of Risley in gradually increasing strengths are placed before one eye until diplopia occurs ("break point"). This is done with both base-in and base-out prism measurements for both near and distance. This measures the fusional convergence and divergence, respectively. Prisms are used base-up or base-down to measure the relative vertical divergence. (Positive vertical divergence if the right eye is directed upward; negative vertical divergence if the left eye is directed upward.) In calculating the numerical results of these tests, one must use the reading for distance heterophoria as a starting point. The normal values for prism vergence at 20 feet are as follows: prism divergence, 7 Δ; prism convergence, 20 Δ; vertical divergence, 5 Δ. Prism vergence at 13 inches: prism divergence, 20 Δ; prism convergence, 20 Δ; vertical divergence, 5 Δ.

DISCUSSION AND TREATMENT OF HETEROPHORIA

Esophoria
Esophoria greater than 3 Δ for near or distance may cause asthenopic symptoms.

A. Significant Esophoria for Near and Distance: If the patient has uncorrected hyperopia, the addition of plus sphere to the correction, or the prescription of eyeglasses if not previously worn, may relieve the symptoms. Less accommodation is thus required both for near and for distance, and so less convergence is induced. If full hyperopic correction still leaves a significant esophoria, base-out prism equally divided in the 2 spectacle lenses may be prescribed. One-half to one-third of the

residual deviation is usually prescribed, although more than a total of 4 prism Δ is usually poorly tolerated. If symptoms persist and
optical methods are unsatisfactory, surgery
is indicated. It is usually necessary to operate on only one muscle, most often a recession of a medial rectus muscle.

B. Significant Esophoria for Near and Not
for Distance: In this instance the complaint
is ''tired eyes'' or other symptoms upon reading or using the eyes for close work. Treatment by optical methods is usually satisfactory. In the case of a hyperope who has been
wearing full correction, the addition of more
plus sphere for reading (up to 2 or 2.5 diopters)
will often be helpful. This reduces necessary
accommodation and accompanying convergence,
so that it is possible to reduce or nullify the
esophoria. In the case of a myopic individual
the same principle can be applied, giving less
minus correction. If significant esophoria
persists, base-out prism may be added to the
prescription and adjusted until the symptoms
disappear. In rare instances, if optical devices fail, a recession of one medial rectus
muscle may be performed.

Exophoria

Larger amounts of exophoria are tolerated
than of esophoria, particularly for near vision
where it is not unusual to have a measurement
of 7-10 Δ without symptoms. Exophoria above
3 Δ for distance is considered abnormal.

A. Significant Exophoria for Near and
Distance: With exophoria it is more difficult
to overcome the phoria by manipulating the
power of the eyeglasses. Undercorrection or
no correction in the hyperope induces more
accommodation and thus convergence, which
helps to nullify exophoria. Similarly, over-
correction in myopes accomplishes the same
result (stimulates accommodation). More
commonly, base-in prism equally divided between the 2 eyes, correcting one-fourth to one-
half of the deviation, is the treatment of choice.
If the deviation is too large, usually above 15 Δ,
or if spectacles with prisms do not relieve
symptoms, recession of a lateral rectus muscle is indicated.

B. Significant Exophoria for Near and Not
for Distance: Base-in prisms are incorporated
in spectacles used only for close work. One-
fourth to one-half of the deviation is neutralized with prisms. If prisms fail, and particularly if poor convergence is also present,
resection of one or both medial rectus muscles
is indicated (depending on the degree of exophoria).

C. Significant Exophoria for Distance and
Not for Near: The same principle applies as
above except that the prism correction must
be placed in the distance glasses and a separate pair of eyeglasses used for near. Occasionally there will be a large exophoric
deviation for distance and a relatively small
one for near. If the deviation for distance is
15 Δ or more, surgery may be indicated,
depending upon the severity of symptoms and
the patient's occupation. The procedure of
choice is recession of one or both lateral
rectus muscles.

Hyperphoria

This is a frequent cause of asthenopia.
Symptoms are often present if the deviation
is 2-4 Δ or more. In very high degrees of
hyperphoria, a paretic muscle may be diagnosed and surgery (as described for hypertropia) is indicated to strengthen the paretic
muscle or weaken its antagonist or yoke muscle. Lesser degrees of deviation can be corrected with prisms. It is important to measure the hyperphoria in the cardinal directions
of gaze for both near and distance. If the
deviation proves to be comitant or nearly
comitant, neutralizing vertical prisms, base-
down in front of the higher eye and base-up in
front of the lower eye, equally divided, are
effective. It is usually necessary to neutralize one-third to one-half the deviation in this
manner. If the deviation is noncomitant, treatment may be difficult. Symptoms will usually
then be produced only under certain conditions.
For example, in driving, if the deviation is
greatest with the eyes straight ahead for distance, special prismatic driving glasses could
be prescribed. In other cases the deviation
is greatest for near in the reading position, in
which case prisms could be incorporated into
reading glasses or into the reading segment of
bifocals.

Double Hyperphoria (Alternating Sursumduc-
tion).

Double hyperphoria is frequently associated with horizontal strabismus, sometimes
combined with vertical muscle imbalance and
occasionally with otherwise normal muscle
balance. The cause is not known. It is important only to differentiate this condition from
true hyperphoria or hypertropia, since in itself
it does not require treatment and usually causes
no symptoms (fusion is normal). The diagnosis
is made by having the patient fix a light at 20
feet and cover one eye. The eye under cover
is noted to deviate upward. Changing the cover,
the opposite eye then takes up fixation and the
other eye, now under cover, deviates upward.
With the cover entirely removed, the eyes regain fusion.

Cyclophoria

Cyclophoria is a rare disorder characterized by abnormal torsional movements held in
check by fusion. There is some dispute about
its importance, but it certainly may cause
asthenopia. Treatment is quite difficult.

• • •

Bibliography

Adler, F. H.: Physiology of the Eye, 5th
ed. Mosby, 1970.

Allen, J. H.: Strabismus Ophthalmic
Symposium II, 2nd ed. Mosby, 1958.

Burian, H. M.: Exodeviations: Their classification, diagnosis and treatment.
Am J Ophth **62**:1161-6, 1966.

Burian, H. M.: Pathophysiologic basis of
amblyopia and of its treatment. Am J
Ophth **67**:1-12, 1969.

Burian, H. M., & others: Symposium on
Strabismus. Mosby, 1971.

Costenbader, F. D.: Symposium: The "A"
and "V" patterns in strabismus. Tr Am
Acad Ophth **68**:354-86, 1964.

Duke-Elder, S.: Text-book of Ophthalmology, Vol. IV. Mosby, 1949.

Dunlap, E. A.: Selection of operative procedures in vertical muscle deviations.
Arch Ophth **64**:167-74, 1960.

Dyer, J. A.: Atlas of Extraocular Muscle
Surgery. Saunders, 1970.

Fink, W. H.: Surgery of the Oblique Muscles
of the Eye, 2nd ed. Mosby, 1962.

Gibson, G. G., & R. D. Harley: Sensori-
motor Anomalies of the Extrinsic Ocular
Muscles. Manual of American Academy
of Ophthalmology and Otolaryngology,
1961.

Linksz, A.: Pleoptics. Internat Ophth
Clin **1**:745-846, 1961.

Scott, A. B.: A and V patterns in exotropia.
An electromyographic study of horizontal
rectus muscles. Am J Ophth **65**:12-9,
1968.

Sugar, H. S.: The Extrinsic Eye Muscles.
Manual of American Academy of Ophthalmology and Otolaryngology, 1955.

Von Noorden, G. K.: Strabismus. Annual
review. Arch Ophth **84**:103-22, 1970.

15...

Glaucoma

Glaucoma includes a complex of disease entities which have in common an increase in intraocular pressure sufficient to cause degeneration of the optic disk and atrophy of the retina. An estimated 50,000 persons in the USA are blind as a result of glaucoma. The incidence of glaucoma in unselected persons over age 40 is between 1 and 2%.

The chief threat of chronic glaucoma is insidious visual impairment. The degree of interference with vision varies from slight blurring to complete blindness. The disease is bilateral and must be genetically determined, probably as an autosomal recessive trait which is so common that it is easily confused with dominant inheritance (pseudo-dominant). Infantile glaucoma usually has an autosomal recessive mode of inheritance, whereas some specific glaucoma syndromes are transmitted as autosomal dominant diseases. Acute glaucoma (angle-closure glaucoma) comprises less than 5% of primary glaucoma cases.

In most cases blindness can be prevented if treatment is instituted early. The objective of therapy is to facilitate the excretion of aqueous through existing outflow channels by the use of miotics, and in some cases to inhibit the secretion of aqueous by the ciliary processes, using systemically and topically administered drugs. The most commonly used miotic is pilocarpine. Operative treatment is sometimes indicated in the later stages when medical management is no longer sufficient to control the intraocular pressure.

The management of glaucoma is best left in the hands of the ophthalmologist, but all physicians should participate in diagnosis by making tonometry and ophthalmoscopy a part of the routine physical examination of all patients over 20 years of age. The procedure is simple and the equipment is not expensive. Tonometry and ophthalmoscopy should be done routinely by the internist and general practitioner, and doubtful cases should be referred to an ophthalmologist for confirmation and management.

Classification

A generally accepted classification of glaucoma is as follows:

A. Primary Glaucoma:
1. Open-angle*(simple, wide-angle, chronic simple)(the most common form).
2. Angle-closure*(narrow-angle, closed-angle, acute congestive) -
   a. Acute.
   b. Subacute or chronic.

B. Congenital Glaucoma:
1. Primary congenital or infantile glaucoma (buphthalmos, hydrophthalmos).
2. Glaucoma associated with congenital anomalies (includes types formerly classified as juvenile glaucoma) -
   a. Pigmentary glaucoma.
   b. Aniridia.
   c. Axenfeld's syndrome.
   d. Sturge-Weber syndrome.
   e. Infantile glaucoma developing late.
   f. Marfan's syndrome.
   g. Neurofibromatosis.
   h. Lowe's syndrome.
   i. Spherophakia.
   j. Microcornea.

C. Secondary Glaucoma:
1. Due to changes of the lens -
   a. Dislocation.
   b. Intumescence.
   c. Phacotoxic or phaco-anaphylactic.
   d. Glaucoma capsulare (pseudoexfoliation of lens capsule).
2. Due to changes of the uveal tract -
   a. Iridocyclitis.
   b. Tumor.
   c. Essential iris atrophy.
3. Due to trauma -
   a. Massive hemorrhage into the anterior chamber.

---

*In 1954 a group of the world's leading ophthalmologists, organized by the Council for International Organization of Medical Sciences, held a symposium on glaucoma. At this meeting, the terms "simple glaucoma" and "closed-angle glaucoma" were chosen to designate the 2 primary types. In the USA the terms "open-angle glaucoma" and "angle-closure glaucoma" are more common and will be retained in this text.

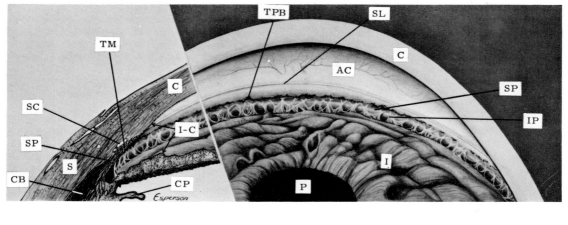

AC = anterior chamber I   = iris   S = sclera   TM = trabecular mesh-
C   = cornea   I-C = iris-corneal angle SC = Schlemm's canal   work
CB = ciliary body   IP = iris processes   SL = Schwalbe's line   TPB = trabecular pigment
CP = ciliary process   P   = pupil   SP = scleral spur   band

Fig 15-1. **Composite illustration showing anatomic (left) and gonioscopic (right) view of normal anterior chamber angle.** (Courtesy of R. Shaffer.)

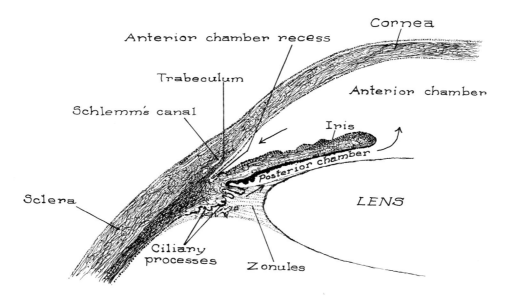
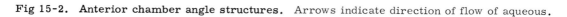

Fig 15-2. **Anterior chamber angle structures.** Arrows indicate direction of flow of aqueous.

b. Massive hemorrhage into the posterior chamber.

c. Corneal or limbal laceration with iris prolapse into the wound.

d. Retrodisplacement of iris root following contusion.

4. Following surgical procedures -

a. Epithelial ingrowth into the anterior chamber.

b. Failure of prompt restoration of the anterior chamber following cataract extraction.

5. Associated with rubeosis (diabetes mellitus and central retinal vein occlusion).

6. Associated with pulsating exophthalmos.

7. Associated with topical use of corticosteroids.

8. Other rare causes of secondary glaucoma.

D. Absolute Glaucoma: The end result of any uncontrolled glaucoma is a hard, sightless, and often painful eye.

PHYSIOLOGY OF GLAUCOMA

Aqueous Humor

The intraocular pressure is determined by the rate of aqueous production by the ciliary body and the resistance to outflow of aqueous from the eye. Some knowledge of the physiology of aqueous is necessary to an understanding of glaucoma.

A. Composition of Aqueous: The aqueous is a clear liquid that fills the anterior and posterior chambers of the eye. Its volume is about 125 μl. The osmotic pressure of aqueous is slightly higher than that of plasma. The total protein content is 0.02% (as compared with 7% in blood serum). The albumin-globulin ratio is the same as that of blood serum (2:1). In general, the same electrolytes and other components are found in the aqueous as in plasma, although the concentrations differ.

Emptying of the anterior chamber, either by surgery or trauma or during intraocular inflammatory conditions, causes the formation of plasmoid aqueous, which closely resembles blood serum and has a much higher protein concentration than normal aqueous.

B. Formation and Flow of Aqueous: A great deal is known about the dynamics of aqueous humor, but the exact mechanism of production and elimination of aqueous is not completely understood. Water, electrolytes, and nonelectrolytes enter and leave the eye at varying rates. Water enters both by diffusion

from the ciliary body and by secretion from the epithelium of the ciliary processes. From the posterior chamber the fluid passes through the pupil into the anterior chamber. The flow in the anterior chamber is peripheral, toward the filtering trabecular meshwork and into Schlemm's canal. Efferent channels from Schlemm's canal (about 30 collector channels and about 12 aqueous veins) conduct the fluid into the venous system. There is also a constant exchange of nonelectrolytes as well as a major exchange of water in and out of the iris stroma. (The vessels of the iris are impermeable to ions.)

SPECIAL DIAGNOSTIC TECHNICS
(See also Chapter 3.)

A number of special diagnostic tests have been developed to help detect, classify, and follow the course of glaucoma.

Tonometry

This is the most important test in establishing the diagnosis of glaucoma since it measures the intraocular pressure. A single normal reading either with the Schiotz or applanation tonometer does not rule out glaucoma, however, as the intraocular pressure may vary within wide limits. A single "high normal" reading (24-32 mm Hg) suggests glaucoma and requires repeated testing before making a diagnosis.

Gonioscopy

This test differentiates angle-closure from open-angle glaucoma, demonstrates the extent of peripheral anterior synechias, and offers the only means of detecting an impending angle closure before there is any rise in intraocular pressure. It is an essential part of any glaucoma evaluation.

Tonography

Tonography aids greatly in detecting early cases of open-angle glaucoma, and is helpful in evaluating the effectiveness of therapy in open-angle glaucoma. It consists of applying the tonometer (usually electronic with a special recording device) to the eye and recording the intraocular tension over a 4-minute period. Mathematical calculations based upon these measurements allow an approximation of the amount of aqueous leaving the eye per unit of time. Comparison of this figure with normal readings gives an index of the outflow mechanism of the eye in question. Low readings are often obtained in open-angle glaucoma before any other signs appear. Readings are normal in acute angle-closure glaucoma between attacks if no synechias have formed and are decreased in subacute angle-closure glaucoma in direct proportion to the amount of angle closure caused by iris apposition to the trabeculum. Tonography may be helpful in the diagnosis of open-angle glaucoma when the pressure is only moderately elevated.

Provocative Tests

A. Dark Room Test of Seidel: The patient sits in a dark room for one hour without going to sleep. A rise in intraocular tension of more than 8 mm indicates that iris blockage is impeding outflow when the pupil is relatively dilated. Positive results are obtained in acute and subacute angle-closure glaucoma. The test is usually negative in open-angle glaucoma. A negative result does not rule out impending angle-closure glaucoma.

B. Mydriatic Test: The same principle is utilized as in the dark room test except that a drug is used to dilate the pupil. Phenylephrine (Neo-Synephrine®), 2.5%, or a similar weak mydriatic solution, is instilled into one eye at a time and tonometric readings are taken at intervals of 10 minutes for one hour. A rise of 5-10 mm Hg constitutes a positive test. The test is hazardous, and miotics must be used immediately if there is any evidence of acute glaucoma.

C. Water Drinking Test: Breakfast is withheld and an initial tonometric pressure is recorded. The patient then drinks one quart of water, and intraocular pressures are recorded after 30, 45, and 60 minutes. A rise of more than 8 mm indicates a poor outflow mechanism. The test is usually negative in acute angle-closure glaucoma but may be positive in subacute angle-closure glaucoma. It is often positive in open-angle glaucoma (30%), although a negative test does not rule out open-angle glaucoma.

D. Tonography Following Water Drinking Test: One of the most reliable provocative tests for open-angle glaucoma is having the patient drink one quart of water and performing tonography 45 minutes later. A calculation involving the intraocular pressure and resistance to aqueous outflow gives results at least 90% reliable in detection of open-angle glaucoma from a single test.

E. Prone Position Test: If a patient lies in the prone position and the intraocular pressure rises 8-10 mm Hg, there may be some significance. This recently conceived provocative test is still in the trial stage.

Visual Fields in Glaucoma

The visual field test is most important in detecting open-angle glaucoma and in following the course of visual deterioration caused by the disease. The tangent screen, using a 2 mm white object at 1 meter, gives important information. Small extensions of the blind spot or early nerve fiber bundle defects not necessarily connected to the blind spot are noted early in the disease. Ideally, the diagnosis is made before visual field loss occurs. Under these circumstances medical control can usually prevent visual loss entirely.

The nerve fibers are arranged in the retina as indicated in the illustration on p 199. Increased intraocular pressure at the nerve head will gradually destroy the function of a bundle of these fibers, and the resulting visual field defect is spoken of as a "nerve fiber bundle defect." As the nerve fiber bundle defect enlarges, it takes an arcuate shape from the blind spot encircling the fixation area. It arches into either the superior or inferior field and ends at the horizontal meridian (Bjerrum scotoma). A double arcuate scotoma (one in the superior and one in the inferior field) forms a full-ring scotoma around the central fixation area.

Loss of peripheral field occurs later in the course of the disease. The nasal and superior fields are usually lost first. The last remnant of the visual field is usually a temporal island.

The field of vision may slowly contract in some cases down to 5° from fixation, leaving the patient with good central vision but no peripheral vision for a long time. Central visual acuity, therefore, is not a reliable index to the progress of the disease. There is no substitute for careful periodic study of the visual field combined with ophthalmoscopic visualization of the optic disks.

OPEN-ANGLE GLAUCOMA

At least 90% of cases of primary glaucoma are of the open-angle type. Open-angle glaucoma is bilateral, insidious in onset, and slowly progressive. There are no symptoms until visual impairment occurs, often too late to salvage useful vision. It is therefore the physician's responsibility to diagnose glaucoma before irreversible optic nerve damage has occurred. Early treatment prevents or delays visual deterioration.

Significant advances in the understanding of the course of open-angle glaucoma have been made in recent years, but unsolved problems remain and there are still differences of opinion among authorities on some issues. It now seems certain that increased intraocular pressure is caused by interference with aqueous outflow due to degenerative changes in the trabeculum, Schlemm's canal, and adjacent channels (see below). There is also a rare type of primary open-angle glaucoma caused by hypersecretion of aqueous humor (confirmed by tonography). Increased pressure, whether caused by faulty excretion or increased produc-

tion of aqueous, affects primarily the retina and optic nerve, the functional elements of the eye.

Some authorities feel that in open-angle glaucoma there is also a primary degenerative disorder of the optic nerve due to vascular insufficiency. This view is supported by the observation that loss of function sometimes continues to progress even after the intraocular pressure has been normalized by miotic therapy or surgery.

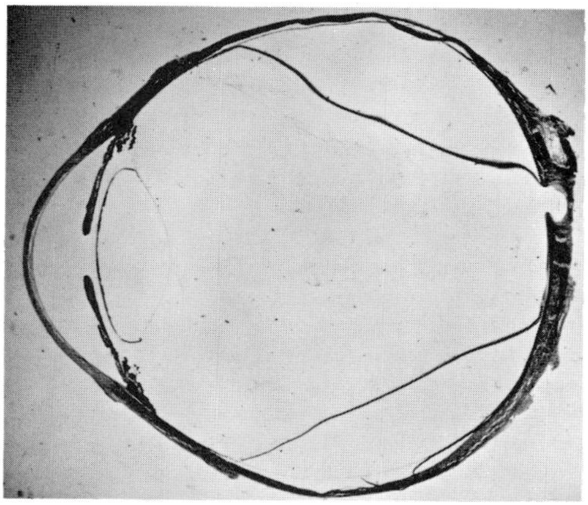

Fig 15-3. Cross section of an eye with open-angle glaucoma. Note open anterior chamber angle (peripheral iris is not in contact with the posterior corneal surface). Deep glaucomatous cupping (bean-pot appearance) shows the process to be well advanced. (Courtesy of R. Carriker.)

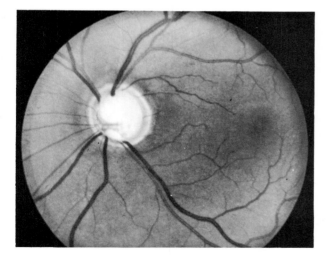

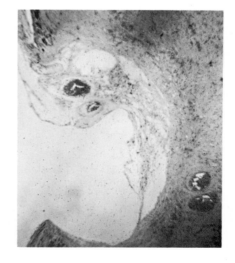

Fig 15-4. Typical glaucomatous cupping. Note the nasal displacement of the vessels and hollowed-out appearance of the optic disk except for a thin border. (Courtesy of Stacey Mettier, Jr.)

Fig 15-5. Glaucomatous ("bean pot") cupping of the optic disk.

There are few detectable histologic changes in the early stages of open-angle glaucoma. In the later stages nonspecific changes occur which are common to all forms of primary glaucoma. Studies upon eyes with early open-angle glaucoma have revealed primary degeneration in the trabecular meshwork, with degeneration of the collagen and elastic fibers of the trabeculum as well as endothelial proliferation and edema. The trabecular spaces tend to be obliterated. The collector channels also undergo degenerative changes.

If the pressure remains elevated, gross damage to the eye occurs. The optic nerve undergoes degeneration, often assuming a typical bean-pot cupping appearance (Fig 15-5). There is degeneration of ganglion cells and nerve fibers in the retina. The iris and ciliary body become atrophic, and the ciliary processes show hyaline degeneration. Chronic edema of the cornea results in loosening of the corneal epithelium and formation of epithelial bullae (bullous keratopathy). Eventually the lens shows cataractous changes.

Genetic aspects: Open-angle glaucoma is a familial, genetically determined disorder. Its hereditary pattern is consistent with autosomal dominant inheritance with decreased penetrance. However, Becker's interpretation of the corticosteroid provocative test suggests to him that open-angle glaucoma may result from a very frequently occurring autosomal recessive gene. He theorizes that eyes giving responses above 31 mm Hg are homozygously affected; that the intermediate group—pressure rises to 20-30 mm Hg—represent the heterozygous carriers; and that the 60-70% whose pressures do not rise to 20 mm Hg have no abnormal glaucoma gene.

Regardless of whether the disorder is a dominant or a frequent recessive, family history and the routine systematic testing of relatives of glaucoma patients are most important in glaucoma detection.

Clinical Findings

Open-angle glaucoma causes no early symptoms. Subjective visual loss is nearly always a late finding. Although the disease is nearly always bilateral, one eye is frequently involved earlier and more severely than the other.

Optic disk changes are important early findings. The temporal disk margin thins (Fig 15-4) and the cup gradually becomes wider and deeper. The large vessels become nasally displaced, and the affected area of the disk becomes atrophic (light gray or white rather than pink).

The intraocular pressure (IOP) is increased. The anterior chamber angle may be normal on gonioscopy. Tonography reveals a decreased rate of aqueous outflow which becomes more marked as the disease progresses.

Visual loss is peripheral until late in the course of the disease. Careful visual field evaluation is most important since it is the only method of accurately following the loss of visual function during the disease.

Treatment

A. Medical Treatment: Miotics facilitate aqueous outflow by increasing the efficiency of the outflow channels. The exact mechanism of their effect is not understood. The drug of choice is pilocarpine, 1-4%, 2 drops in each eye up to 5 times daily. Physostigmine, 0.2-0.5%, may also be used, sometimes in combination with pilocarpine. Physostigmine ointment is sometimes used just before bedtime to supplement daytime drop medication. In general, the smallest dosage that will control tension and prevent visual field loss is used.

Isoflurophate (diisopropyl fluorophosphate, DFP, Floropryl®), 0.1%, 1 drop once or twice a day, and echothiophate (Phospholine®) iodide are the longest-acting miotics available. **Caution:** These drugs should not be used in the presence of a narrow anterior chamber angle or in chronic angle-closure glaucoma since the extreme miosis increases relative pupillary block and can lead to acute angle closure. They are useful mainly to control open-angle glaucoma which is refractory to other forms of medical therapy.

Miotics frequently cause a temporary dimness of vision for 1-2 hours after instillation. Younger glaucoma patients or those with early cataract change are most prone to this unpleasant side effect.

There are now confirmed reports that the stronger miotics such as isoflurophate and echothiophate can cause insidious cataract development.

Epinephrine hydrochloride or borate instilled locally supplements the action of miotics by decreasing aqueous production. Tonography often reveals an improved facility of aqueous outflow while a patient is on epinephrine therapy.

Carbonic anhydrase inhibitors such as acetazolamide (Diamox®), 125-250 mg 4 times daily, are occasionally used in open-angle glaucoma if strong miotics and epinephrine do not adequately control intraocular tension. Dichlorphenamide (Daranide®), methazolamide (Neptazane®), and ethoxzolamide (Cardrase®, Ethamide®) are similarly effective carbonic anhydrase inhibitors and usually suppress aqueous production from 40-60%. Complications of long-term therapy with carbonic anhydrase inhibitors include renal calculi (see also p 292). Nevertheless, these drugs are occasionally indicated to avoid glaucoma surgery.

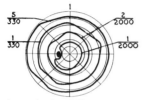

Baring of the blind spot. The earliest nerve fiber bundle defect.

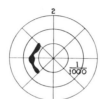

Incipient double nerve fiber bundle defect (Bjerrum Scotoma)

Bjerrum Scotoma isolated from blind spot.

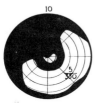

End stages in glaucoma field loss. Remnant of central field still shows nasal step

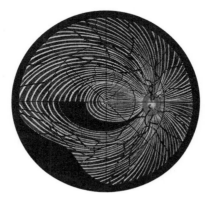

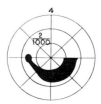

Fully developed nerve fiber bundle defect with nasal step. (Arcuate Scotoma)

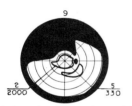

Peripheral depression with double nerve fiber bundle defect. Isolation of central field.

The basic visual field loss in glaucoma is the nerve fiber bundle defect with nasal step and peripheral nasal depression. It is here shown superimposed upon the nerve fiber layer of the retina and the retinal vascular tree. All perimetric changes in glaucoma are variations of these fundamental defects.

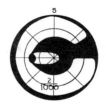

Double Arcuate Scotoma with peripheral break through and nasal step.

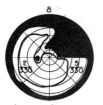

Nasal depression connected with Arcuate Scotoma. Nasal step of Ronne

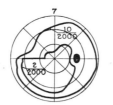

Peripheral break through of large nerve fiber bundle defect with well developed nasal step

Seidel Scotoma. Islands of greater visual loss within a nerve fiber bundle defect.

Fig 15-6. Visual field changes in glaucoma. (Reproduced, with permission, from Harrington: The Visual Fields, 2nd ed. Mosby, 1964.)

B. Surgical Treatment: (See p 207.) Filtering operations may be performed if the intraocular pressure is not maintained within normal limits by medical therapy and there is progressive visual field loss. As a rule these procedures are delayed as long as possible, since at best they are mutilating and unphysiologic. A reliable operation for open-angle glaucoma is not available. Iridencleisis, trephine, sclerectomy, and cyclodialysis all have their advocates. Cyclodiathermy and cyclocryosurgery, which directly reduce the amount of aqueous formation by damaging the ciliary body, are generally used only in otherwise hopeless cases of advanced glaucoma.

Any of these operations may hasten the formation of cataract. For this reason some authorities advocate lens extraction as the primary glaucoma operation if significant lens opacity is present. Lens extraction alone often has a favorable effect upon the course of the glaucoma, and miotics may control the intraocular pressure after cataract surgery when they have failed to do so before surgery was performed. If the pressure is still uncontrolled after cataract surgery, cyclodialysis is the procedure of choice.

In general, the modern trend is to delay surgery as long as possible in open-angle glaucoma if the patient is faithful in adhering to his medical regimen and there is no evidence of damage to the optic nerve.

Course and Prognosis

Without treatment, open-angle glaucoma is insidiously progressive to complete blindness. If miotics control the intraocular pressure in an eye which has not had extensive glaucomatous damage, the prognosis is good (although visual field loss sometimes continues to progress in spite of normalized intraocular pressure. Response to medical treatment cannot be predicted initially. Tonographic studies are helpful prognostically.

LOW PRESSURE GLAUCOMA
(Pseudoglaucoma)

''Low pressure glaucoma'' and ''pseudoglaucoma'' are terms used to denote a number of conditions in which there is evidence of intraocular glaucomatous damage (cupping of the optic disk, visual field defects, etc) with normal or low intraocular pressure. Most such cases can be classified in the following groups:

(1) Cases of open-angle glaucoma in which reduced scleral rigidity causes falsely low pressure readings by Schiotz tonometry. The truly elevated intraocular pressure is determined by use of the applanation tonometer (see p 23). These cases are being recognized with increasing frequency as applanation tonometry becomes more widely used in glaucoma evaluation. Low scleral rigidity is particularly common following intraocular surgery, in association with myopia, and in patients receiving miotic therapy.

(2) Cases in which some type of glaucoma, usually secondary, has caused permanent changes and then regressed spontaneously.

(3) Cases of open-angle glaucoma with hyposecretion of aqueous as well as decreased facility of aqueous outflow. Such cases can be diagnosed by tonography.

(4) **Hypersecretion glaucoma:** The pressure is usually normal when taken but is elevated at other times. This may be due to diurnal variation, so that if the pressure is always measured at the same time of day it seems to be normal. Tonography studies disclose the real diagnosis.

(5) A variety of miscellaneous cases of damage to the optic nerve and retina due to vascular, congenital, degenerative, and other causes. Some of these are apparently due to reduced blood pressure and blood flow to the optic nerve.

ANGLE-CLOSURE GLAUCOMA
(Acute Glaucoma)

Angle-closure glaucoma occurs when there is a sudden increase in the intraocular tension due to a block of the anterior chamber angle by the root of the iris which cuts off all aqueous outflow, causing severe pain and sudden visual loss.

An acute attack of angle-closure glaucoma can develop only in an eye in which the anterior chamber angle is anatomically narrow. Such eyes often have shallow anterior chambers and tend to have a short axial length (hyperopic eyes). The factors listed below may cause further encroachment upon the anterior chamber angle, setting the stage for angle closure glaucoma.

(1) **Physiologic iris bombé:** In eyes which tend to have the above-listed anatomic configurations, the iris has a relatively large arc of contact with the anterior surface of the lens. This may obstruct the free passage of aqueous from the posterior to the anterior chamber. As pressure builds up in the posterior chamber, the peripheral iris is pushed forward. If the iris is pushed forward far enough so that it lies against the trabeculum, an attack of acute angle-closure glaucoma occurs.

(2) **Increased size of the lens:** Normally the lens continues to enlarge slightly with age. During the act of accommodation there may be a further increase in the forward displacement of the lens, pushing the iris against the trabeculum.

(3) **Increased thickness of the iris:** This is greatly increased during pupillary dilatation and may be a contributing factor in blocking an anatomically predisposed angle.

Precipitating factors: A sudden increase in the volume of the posterior chamber may push the iris forward against the trabeculum. This results from congestion or edema of the iris, ciliary body, or choroid or from a sudden increase in aqueous production. The causes of these changes are not known.

Therapeutic or physiologic mydriasis occasionally bunches the iris into the chamber angle sufficiently to precipitate an acute attack of angle-closure glaucoma. **Caution:** Dilation of the pupil should be avoided if the anterior chamber is shallow. This is easily determined by oblique illumination of the anterior segment of the eye (Fig 15-7).

An eye which is predisposed to acute angle-closure glaucoma has a shallow anterior chamber. Otherwise the eye is normal, with complete permeability of the trabeculum, Schlemm's canal, and the aqueous veins. A rapid increase in intraocular pressure occurs when the peripheral iris is forced against the trabeculum, occluding the outflow channels.

The pathologic changes in acute glaucoma include peripheral anterior synechias and edema and congestion of the ciliary processes and iris. These are secondary to the vascular strangulation which results from the high pressure. Late changes are the result of interference with circulation and the continued high pressure. The iris and ciliary body become atrophic, and the ciliary processes show hyaline degeneration. Chronic edema of the cornea results in loosening of the corneal epithelium and the formation of epithelial bullae (bullous keratopathy). The only important pathologic change is damage to the nerve elements: degeneration of nerve fibers and a loss of substance of the optic cup associated with a backward bowing of the cribriform plate. The ganglion cell layer and the nerve fiber layer of the retina undergo degeneration. Eventually the lens may show cataractous change. In the later stages these eyes are similar to eyes in the late stages of open-angle glaucoma.

Clinical Findings

Angle-closure (acute) glaucoma is characterized by a sudden onset of blurred vision followed by excruciating pain. Nausea and vomiting are often present. The pain is usually localized in and around the eye. Other findings include markedly increased intraocular pressure, a shallow anterior chamber, an edematous cornea, decreased visual acuity (at times limited to light perception only), a fixed, moderately dilated pupil, and ciliary injection.

Differential Diagnosis

Acute iritis and conjunctivitis must be considered with acute angle-closure glaucoma

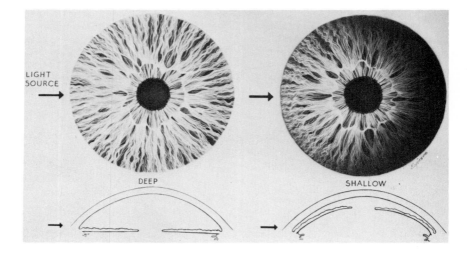

Fig 15-7. Estimation of depth of the anterior chamber by oblique illumination (diagram). (Courtesy of R. Shaffer.)

in the differential diagnosis of any acutely inflamed eye. (1) Acute iritis causes more photophobia and less pain than acute glaucoma. Intraocular pressure is normal, the pupil is constricted, and the cornea is not edematous. Marked flare and cells are present in the anterior chamber, and there is deep ciliary injection. (2) In acute conjunctivitis there is little or no pain and no visual loss. There is discharge from the eye and an intensely inflamed conjunctiva, but no ciliary injection. The pupillary responses are normal, the cornea is clear, and intraocular pressure is normal. (3) Iridocyclitis with secondary glaucoma occasionally presents a difficult problem of differentiation. Gonioscopy to define the type of angle is most helpful. If corneal or anterior chamber haze prevents good visibility, gonioscopy of the other eye will usually confirm the diagnosis.

Complications and Sequelae

A. Formation of Peripheral Anterior Synechias: The peripheral iris adheres to the posterior corneal surface in the trabecular area and blocks the outflow of aqueous.

B. Cataract Formation: The lens sometimes swells, and a cataract may develop. The enlarged lens pushes the iris even farther anteriorly; this increases the pupillary block, which in turn increases the degree of angle block.

C. Atrophy of the Retina and Optic Nerve: The nerve elements of the eye withstand increased intraocular pressure poorly. Glaucomatous cupping of the optic disk and retinal atrophy, particularly of the ganglion cell layer, occur. Neurovascular changes in the posterior segment of the eye may contribute to this process.

D. Absolute Glaucoma: The end result of uncontrolled angle-closure glaucoma is the same as that of any other uncontrolled glaucoma, ie, absolute glaucoma. The eye is stony hard, sightless, and often quite painful, in which case enucleation or retrobulbar alcohol injection is necessary.

Treatment

Angle-closure glaucoma is an ophthalmic surgical emergency.

A. Medical Treatment: Before surgery, every effort must be made to reduce the intraocular pressure by medical means. The combination of an osmotic agent and a miotic is the medical treatment of choice. The immediate administration of oral glycerine (glycerol), 1 ml/kg body weight in a 50% solution mixed with chilled lemon juice, nearly always interrupts the acute attack by making the blood hypertonic and drawing fluid from the eye. Pilocarpine, 4%, 2 drops every 15 minutes for several hours, will usually constrict the pupil and pull the iris away from the trabeculum, allowing aqueous outflow to be reestablished (unless permanent adhesions have formed).

If treatment with glycerine is not successful, intravenous hypertonic mannitol (20%) may be effective in total doses of 1.5-3 gm/kg. Intravenous urea (Urevert®), 1 gm/kg body weight, is also an effective osmotic agent.

Meperidine (Demerol®), 100 mg IM, or other systemic analgesics should be given as necessary to relieve pain.

B. Surgical Treatment: (See p 207.) In general, if the pressure has not begun to recede within 4-6 hours of medical treatment as outlined above, surgical intervention is mandatory. Peripheral iridectomy is the procedure of choice. It is often performed on the fellow eye within a week to prevent an acute attack.

Course and Prognosis

An acute attack of glaucoma may terminate without treatment, but if the pressure remains at a high level the eye soon undergoes irreparable damage. Medical or surgical intervention is usually required to reduce the pressure to normal if eye function is to be preserved.

Miotics may prevent attacks of acute glaucoma indefinitely in predisposed individuals. More commonly, however, acute attacks occur despite miotics. An acute attack occurs in the second eye in at least 50% of cases even when miotic prophylactic treatment has been conscientiously carried out. Well controlled peripheral iridectomies have little operative risk and result in true cure of angle-closure glaucoma if permanent anterior synechias have not formed. Acetazolamide (Diamox®) is contraindicated between attacks since its action could easily mask the extension of peripheral anterior synechias until involvement is so severe that iridectomy would not be effective.

SUBACUTE OR CHRONIC ANGLE-CLOSURE GLAUCOMA

Chronic angle-closure glaucoma is caused by the same etiologic factors as acute angle-closure glaucoma. The difference is that there is no sudden complete block to aqueous outflow by the iris being pushed against the trabeculum. The iris extends its arc of contact with the trabeculum gradually until an adequate area of angle is no longer available for aqueous outflow. The pressure rises and glaucoma results which may be clinically similar to open-angle glaucoma.

Clinical Findings

Symptoms are minimal or absent. Occasional mild attacks of increased intraocular pressure cause transient blurring of vision, halos around lights, and possibly slight pain in or about the eyes. On examination one finds a shallow anterior chamber, high intraocular pressure (25-50 mm Hg Schiotz), and a gonioscopically narrow chamber angle. The iris is in apposition to the trabeculum except in an area covering one-fifth or less of the chamber angle. Tonography indicates decreased facility of aqueous outflow. Not until late in the disease are typical glaucomatous visual field changes and cupping of the optic disk observed. Provocative tests are not necessary since the glaucoma is obvious from tonometric study.

Complications and Sequelae

A. Acute Attack: If the last open segment of the chamber angle is suddenly blocked, a full-blown attack of glaucoma occurs. Untreated cases which escape an acute attack undergo slow degeneration much like that which occurs in open-angle glaucoma. The end result is absolute glaucoma: a sightless, stony-hard, and often painful eye.

B. Malignant Glaucoma: Unavoidable surgery upon an eye with markedly increased tension can lead to malignant glaucoma, a severe disorder which is not fully understood. Immediately after surgery the intraocular tension increases markedly and the lens-iris diaphragm is pushed forward as a result of the collection of aqueous in and behind the vitreous body. Both angle block and pupillary block make effective treatment difficult. Maximum dilatation of the iris will at times break the pupillary block and cure the attack. If this fails, surgical intervention is mandatory. Intracapsular lens extraction is the procedure of choice even if no cataract is present. This should be done as soon as possible, preferably after the pressure has been temporarily lowered by the systemic administration of urea, mannitol, or glycerol (see p 202). If the pressure cannot be lowered before surgery, vitreous aspiration through a posterior scleral incision should be performed before lens extraction.

C. Other complications and sequelae include cataract and atrophy of the optic nerve and retina as described for acute angle-closure glaucoma.

Treatment

A. Medical Treatment: Pilocarpine, 1-4%, or carbachol (Doryl®), 0.5-2%, 2 drops in the affected eye 5 times daily as necessary, may reduce the base pressure and prevent transient rises in intraocular pressure.

B. Surgical Treatment: Once the diagnosis of chronic angle-closure glaucoma is made, surgical intervention is indicated. Peripheral iridectomy (see p 207) may allow the iris to fall away from the posterior corneal surface if the iris is not permanently adherent to the trabeculum. This also relieves whatever physiologic pupillary block is present. Iridectomy may prove to be inadequate if too great an area of the filtration angle is blocked by permanent anterior synechias. In these cases, a filtering operation is performed.

Course and Prognosis

Chronic angle-closure glaucoma causes transient episodes of relatively slight elevations in intraocular tension (25-40 mm Hg Schiotz). During these periods insidious damage occurs to the nerve elements of the eye. Anterior peripheral synechias slowly extend and further impede the aqueous outflow.

Permanent medical control of chronic angle-closure glaucoma is usually not possible. The sooner peripheral iridectomy is performed, the better the ultimate visual prognosis will be. When the disease has progressed to the point that a filtration operation is necessary, the long-term visual prognosis becomes much more guarded.

PRIMARY CONGENITAL OR INFANTILE GLAUCOMA

Infantile glaucoma can be defined as that form of increased intraocular pressure (bilateral) which has its onset at birth or in the first 3 years of life. It is usually an autosomal recessive trait. The filtration angle forms by a cleavage between the corneal elements and the less rapidly growing iris elements in the embryo. Incomplete cleavage, preventing normal angle development, prevents normal outflow of aqueous and causes infantile glaucoma.

The insertion of the iris onto the trabeculum is abnormally high. The scleral spur is poorly developed and is more posterior than normally. Because aqueous is unable to reach it, Schlemm's canal is usually collapsed.

Clinical Findings

The earliest and most constant symptom is epiphora. Photophobia may be present.

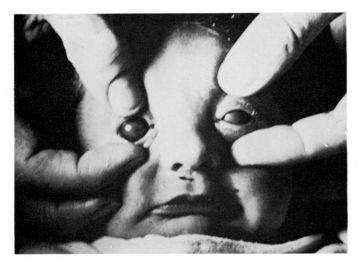

Fig 15-8. Infantile glaucoma
(buphthalmos).

Increased intraocular pressure is the cardinal
sign. Glaucomatous cupping of the optic disk
is a relatively early and most important change.
Later findings include increased corneal diameter (above 11.5 mm is considered significant),
epithelial edema, tears of Descemet's membrane, and increased depth of the anterior
chamber (associated with general enlargement
of the anterior segment of the eye), as well as
edema and opacity of the corneal stroma. The
iris inserts anteriorly onto the trabeculum instead of into the ciliary body.

Differential Diagnosis
Megalocornea, secondary glaucoma, and
traumatic corneal haze should be ruled out.
Measurement of intraocular tension is the key
to differential diagnosis.

Treatment
Unlike open-angle glaucoma, in which the
best treatment is often nonsurgical, infantile
glaucoma must be treated surgically to obtain
lasting results. Medical treatment with miotics is at best a preoperative adjunctive
measure.
Goniotomy is the treatment of choice. If
repeated goniotomies fail, a filtering operation
(eg, sclerectomy, trephine, iridencleisis) is
used. The long-term visual prognosis is then
much less favorable.

Course and Prognosis
In untreated cases, blindness occurs early.
The eye undergoes marked stretching and may
even rupture with minor trauma. Typical
glaucomatous cupping occurs relatively soon,
emphasizing the necessity of early effective
treatment.

The earlier the disease becomes manifest,
the less favorable the prognosis, since the
early appearance of symptoms implies a more
severe defect of aqueous drainage. Over 80%
of cases are evident by age 3 months. Goniotomy controls the tension permanently in 70-
80% of cases. A recent follow-up series shows
somewhat disappointing long-term visual results despite effective control of intraocular
tension. This may be due in part to amblyopia caused by anisometropia and failure to
correct refractive errors adequately prior to
age 7.

CONGENITAL GLAUCOMA ASSOCIATED
WITH OTHER CONGENITAL ANOMALIES
(Formerly classified as Juvenile Glaucoma)

A number of syndromes characterized by
increased intraocular pressure occurring in
persons under 40 have been arbitrarily grouped
under this broad heading, which includes late-
developing infantile glaucoma.

Pigmentary Glaucoma
This syndrome seems to be primarily a
degeneration of the pigmented epithelium of
the iris and ciliary body. The pigment granules
flake off and are deposited on the posterior corneal surface (Krukenberg's spindle). The pigment becomes lodged in the trabecular meshwork and impedes the normal outflow of aqueous. The syndrome occurs most often in young
myopic males between the ages of 25 and 40
who have a deep anterior chamber with a wide
anterior chamber angle.

A number of pedigrees of autosomal dominant inheritance of pigmentary glaucoma have been reported. The pigmentary changes may be present without glaucoma, but such persons must be considered "glaucoma suspects."

This type of glaucoma responds to miotics fairly well, but the prognosis is not favorable if the process is severe enough to require surgery. A filtering operation such as trephine or sclerectomy is the procedure of choice.

Aniridia

The distinguishing feature of aniridia, as the name implies, is the vestigial iris. Often little more than the root of the iris or a thin iris margin is present. Other deformities of the anterior segment of the eye may be present, most often congenital cataract. Glaucoma frequently develops before adolescence and is usually refractory to medical or surgical management.

The syndrome is genetically determined. Numerous examples of both autosomal dominant and recessive inheritance have appeared in the literature.

If medical therapy is ineffective, goniotomy may occasionally normalize the intraocular pressure. More often, filtering operations such as sclerectomy or trephine are necessary, but the long-term prognosis for retention of good visual function is poor.

Axenfeld's Syndrome (Rieger's Syndrome)

This rare syndrome is characterized by the presence of a posterior embryotoxon: prominent Schwalbe's line and iris adhesions to Schwalbe's line. It appears much like arcus senilis except that there is no clear zone at the limbus. Anomalies of the iris and anterior chamber angle are frequently associated, often resulting in increased resistance to aqueous outflow and therefore increased intraocular pressure. The glaucoma is apparent by adolescence or early adulthood.

This disease is genetically determined, most frequently as a dominant, but some sporadic cases are also seen, indicating a recessive pattern.

Treatment is the same as for open-angle glaucoma. If surgery is indicated, sclerectomy or trephine is the procedure of choice. The prognosis is poor for long-term retention of good visual function.

Other Rare Glaucoma Syndromes

Glaucoma is frequently associated with Sturge-Weber or Marfan's syndrome and rarely with neurofibromatosis, Lowe's syndrome, spherophakia with microcornea, and many other ocular syndromes.

SECONDARY GLAUCOMA

Increased intraocular tension occurring as one manifestation of intraocular disease is called secondary glaucoma. These diseases are difficult to classify satisfactorily.

In addition to treatment of the underlying disease, several drugs are of value in control of secondary glaucoma. With moderate elevation of intraocular tension, reduction of aqueous production with epinephrine, with or without carbonic anhydrase inhibitors, is adequate. With extreme elevations, osmotic agents are indicated. These antihypertensive drugs may prevent permanent damage due to increased intraocular pressure until the underlying cause of secondary glaucoma can be controlled.

GLAUCOMA SECONDARY TO CHANGES IN THE LENS

Lens Dislocation

The lens may dislocate anteriorly, pressing the iris against the posterior cornea and blocking aqueous outflow, or it may dislocate posteriorly. Secondary glaucoma is a frequent complication of posterior dislocation of the lens and is not easy to explain. Tonography at times reveals decreased facility of aqueous outflow for no obvious reason. In other cases pupillary block occurs when a wedge of vitreous curls around the dislocated lens and plugs the pupillary opening. Whatever the mechanism, lens extraction is indicated if the intraocular pressure cannot be controlled medically.

Intumescence of the Lens

The lens may take up considerable fluid during cataractous change, increasing its size markedly. It may then encroach upon the anterior chamber, produce a pupillary block, or cause angle occlusion, resulting in angle-closure glaucoma. Treatment consists of lens extraction.

Phacotoxic and Phaco-anaphylactic Glaucoma

As cataract formation proceeds, the lens cortex elements may undergo liquefaction and seep out through the lens capsule. These protein products are often toxic or may cause an anaphylactic reaction within the eye. In either event uveitis occurs, and the protein and cellular debris lodge in the outflow system to obstruct the free passage of aqueous. Edema of the trabeculum itself is probably associated, further decreasing the facility of aqueous outflow. Lens extraction is indicated.

Glaucoma Capsulare (Pseudo-exfoliation of the Lens Capsule)

In pseudo-exfoliation of the lens capsule (glaucoma capsulare), deposits of unknown origin and composition are seen on the lens surface, ciliary processes, lens zonules, posterior iris surface, loose in the anterior chamber, and in the trabecular meshwork. Glaucoma and sometimes cataract eventually develop. Lens extraction has no effect on the glaucoma. Miotics are moderately effective, but a filtering operation may be necessary.

GLAUCOMA SECONDARY TO CHANGES IN THE UVEAL TRACT

Uveitis

Often the intraocular pressure is below normal early in uveitis. This is because the inflamed ciliary body is functioning poorly and does not secrete the elements which produce the difference in osmotic pressure between aqueous and plasma. There is edema of the trabeculum as well as the ciliary body and iris, and this may result in a decreased facility of aqueous outflow. As long as there is no osmotic difference between blood and aqueous there will be no rise in tension, but when the ciliary body begins secreting there will be an abrupt rise of pressure unless there has been a simultaneous improvement in the patency of the outflow channels. Long-standing or repeated attacks of iridocyclitis cause permanent damage to the trabeculum or extensive permanent anterior synechias. In these cases, after the inflammatory reaction has subsided, miotics or even filtering procedures may be needed to control the intraocular pressure.

Tumor

Rapidly growing melanomas originating in the uveal tract can cause increased intraocular pressure by volume replacement, encroachment on the filtration angle, or by blocking of a vortex vein. Enucleation is indicated.

Essential Atrophy of the Iris

Slowly progressive atrophy of iris tissue is a rare disorder of unknown etiology which is almost always associated with glaucoma. Anterior synechias form and the degenerated iris elements block the trabecular meshwork, creating a glaucoma that is very difficult to control either medically or surgically. The condition is nearly always unilateral.

GLAUCOMA SECONDARY TO TRAUMA

Massive Hemorrhage Into the Anterior Chamber

Contusion or penetrating injuries of the globe can cause tears in the iris or ciliary body and thus massive hemorrhage into the anterior chamber. The intraocular tension is immediately elevated, and blood breakdown products or organized clots lodge in the outflow mechanism. One serious complication is blood staining of the cornea. Once well established the staining may require several years to absorb. If the intraocular pressure cannot be controlled with systemic hypotensive drugs the hyphema should be evacuated through a limbal incision.

Corneal or Limbal Laceration With Prolapse of Iris Into the Wound

Lacerations of the anterior eye or contusions causing anterior rupture of the eye are sealed spontaneously by prolapse of uveal tissue into the wound. This ordinarily causes loss of the anterior chamber and the rapid closure of the chamber angle by the adherence of the iris to the cornea. The primary objective of treatment is the re-formation of the anterior chamber to prevent permanent anterior peripheral synechias. Excision of prolapsed uvea, tight closure of the wound, and injection of saline into the anterior chamber are of paramount importance.

Contusion Causing Retrodisplacement of the Iris Root and Deepening of Anterior Chamber Angle (Angle Recession Glaucoma)

A number of clinicians have called attention to this type of trauma-induced unilateral secondary glaucoma. Following a contusion injury, the anterior chamber is observed to be significantly deeper than in the uninjured eye. Gonioscopically one sees a recession of the angle with exposed ciliary body. Glaucoma occurs if there is sufficient associated damage to the trabecular meshwork to interfere with aqueous outflow. The condition often responds to standard open-angle glaucoma therapy, although occasionally a filtering operation is necessary.

GLAUCOMA FOLLOWING SURGERY

Epithelial Ingrowth Into the Anterior Chamber

Following cataract surgery with resultant poor healing of the wound edges, epithelium may grow into the anterior chamber and eventually line the anterior chamber angle structures, preventing normal outflow of aqueous. This is a difficult complication to treat once it is well established. An effort can be made to scrape the newly deposited epithelium off of the angle structures. The problem is primarily one of prevention.

Failure of Prompt Restoration of the Anterior Chamber Following Cataract Extraction

Following cataract extraction, the anterior chamber may remain flat as a result of a leaking corneal wound which allows aqueous to escape. If this persists longer than 5-7 days postoperatively, permanent anterior synechias may form.

GLAUCOMA SECONDARY TO RUBEOSIS IRIDIS

Rubeosis often follows central vein occlusion and occurs frequently in advanced diabetes mellitus. Small vessels grow on the anterior surface of the iris and into the anterior chamber angle, interfering with normal aqueous outflow. Miotics are of little value. Cyclodiathermy and cyclocryosurgery are the best therapeutic technics available, but results are poor.

GLAUCOMA SECONDARY TO PULSATING EXOPHTHALMOS

Pulsating exophthalmos from arteriovenous fistula is usually accompanied by a slightly elevated intraocular pressure due to increased venous pressure. Treatment is directed at the underlying condition.

GLAUCOMA SECONDARY TO THE USE OF TOPICAL CORTICOSTEROIDS

Much interest has been aroused by the observation that topically administered corticosteroids may produce a type of glaucoma that simulates open-angle glaucoma. Most persons do not develop significant intraocular pressure elevations while on such treatment. In those that do, withdrawal of the medication eliminates the glaucoma; but permanent damage can occur if the condition goes unrecognized too long. If topical steroid therapy is absolutely necessary, miotics or other open-angle glaucoma therapy

usually will control the glaucoma. It is imperative that patients receiving long-term topical steroid therapy should have periodic tonometry. It is equally important to beware of topical administration of corticosteroids in the eyes of patients known to have glaucoma or a family history of glaucoma. Less commonly, glaucoma can occur in patients on long-term systemic corticosteroids.

SURGICAL PROCEDURES USED IN THE TREATMENT OF THE GLAUCOMAS

PERIPHERAL IRIDECTOMY

In acute or chronic angle-closure glaucoma when extensive peripheral anterior synechias have not formed, peripheral iridectomy is the operation of choice. It offers the one hope of a permanent cure by reestablishing ready communication between the posterior and anterior chambers. This relieves pupillary block and allows the iris root to drop away from the filtration angle, thus reestablishing the outflow of aqueous by normal channels.

Technic

Under local anesthesia (including akinesia and retrobulbar injection as for cataract surgery), a small limbal-based conjunctival flap is turned down 4 mm behind the limbus. A scratch incision (ab externo) 4 mm long is used to enter the anterior chamber. By counterpressure at the opposite limbus a small wedge of iris is prolapsed into the scleral wound. The iris is picked up with a smooth forceps and a small piece cut out in its periphery. One preplaced suture is used to secure the limbal wound, and the conjunctival flap is sutured in place with a running suture.

Postoperative Care, Complications, and Prognosis

Postoperatively the eye is bandaged for one week, with daily changes. Posterior synechias develop easily, and care must be taken to keep the pupil dilated. There is no cosmetic blemish, and little or no change in visual acuity. Complications are rare if care is taken to prevent the development of synechias. In properly selected cases the results are excellent. If iridectomy does not normalize the intraocular pressure, then iridencleisis or some other filtering operation (ie, trephine or sclerectomy) is indicated.

IRIDENCLEISIS

Iridencleisis is used in open-angle glaucoma but more particularly in acute and sub-acute angle-closure glaucoma in patients whose eyes have narrow anterior chamber angles when extensive anterior synechias have formed. Like all filtering operations, it is unphysiologic in that it establishes an artificial way of draining aqueous. Here the iris is used as a wick in a limbal incision to allow aqueous to drain into the subconjunctival space for reabsorption there by the blood stream and diffusion through the conjunctival bleb into the tear film.

Technic

Under local anesthesia, a large conjunctival flap is turned down, usually centered at 12 o'clock, and an ab externo incision is used to enter the anterior chamber. The iris is then drawn into the wound and a complete radial iridotomy is performed. The 2 pillars of iris are pulled into the scleral wound and separated as much as the wound allows. The pillars lie on the sclera with the pigmented epithelial surfaces adjacent. The conjunctival wound is closed with a continuous suture. Postoperatively the aqueous flows through the limbal wound and is absorbed in the subconjunctival space or escapes through the bleb into the tear film. The incarcerated iris tends to keep the iridencleisis functioning, although 25-35% prove to be nonfunctioning within 6 months. Those still functioning at 6 months usually function permanently.

Postoperative Care, Complications, and Prognosis

The postoperative care is similar to that for iridectomy. Some surgeons advise daily massage for 1-2 weeks postoperatively at the iridencleisis site to help maintain patency of the filtering area. A noticeable surgical iris coloboma is present, and often there is an immediate decrease in visual acuity due to irregular astigmatism. Cataract formation is often hastened.

TREPHINE WITH IRIDECTOMY

This operation is similar to iridencleisis in that it establishes an abnormal aqueous drainage for subconjunctival absorption. The iridectomy relieves any pupillary block present. The operation is used primarily for open-angle glaucoma; it is technically more difficult for angle-closure glaucoma.

Technic

Under local anesthesia, a large limbal-based conjunctival flap is made in one quadrant of the eye. A small (1-2 mm) trephine is used to cut out a small button of tissue (ideally, half cornea and half sclera). An iridectomy, either full or peripheral, is performed

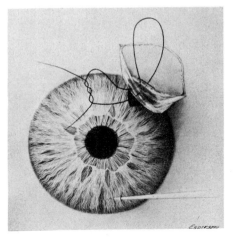 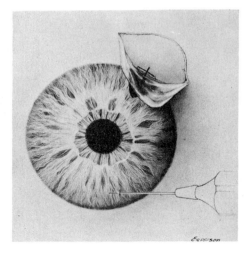

Fig 15-9. Peripheral iridectomy. Left: Position of iridectomy, conjunctival flap with McLean preplaced suture in place. Below, a tract through the cornea is made to allow re-formation of the anterior chamber at conclusion of operation if necessary. **Right:** Corneoscleral suture has been tied. If the anterior chamber is not re-formed, a small needle on a syringe is introduced through the corneal tract previously made with a Wheeler knife, and saline injected. Gonioscopy at this time determines if iridencleisis is necessary. (Courtesy of R. Shaffer.)

by picking up the iris through the trephine opening. The conjunctival flap is then resutured in place. The aqueous escapes through the trephine hole into the subconjunctival space, where some is absorbed into the blood stream and some diffuses through the conjunctiva into the tear film.

Postoperative Care, Complications, and Prognosis

This operation is somewhat more difficult to perform than iridencleisis and has more serious immediate complications, such as loss of vitreous, dislocated lens, and trauma to the lens leading to cataract formation. The conjunctiva tends to be thin over the bleb, so that intraocular infection occurs fairly frequently as a late complication. Nevertheless, it is preferred in many parts of the country as the primary operation in open-angle glaucoma as well as some types of secondary glaucoma.

SCLERECTOMY

This filtering operating has the same indications and is based upon the same principles as trephine.

After making a limbal-based conjunctival flap under local anesthesia, a scratch incision is made into the anterior chamber just behind the limbus. A short strip of sclera 1 mm wide is then removed from the anterior or posterior lip of the scleral incision. A full or peripheral iridectomy is performed and the flap reapproximated with a running conjunctival suture. Drainage is effected in the same way as after trephine, and the results are similar. The procedure is somewhat safer to perform than trephine but may have a lower percentage of effective postoperative filtration. The cosmetic blemish consists of a surgical iris coloboma. The procedure may be repeated if unsuccessful, but most surgeons prefer to select another type of glaucoma surgery, such as cyclodialysis, for the second operation. Another technic can be used to accomplish the same result. Cautery may be used on the scleral lip edges which causes scleral shrinkage and the permanent maintenance of a scleral opening (Scheie operation). This operation has proved quite effective, particularly in open-angle glaucoma.

CYCLODIALYSIS

This filtering operation uses another artificial route for aqueous escape, absorption into the suprachoroidal space. It is the operation of choice in aphakic glaucoma. It is used less frequently in open-angle glaucoma.

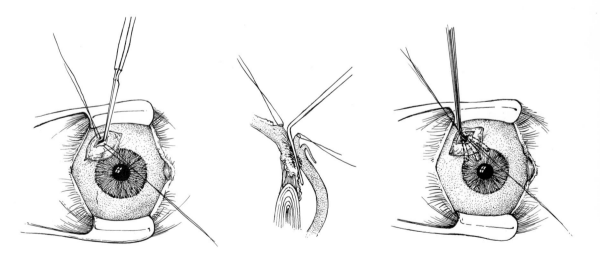

Fig 15-10. Cyclodialysis. Left: Incision through the conjunctiva and sclera 4 mm behind the limbus away from the rectus muscles. **Center:** Blunt cyclodialysis spatula inserted into the suprachoroidal space. The ciliary body is detached from the scleral spur. **Right:** Spatula carried around 90-180° of surface. (Reproduced, with permission, from Callahan: Surgery of the Eye: Diseases. Thomas, 1956.)

Technic

Under local anesthesia a conjunctival incision is made 4-6 mm behind the limbus in one of the 4 quadrants as shown below (to avoid the ciliary arteries). A scratch incision is made perpendicular to the limbus through the sclera. A spatula is then introduced into this opening and, carefully hugging the inner scleral surface, is passed just posterior to the scleral spur. The spatula is then passed into the anterior chamber, detaching the scleral spur from its ciliary body attachment. The spatula then sweeps up to 90° of the circumference of the chamber angle. The spatula can be withdrawn and introduced in the opposite direction to detach another quadrant if desired. The conjunctival wound and scleral wounds are then sutured. Sterile saline solution is sometimes injected through the cyclodialysis cleft to re-form the anterior chamber if necessary. Avoiding anterior chamber hemorrhage improves the chances of a filtering cyclodialysis cleft. Postoperatively the aqueous escapes through the cleft between the detached ciliary body and sclera, to be absorbed in the suprachoroidal space.

Postoperative Care and Prognosis

The postoperative care is the same as for the other filtering operations. It is technically easy to perform and leaves no cosmetic defect. It is repeatable, and does not alter the structure of the eye as much as the other filtering operations. About 60% of such operations are effective in controlling the intraocular pressure.

CYCLODIATHERMY

Cyclodiathermy is generally reserved for advanced cases, especially of secondary glaucoma, in which other glaucoma surgery has failed. It is technically easy to perform and repeatable.

Under local anesthesia, coagulating electrodiathermy is applied to the sclera either directly or through a conjunctival opening. Two or 3 10-second applications are placed 4-6 mm behind the limbus in each quadrant of the eye (superior nasal, superior temporal, inferior nasal, and inferior temporal). The procedure is designed to damage the underlying ciliary body and thus decrease aqueous secretion.

The patient may be ambulatory immediately after the operation, and requires an eye dressing for only a few days. There is no cosmetic blemish and no loss of vision due to the surgery.

CYCLOCRYOSURGERY

Cyclocryosurgery is presently undergoing intensive clinical study, and the indications are that it will replace cyclodiathermy in the treatment of glaucoma. It has the unique advantage of destroying the ciliary body without much damage to either the conjunctiva or the sclera. No cutting is required. The cryoprobe is applied directly to the conjunctiva over several areas 4-5 mm posterior to the limbus. The highly vascular reaction in the ciliary body leads to fibrosis, decreased ciliary body function, and consequent decreased aqueous production.

Cyclocryosurgery is presently being used as a secondary procedure in advanced open-angle glaucoma. It is not a substitute for iridectomy or filtering operations when they are indicated.

GONIOTOMY

Infantile glaucoma and occasionally some forms of juvenile glaucoma are best treated by goniotomy. Goniotomy was introduced into the treatment of infantile glaucoma about 1938 and changed the prognosis of this disease from very bad to good (70-80% cure). Unlike all other glaucoma surgery except iridectomy, this operation seeks to establish normal aqueous outflow through regular channels.

Under general anesthesia and utilizing a contact lens which allows direct visualization of the chamber angle structures, a special goniotomy knife is introduced 1 mm anterior to the temporal limbus. The knife is passed across the anterior chamber to engage the opposite trabecular area just below Schwalbe's line. A sweep of about 50° is made in each direction. The knife is withdrawn with occasional loss of aqueous humor. The anterior chamber is re-formed by the injection of saline solution through the original tract. Postoperatively, aqueous humor has a more ready access to the area of Schlemm's canal for outflow through normal channels once the trabecular area block has been overcome by goniotomy. The operation is reported to permanently normalize intraocular pressure in 70-80% of cases of infantile glaucoma. It can be repeated in other quadrants of the chamber angle if necessary, and leaves no cosmetic blemish.

Postoperatively the child should be kept quiet for one day, but after that can return to normal activity without an eye dressing.

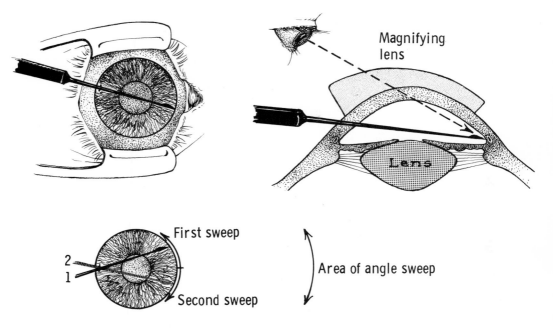

First sweep

Area of angle sweep

Second sweep

Fig 15-11. Goniotomy. Above, left: Goniotomy knife introduced into anterior chamber through the limbus. **Above, right:** Knife passed straight across the anterior chamber under direct visualization until trabecular area is engaged. **Below:** Knife is swept approximately 50° in each direction and then withdrawn. (Courtesy of R. Shaffer.)

•   •   •

Bibliography

Ballintine, E. J., & L. L. Garner: Improvement of the coefficient of outflow in glaucomatous eyes. Prolonged local treatment with epinephrine. Arch Ophth **66:** 314-8, 1961.

Becker, B.: Diabetes mellitus and primary open-angle glaucoma. Am J Ophth **71:** 1-16, 1971.

Becker, B.: The genetic problem of chronic simple glaucoma. Annals of Ophth **3:** 351-4, 1971.

Becker, B. C.: Decrease in tension by carbonic anhydrase inhibitor, Diamox. Am J Ophth **37:**13-6, 1954.

Becker, B., & L. Chevrette: Topical corticosteroid testing in glaucoma siblings. Arch Ophth **76:**484-8, 1966.

Begg, I. S., Drance, S. M., & V. P. Sweeney: Ischaemic optic neuropathy in chronic simple glaucoma. Brit J Ophth **55:**73-90, 1971.

Calhoun, F. P., Jr.: Pigmentary glaucoma and its relationship to Krukenberg's spindles. Am J Ophth **36:**1398-415, 1953.

Chandler, P. A.: Glaucoma from pupillary block in aphakia. Tr Am Ophth Soc **59:** 96-105, 1961.

Chandler, P. A.: Long-term results in glaucoma therapy. The Sanford R. Gifford Memorial Lecture. Am J Ophth **49:**221-46, 1960.

Chandler, P. A., & W. M. Grant: Lectures in Glaucoma. Lea & Febiger, 1965.

Cristiansson, J.: Glaucoma simplex in diabetes mellitus. Acta Ophth **43:**224-34, 1965.

DeRoetth, A., Jr.: Cryosurgery for glaucoma. Tr Am Acad Ophth **73:**1041-3, 1969.

Fisher, R. F., Carpenter, R. G., & C. Wheeler: Assessment of established cases of chronic simple glaucoma. Brit J Ophth **54:**217-28, 1970.

Francois, J., Heintz-De Bree, C., & R. C. Tripathi: Primary open-angle glaucoma. Am J Ophth **62:**844-52, 1966.

Goldmann, H.: Some basic problems of simple glaucoma. The Proctor Medal Lecture. Am J Ophth **48:**213-9, 1959.

Goldmann, H.: Cortisone glaucoma. Arch Ophth **68**:621-7, 1962.

Hansen, E., & O. J. Sellevold: Pseudoexfoliation of the lens capsule: Development of the exfoliation syndrome. Acta Ophth **47**:161, 1969.

Harrington, D. O.: The Visual Fields, 2nd ed. Mosby, 1964.

Hayreh, S. S.: Blood supply of the optic nerve head and its role in optic atrophy, glaucoma, and oedema of the optic disc. Brit J Ophth **53**:721-48, 1969.

Kinsey, V. E.: Unified concept of aqueous humor dynamics and the maintenance of intraocular pressure. Arch Ophth **44**: 215-35, 1950.

Kitazawa, Y.: Primary angle-closure glaucoma. Arch Ophth **84**:724-7, 1970.

Kolker, A. E.: Hyperosmotic agents in glaucoma. Invest Ophth **9**:418, 1970.

Kronfeld, P. C.: Eserine and pilocarpine: Our 100-year-old allies. Survey Ophth **14**:479-85, 1970.

Kronfeld, P. C.: Functional characteristics of surgically produced outflow channels. Tr Am Acad Ophth **73**:176-93, 1969.

Lee, P.: Importance of status of visual field and optic disc in management of open-angle glaucoma. Am J Ophth **53**: 435-42, 1962.

Levene, R.: Glaucoma. Annual review. Arch Ophth **85**:227-51, 1971.

Lichter, P. R., & R. N. Schaffer: Diagnostic and prognostic signs in pigmentary glaucoma. Tr Am Acad Ophth **74**:984-98, 1970.

Podos, S. M., Becker, B., & W. R. Morton: High myopia and primary open angle glaucoma. Am J Ophth **62**:1039-43, 1966.

Podos, S. M., Krupin, T., & B. Becker: Effect of small-dose hyperosmotic injections on intraocular pressure of small animals and man when optic nerves are transected and intact. Am J Ophth **71**: 898-903, 1971.

Richardson, K. T.: Parasympathetic physiology and pharmacology. Survey Ophth **14**:461-76, 1970.

Scheie, H. G.: Filtering operations for glaucoma. A comparative study. Am J Ophth **53**:571-90, 1962.

Shaffer, R. N.: Goniotomy technique in congenital glaucoma. Am J Ophth **47**:90-7, 1959.

Shaffer, R. N.: Open-angle glaucoma. Tr Am Acad Ophth **67**:467-75, 1963.

Shaffer, R. N.: Autonomic ocular drugs. Invest Ophth **3**:498-503, 1964.

Shaffer, R. N.: Stereoscopic Manual of Gonioscopy. Mosby, 1962.

Sugar, H. S.: Pigmentary glaucoma: A 25 year review. Am J Ophth **62**:499-506, 1966.

Swan, K. C.: Iridectomy for closed- (narrow) angle glaucoma: Anatomic considerations. The 26th deSchweinitz Lecture. Am J Ophth **61**:601-19, 1966.

Symposium on glaucoma. Joint Meeting With the National Society for the Prevention of Blindness. Invest Ophth **5**: 115-51, 1966.

Teng, C. C., Paton, R. T., & H. M. Katzin: Primary degeneration in the vicinity of the chamber angle as an etiologic factor in wide-angle glaucoma. Am J Ophth **40**: 619-31, 1955.

Theobald, G. D.: Pseudo-exfoliation of the lens capsule. Am J Ophth **37**:1-15, 1954.

Virno, M.: Intravenous glycerol-vitamin C (sodium salt) as osmotic agents to reduce intraocular pressure. Am J Ophth **62**: 824-33, 1966.

Weiss, D. I., Cooper, L. Z., & R. H. Green: Infantile glaucoma: A manifestation of congenital rubella. JAMA **195**:725-7, 1966.

Wolff, S. M., & L. E. Zimmerman: Chronic secondary glaucoma. Am J Ophth **54**: 547-63, 1962.

16...

Tumors

Both benign and malignant tumors are encountered in the eye and its related structures. Most can be diagnosed early since they are visible, interfere with vision, or displace the eyeball. Care must be taken not to overlook the possibility of malignancy. Fluorescein angiography is helpful in the detection of intraocular tumors but may fail to differentiate benign from malignant lesions. Delay in diagnosis makes curative surgery technically more difficult and may result in loss of all useful vision. As far as possible, biopsies should be taken of all accessible suspicious lesions, excising completely the smaller lesions, since a positive diagnosis of malignancy can only be made by histologic examination. Accurate diagnosis of intraocular and retrobulbar tumors is difficult but vital, since curative therapy can only be given early; later, only palliation is possible.

Secondary (metastatic) ocular malignancies do occur but are quite rare. The most frequent site of metastasis is the choroid. The ophthalmoscopic appearance may be difficult to differentiate from that of primary malignancies of the choroid, and finding the primary tumor elsewhere is of the greatest diagnostic importance. The prognosis for cure of metastatic cancer by enucleation is of course hopeless. X-ray or other treatment may relieve the ocular condition.

Physiology of Symptoms

Small tumors of the lids are asymptomatic except in the case of verrucae and molluscum contagiosum, which occasionally shed a toxic substance into the eye to cause chemical conjunctivitis. There may be no complaints until the late stages, when the lesion is large enough to cause pressure or displacement. Tumors of the conjunctiva are painless unless there is lid irritation. A central corneal lesion causes blurring of vision. An intraocular lesion involving the macula causes blurring of vision as a presenting symptom. Extramacular tumors are not manifested until they become large enough to obstruct vision or produce secondary changes in the eye such as retinal detachment or a rise in intraocular pressure.

A history of recent change in size or appearance of an external ocular growth should call for careful observation, including photographs. If there is any suspicion of malignancy, biopsy or total removal is indicated for microscopic examination.

LID TUMORS

BENIGN TUMORS OF THE LIDS
(Nevus, Verruca, Molluscum Contagiosum, Xanthelasma, Hemangioma)

Nevus

Nevi of the eyelids are common congenital benign pigmented tumors having the same pathologic structure as nevi found elsewhere. They are usually congenital but may be relatively unpigmented at birth, enlarging and darkening during later life. Nevi rarely become malignant.

Nevi may be removed by shave excision if desired for cosmetic reasons.

Verrucae (Warts)

Warts commonly appear along the margins of the lids as fleshy, multilobulated, flat-based to pedunculated lesions. They are thought to be caused by viruses.

If treatment is indicated for cosmetic reasons, verrucae may be removed by excision with cauterization at the base of the lesion. Care must be exercised to avoid producing a marginal notch in the eyelid.

Molluscum Contagiosum

The typical lesion of this unusual disorder is a small, flat, symmetrical, centrally umbilicated growth along the lid margin. It is caused by a large virus and may produce toxic conjunctivitis if the lesion sheds into the conjunctival space.

Cure can be obtained in many cases by merely incising the lesion and allowing blood to permeate the central portion, or by cautery.

213

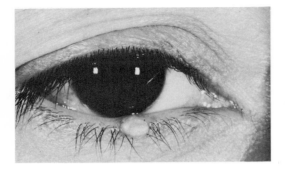

Fig 16-1. **Molluscum contagiosum.** Note central umbilication.

Xanthelasma

Xanthelasma is a common disorder that occurs on the anterior surface of the eyelid, usually bilaterally near the inner angle of the eye. The lesions appear as yellow, wrinkled patches on the skin, and occur more often in elderly people. Xanthelasma represents lipid deposits in histiocytes in the dermis of the lid. Clinical evaluation of serum cholesterol levels is indicated, but only rarely is a direct relationship found.

Treatment is indicated for cosmetic reasons. Surgical removal is simple. Cauterization of the smaller lesions is sometimes effective.

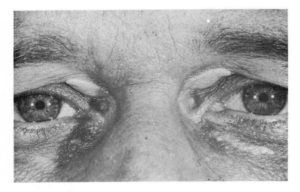

Fig 16-2. **Xanthelasma.** (Courtesy of M. Quickert.)

Hemangioma

Two main types of vascular tumors occur in the lids: cavernous hemangiomas and telangiectases. Cavernous hemangiomas are composed of large venous channels lying in the subcutaneous tissue; they are bluish in color and change in size according to their distention with blood. Telangiectases are bright red spots composed of dilated capillaries. They are painless unless spontaneous hemorrhage occurs, causing marked swelling.

Various types of treatment have been used, eg, surgical excision of the smaller lesions, freezing with CO_2, and x-ray radiation. Hemangiomas may be disregarded if they are not cosmetically disturbing, and usually fade after a child is a few years old. They should not be treated before 8 years of age.

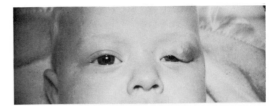

Fig 16-3. **Cavernous hemangioma** of left upper lid.

PRIMARY MALIGNANT TUMORS OF THE LIDS
(Carcinoma, Xeroderma Pigmentosum, Sarcoma, Malignant Melanoma)

Carcinoma

Carcinoma of the lids has the highest incidence of any malignant ocular tumor. The average age at onset is 50-60 years. Men are more commonly affected than women.

The commonest site of the tumor is near the margin of the lower lid near the inner canthus. Ninety-five percent of lid carcinomas are of the basal cell type. The remaining 5% consist of squamous cell carcinomas and sebaceous (meibomian gland) carcinomas. Keratoacanthomas and inverted follicular keratoses are benign lesions which resemble squamous cell carcinomas. In the past this was not recognized, and the incidence of squamous cell carcinomas was thought to be higher than it actually is. Basal cell carcinoma is much more common in the lower lid; squamous cell carcinoma in the upper lid. Diagnosis is based upon clinical appearance and biopsy.

Squamous cell carcinoma tends to spread via the lymphatic system. On the upper lid it drains into the preauricular nodes; on the lower lid, into the submaxillary node. Basal cell tumors grow very slowly and do not spread to the regional lymph nodes. Systemic metastases are extremely rare in basal cell carcinoma but do occur in squamous cell carcinomas.

Squamous cell carcinoma grows slowly and painlessly, and may be present for many months before it is noted. It usually begins as a small warty growth with a keratotic covering, gradually eroding and fissuring until an ulcer develops. The base of the ulcer is indurated and hyperemic and the edges hard. Unless the tumor is excised early it grows through the skin, connective tissue, cartilage, and bone until large areas are destroyed in a fungating crater which may eventually reach the cranial cavity. Pain then becomes severe and constant. When sensory nerves are involved, the pain may be excruciating. The patient may die of hemorrhage, meningitis, or general debility.

Basal cell carcinoma begins in a similar manner, eventually forming the typical rodent ulcer with a raised nodular border and indurated base. It eventually erodes the surrounding tissue in somewhat the same way as squamous cell carcinoma, but much more slowly. Biopsy of the tumor itself is a simple office procedure, and is the only sure method of diagnosis.

Basal cell tumors of the lower lid near the inner canthus tend to invade the structures of the inner canthus and the orbit. Complete eradication of these tumors is important.

Any suspicious warty growth on the lids should be removed and submitted for pathologic examination.

The objective of treatment is the complete destruction of the tumor. The squamous cell type is resistant to x-ray radiation, and the only effective means of treatment is complete surgical excision. If the diagnosis is made while the growth is still a local nodule in the eyelid, a large "V" resection may be performed well beyond the limits of the tumor. Plastic repair of the deformity should be done concurrently.

Basal cell carcinomas are more radiosensitive, but each case should be evaluated individually. Simple excision and electrodesiccation of the small lesion is usually quite effective and avoids the complication of radiation burns. Good results have been reported with a combination of surgery and irradiation.

Carcinoma Associated With Xeroderma Pigmentosum

This rare congenital disease is characterized by the appearance of a large number of freckles in the areas of the skin exposed to the sun. These are followed by telangiectases, atrophic patches, and eventually a warty growth which may undergo carcinomatous degeneration. The eyelids are frequently affected, and may be the first area to show degenerative changes. The malignant change may be of either the squamous cell or basal cell type (usually the former). This condition is inherited as an autosomal recessive trait. Carriers can often be identified by excessive freckling.

The disease usually appears early in life and in most cases is fatal within a few years as a result of metastasis. Life may be prolonged by carefully protecting the skin from actinic rays and treating carcinomatous tumors as rapidly as they appear.

Sarcoma

Sarcoma of the lids is rare and usually represents an anterior extension of an orbital sarcoma. Rhabdomyosarcomas involving the orbit and lids represent the most common malignant tumor in these tissues in the first decade of life. Other sarcomas (usually named after the predominant type of cell) also occur. Most are radiosensitive, but a combination of surgery and radiation is often required. They may be associated with similar lesions elsewhere in the body.

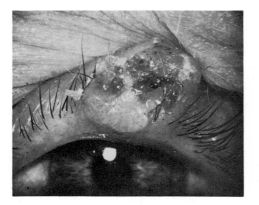

Fig 16-4. Squamous cell carcinoma of upper lid. (Courtesy of A. Rosenberg.)

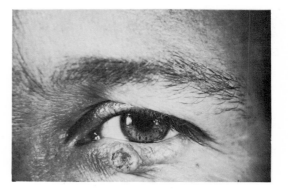

Fig 16-5. Basal cell carcinoma of left lower lid. (Courtesy of S. Mettier, Jr.)

Malignant Melanoma

Contrary to general belief, nevi rarely undergo malignant change. Malignancy should be suspected when a lesion enlarges or becomes darker.

Treatment must be radical, and is of value only if performed early. If the lesion is small and seems to be circumscribed, widespread local excision may be used. If there is any evidence of spread, total exenteration of the orbit with sacrifice of the lids is advocated by many authorities. The prognosis with any form of therapy is poor.

CONJUNCTIVAL TUMORS

PRIMARY BENIGN TUMORS OF THE CONJUNCTIVA
(Nevus, Papilloma, Granuloma, Dermoid, Dermolipoma, Lymphoma, Fibroma, Angioma)

Nevus

Conjunctival nevi are common congenital pigmented tumors, although the pigment may not become visible until puberty or later. They usually appear as brownish or black, flat lesions which move with the conjunctiva and are most frequently located in the caruncle or on the bulbar conjunctiva near the limbus. Bleb-like or cystic elevated forms which have a gelatinous appearance (cystic nevus) occur less commonly.

Histologically, the nevi are composed of nests or sheets of typical pigmented nevus cells which theoretically may be derived from nerve tissue (possibly from the sheath of Schwann). Malignant changes are rare.

Conjunctival nevi should be observed for rare malignant change, but excision is not required unless they become cosmetically disfiguring. If removal is indicated, excision should be well outside the possible area of extension of unpigmented cells.

Granuloma

Granulomas are seen as vascular fungating masses protruding from areas in which the palpebral conjunctiva (usually at the lid margins) has been broken or incised, as in draining chalazions, open conjunctival wounds, or conjunctival foreign bodies. Occasionally, specific etiologic agents such as the tubercle bacillus or cysts containing Coccidioides immitis are identified histologically. They can attain large size rapidly, and may outgrow their blood supply and strangulate, with spontaneous recovery. Treatment is by surgical excision and cleansing of the base. The wound may have to be closed with sutures.

Dermoid Tumor (Fig 16-7)

This rare congenital tumor appears as a smooth, rounded, yellow elevated mass, frequently with hairs protruding. A dermoid tumor may remain quiescent throughout life, although it often increases in size during puberty. Removal is indicated only if cosmetic deformity is severe or if vision is impaired or threatened.

Dermolipoma

Dermolipoma is a common congenital tumor which usually appears as a smoothly rounded growth in the upper temporal quadrant of the bulbar conjunctiva near the lateral canthus. Treatment is usually not indicated, but removal should be attempted if the growth is

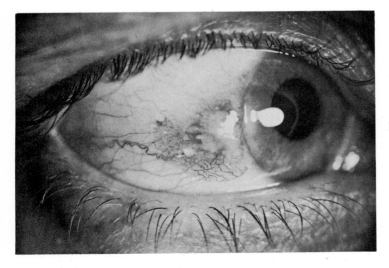

Fig 16-6. Conjunctival nevus.
(Courtesy of A. Irvine, Jr.)

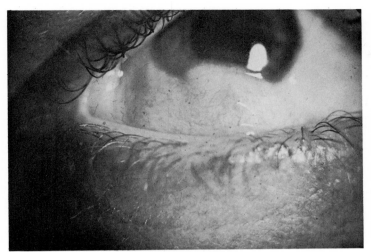

Fig 16-7. Dermoid tumor at the inferior limbus. (Courtesy of A. Irvine, Jr.)

enlarging or is cosmetically disfiguring. Posterior dissection must be undertaken with extreme care (if at all) since this lesion is frequently continuous with orbital fat; orbital derangement may cause scarring and complications far more serious than the original lesion.

Lymphoma

Conjunctival lymphoma is an uncommon local lesion which may appear in adults without evidence of systemic disease or as part of the clinical picture of lymphosarcoma, lymphatic leukemia, Hodgkin's disease, or other related conditions. Lymphomas appear most often at the fornices on the bulbar conjunctiva as firm, reddish, slowly encircling lesions.

Histologically, lymphomatous tissue is composed of dense masses of lymphocytes without germinal centers and with a sparse connective tissue framework and abundant blood vessels. The differential diagnosis between lymphoma and lymphosarcoma may be difficult.

Treatment is by x-ray radiation if malignancy is proved by biopsy, and is remarkably effective.

Fibroma

Fibromas are rare small, smooth, pedunculated, transparent growths which may appear anywhere in the conjunctival tissues but are most often seen in the lower fornix. Histologically they consist of fibrous overgrowths covered by epithelium. Treatment is by excision.

Angioma

Conjunctival angiomas may take 2 forms: hemangioma or lymphangioma. Conjunctival hemangiomas may appear as diffuse telangiectases or capillary nevi, or as encapsulated cavernous hemangiomas. The latter consist of large communicating, fairly well encapsulated vascular spaces which have a tendency to enlarge. Treatment is by excision, x-ray radiation, or electrocoagulation.

PRIMARY MALIGNANT TUMORS OF THE BULBAR CONJUNCTIVA (Epithelioma, Malignant Melanoma, Lymphosarcoma)

Epithelioma (Carcinoma)

Epithelioma is an uncommon tumor which arises most commonly from the limbal transition zone, less frequently from the mucocutaneous juncture at the lid margin and caruncle. It appears initially at the limbus as a small opaque elevation firmly fixed to the underlying tissue. In many instances growth is rapid. Extension can occur through the perivascular and perineural lymphatics into the suprachoroidal space and Schlemm's canal. Eventually the entire eyeball may be destroyed by tumor tissue. Death may ultimately occur as a result of distant metastases.

Histologically, all conjunctival epitheliomas are squamous cell in type since there are no basal cells in the conjunctiva.

Small epitheliomas may be safely excised. If the tumor is large or if there is any possibility of extension, enucleation is indicated. If extension is widespread, exenteration may be required. Irradiation is sometimes used as a routine measure following surgical excision.

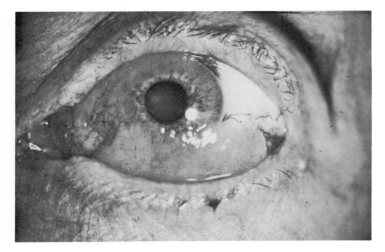

Fig 16-8. Intraepithelial epithelioma. (Courtesy of A. Irvine, Jr.)

Intraepithelial epithelioma (carcinoma in situ) is a type of epibulbar tumor which may begin at the limbus and involve the cornea to a greater extent than the conjunctiva. It is typically a smooth, flat opaque growth over the surface of the cornea and is considered to be carcinoma in situ, although a typical infiltrating squamous cell tumor may develop from it. It is resistant to x-ray radiation so that surgical excision is required.

Malignant Melanoma

Malignant melanoma of the conjunctiva is rare. It may arise from a preexisting nevus, from an area of acquired melanosis, or de novo from normal conjunctiva. Its pigmentation may vary greatly, and its clinical course is often unpredictable. Eventually, most conjunctival melanomas enlarge but do not usually invade the interior of the eye.

Histologically, these tumors have the same structure as other malignant melanomas.

Simple excision is often impossible but may be successful if the lesion is small enough. X-ray radiation is of no benefit. Exenteration of the orbit is advocated, but the prognosis is poor.

Lymphosarcoma

Conjunctival lymphosarcoma is rare. Histology, course, and management are the same as for lymphosarcomas of the lids.

CORNEAL TUMORS

PRIMARY MALIGNANT TUMORS OF THE CORNEA
(Epithelioma, Melanoma)

Only a few cases of epithelioma and melanoma of the cornea are on record. They appear as irregular masses of gray epithelium over the surface of the cornea.

INTRAOCULAR TUMORS

PRIMARY BENIGN INTRAOCULAR TUMORS
(Nevus, Neurofibromatosis, Angioma, Tuberous Sclerosis, Hemangioma of Choroid, Glioma of Retina)

Nevus

Nevi may occur on any of the 3 portions of the uvea: the iris, ciliary body, or choroid. They are usually flat pigmented lesions lying in the stroma of the tissue but not interfering with the function of the tissue itself. On the anterior surface of the iris they may be noted as iris "freckles." Posteriorly in the choroid one may see flat pigmented areas. Large choroidal nevi are difficult to differentiate from malignant melanomas. Their unchanging slate-gray color and flat appearance and the lack of extension are important in the differential diagnosis from malignant melanoma.

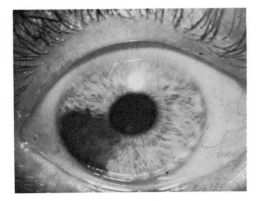

Fig 16-9. Nevus of iris. (Courtesy of A. Rosenberg.)

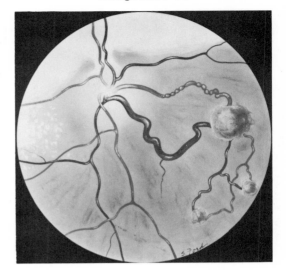

Fig 16-11. **Hemangiomas of the retina** (drawing). (Courtesy of F. Cordes.)

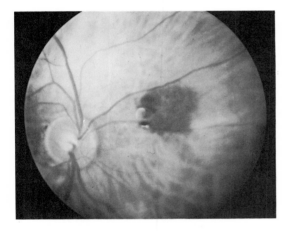

Fig 16-10. **Nevus of choroid.** (Photo by Diane Beeston.)

Tuberous Sclerosis (Bourneville's Disease)

The rare intraocular tumor associated with tuberous sclerosis varies in size and color but is often described as a yellow or white nodular swelling, frequently mulberry in appearance, located in any portion of the posterior fundus but with a predilection for the area near the optic nerve. Other manifestations of tuberous sclerosis include skin changes (adenoma sebaceum), intracranial changes causing epilepsy and mental retardation, and other neurologic symptoms.

There is no treatment.

Because of the difficulties in differentiation from malignant melanomas, fundus photographs (including fluorescein angiography) or careful line drawings should be made of all suspicious lesions. Observations should be made periodically for changes.

Angioma

Angioma of the retina is a rare congenital disorder. Blurring of vision may result if bleeding occurs or if the retina is secondarily detached. Occasionally, angioma is associated with angioma in the cerebral cortex (Lindau's disease). The tumor occurs in the posterior fundus, often in the lower temporal quadrant. It is globular in outline and may be located near one of the pairs of enlarged retinal vessels. Angiomas may enlarge. Photocoagulation therapy (xenon or argon laser) and cryotherapy are currently utilized to eradicate these lesions.

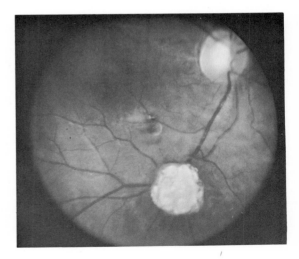

Fig 16-12. **Tuberous sclerosis.**

PRIMARY MALIGNANT TUMORS
OF THE INTRAOCULAR STRUCTURES
(Malignant Melanoma,
Retinoblastoma, Diktyoma)

Malignant Melanoma

It has been estimated that intraocular malignant melanoma occurs in 0.02-0.06% of the total eye patient population. It is seen only in the uveal tract, and is the most common intraocular malignant tumor. The average age of patients with this disorder is 50 years. It is almost always unilateral. Eight-five percent appear in the choroid, 9% in the ciliary body, and 6% in the iris. Most of the choroidal tumors are in the posterior portion of the eye, especially on the temporal side. In the iris, the lower half is most often affected. Intraocular malignant melanoma is rare in Negroes, although uveal nevi are common.

This tumor may be seen in its early stages only accidentally during routine ophthalmoscopic examination or because of blurring due to macular invasion. Blood-borne metastases may occur at any time, and death may occur before local spread occurs or ocular symptoms appear. Glaucoma may occur as a late manifestation.

Histologically, these tumors present a variable cellular picture of spindle cells, epithelioid cells, and reticulum. When properly catalogued, these features have prognostic significance.

Intraocular malignant melanomas may spread directly through the sclera, by local invasion of intraocular structures, or by metastasis.

Clinical manifestations are usually absent unless the macula is involved. In the later stages, growth of the tumor may lead to retinal detachment with loss of a large amount of visual field. A tumor located in the iris may be large enough to change the color of the iris or deform the pupil. Pain does not occur in the absence of glaucoma.

The first step in diagnosis is to suspect the lesion. Most intraocular malignant melanomas can be seen ophthalmoscopically. Transillumination is of some value in differentiation from serous retinal detachment.

A high incidence of intraocular tumors has been found in the study of blind, painful, phthisical (atrophic) eyes, one writer reporting that 10% of such eyes contained previously unsuspected malignant melanomas.

Enucleation is indicated if the tumor is contained within the eyeball. If there is any evidence of extraocular extension, exenteration of the orbit is usually indicated. If distant metastases have occurred, enucleation is not indicated unless the eye becomes painful or unsightly. Small melanomas of the iris which have not invaded the root can be successfully removed by iridectomy. In recent years lesions which invade the iris root have been excised by iridocyclectomy.

The prognosis of malignant melanoma is only fair. Removal of the eye may appear to have eradicated the primary lesion, but distant metastases have been reported 20 years after removal of the primary tumor. Five-year survival (about 50%) is thus of less long-

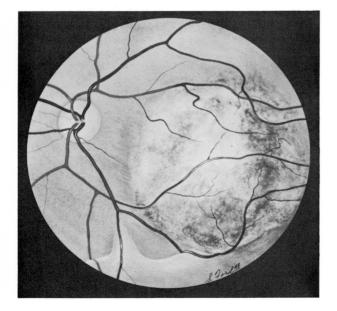

Fig 16-13. Malignant melanoma of the choroid, macular area, left eye (drawing). (Courtesy of F. Cordes.)

term prognostic significance in malignant melanoma than in other malignancies. The prognosis for iris melanoma is far better than for choroidal tumors.

Retinoblastoma

Retinoblastoma is a rare but life-endangering tumor of childhood. Two-thirds of cases appear before the end of the third year; rare cases have been reported at almost every age. Retinoblastoma occurs less frequently in Negroes than in whites. It is bilateral in about 30% of cases. The tumor results from mutation of an autosomal dominant gene. Children of parents who have produced one child with retinoblastoma have about a 4-7%

chance of having retinoblastoma. Persons who have been cured of retinoblastoma should be told that any children produced will have a 50% chance of being affected by retinoblastoma (autosomal dominant inheritance).

Retinoblastomas usually arise from the posterior retina. Growth tends to be nodular, with numerous satellite or seeding nodules which may produce multiple secondary tumors. They gradually fill the eye and extend through the optic nerve to the brain and along the emissary vessels and nerves in the sclera to the orbital tissues. Microscopically, most retinoblastomas are composed of small, closely-packed round or polygonal cells with large, darkly staining nuclei and scanty cytoplasm.

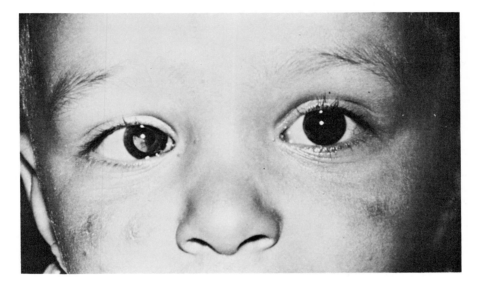

Fig 16-14. Retinoblastoma visible through pupil.

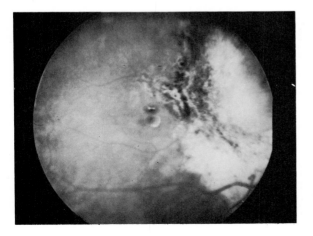

Fig 16-15. Retinoblastoma after x-ray radiation.

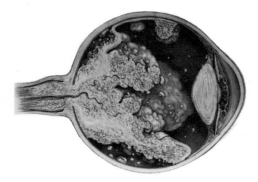

Fig 16-16. Retinoblastoma with multiple seedings and optic nerve invasion. (Courtesy of B. Crawford and W. Spencer.)

A radial "pseudorosette" arrangement around blood vessels is common. Degenerative changes are frequent, with necrosis and calcification. A few spontaneous cures have been reported.

Retinoblastoma usually remains unnoticed until it has advanced far enough to produce a white pupil. The tumor is usually seen in the early stages only when sought for, as in children having a hereditary background or where the other eye has been affected. In the early stages small, yellowish-white nodular masses may be seen protruding into the vitreous from the retina. Infants and children with esotropia should be examined to rule out retinoblastoma, since blind eyes of children will often turn inward.

Retrolental fibroplasia and persistence of the primary vitreous may simulate retinoblastoma.

In general, the earlier the discovery and treatment of the tumor, the better the chance to prevent spread through the optic nerve and orbital tissues.

Immediate enucleation is the treatment of choice in all unilateral cases. The mortality rate is about 20%. In bilateral cases, Reese has suggested enucleating the more involved eye and massively irradiating the other, using radioactive cobalt and follow-up treatment with triethylenemelamine (TEM).

Cryosurgery has been tried in various types of intraocular tumors. The results have been disappointing except in the case of some retinoblastomas which are sensitive to temperatures of -100° C. Further investigations in this field are being pursued by Lincoff and others.

Epithelial Tumor of the Ciliary Body (Diktyoma)

Diktyoma is an extremely rare epithelial tumor growing from the ciliary body and having the histologic characteristics of undifferentiated embryonic retinal tissue. It occurs only in young children. Diktyomas may be visualized as they grow over the posterior surface of the iris between the iris and the lens, and may be present at the pupillary border as a white, irregular nodular sheet. Growth may be very slow, but it is inevitable, and the tumor is said to be locally malignant without metastasizing. Eventually it may fill the entire globe and perforate the sclera.

Enucleation is the only treatment.

Malignant epithelioma of the ciliary epithelium is a rare tumor seen in adults. It also is treated by enucleation. Cyclectomy may be successful.

ORBITAL TUMORS

BENIGN TUMORS OF THE ORBIT
(Vascular Tumors, Neurofibromas, Fibromas, Lymphangiomas, Lymphomas, Osteomas, Dermoids)

Gradually enlarging orbital tumors may attain a diameter of 1 cm before any displacement of the eyeball is noted. The direction of displacement offers a clue to the location of the tumor: posterior tumors tend to displace the eyeball anteriorly, whereas tumors between the eyeball and one of the walls of the orbit will cause lateral displacement. These observations indicate the site of exploration when biopsy is indicated.

With displacement of the eyeball, diplopia is a common symptom. Pressure resulting from marked exophthalmos may interfere with blood supply to the optic nerve and retina, causing blurred vision. Exposure of the eye due to inability to close the lids causes corneal epithelial damage with resultant pain and irritation.

Vascular Tumors

Hemangioma (usually of the cavernous type) is the most common of the orbital tumors. Others include telangiectases (congenital and acquired), aneurysms, and fibroangiomas. At surgery these tumors collapse and are difficult to identify. They are treated satisfactorily by surgical excision.

Cavernous hemangiomas consist of large vascular spaces with an endothelial lining. They are usually localized and encapsulated. Most of the **telangiectatic** lesions appear in the skin surfaces of the lids, nose, and cheek. Congenital telangiectases often disappear a few years after birth, and many authorities believe that treatment is rarely required. **Fibroangiomas** may be diffuse or encapsulated. They occur in the soft tissues of the orbit. If allowed to increase in size they may develop into cavernous hemangiomas as the venous channels are dilated by continuous pressure of the arterial blood. **Arteriovenous aneurysms** are suggested by exophthalmos with dilated conjunctival and lid vessels and pulsation of the eyeball and contents on palpation. Visual acuity may be reduced and the retinal blood vessels engorged. A frequent cause is the rupture of the carotid artery into the cavernous sinus following a skull fracture. Deep penetrating injuries can also produce arteriovenous aneurysms.

Neurofibromas

Any of the nerve structures within the orbit, including the optic nerve, may rarely become involved by neurofibromatosis (Recklinghausen's disease). If an annular tumor compresses the optic nerve, vision is affected. These tumors are not susceptible to radiation therapy, and excision is required if symptoms warrant.

Fibromas

Simple fibromas are rare. The tumor usually develops from a combination of elements, eg, angiofibroma, myxofibroma, fibrolipoma, and neurofibroma. Fibromas are more common in the upper and inner portions of the orbit than elsewhere, and occur most frequently in the third decade. Exophthalmos, diplopia, and displacement of the eyeball are the first symptoms.

Fibromatous tumors are usually encapsulated, firm, and have a meager blood supply. Simple excision is feasible in many cases if necessary to relieve symptoms.

Lymphangiomas

Lymphangioma is a rare tumor which is thought to be congenital in origin. It resembles cavernous hemangioma in structure except that the spaces are filled with lymph instead of blood. Complete excision is often difficult.

Osteomas

These are rare bony tumors originating in the paranasal sinuses and invading the orbit. The frontal and ethmoid sinuses are the most common sources, and the lesion gradually invades the orbit by bony erosion. Osteomas grow slowly from a single pedicle and are covered by mucous membrane continuous with that of the sinus wall. This is in contrast to hyperostosis, which originates in the orbital bone and is covered by periosteum continuous with the periorbita. Both of these lesions are visible and may be differentiated on x-ray.

Treatment consists of surgical removal if symptoms become severe.

Dermoids

Dermoids are congenital tumors that occur only rarely in the orbit, where they are found as solid tumors or cysts. (They are more common in the eyelids and conjunctiva.) In the orbit, they are most frequently found in the superior temporal portion, usually anterior to the lacrimal gland. It is not always possible to differentiate tumors of the lacrimal gland and dermoids on clinical grounds. Hair, cartilage, teeth, bone, and other tissues may be found in varying degrees. Dermoids seldom metastasize or show malignant changes, and show little tendency to grow.

MALIGNANT TUMORS OF THE ORBIT
(Carcinoma, Adenocarcinoma, Sarcoma)

Malignant tumors of the orbit may be primary or metastatic. The orbit may also be secondarily invaded by malignant melanomas (from the eyelids, conjunctiva, uveal tract, paranasal sinuses, brain, or eyeball) or by carcinomas (from various distant tissues).

Malignant tumors of the orbit produce the same clinical picture as benign tumors of the orbit, with proptosis or displacement of the eyeball. The usual rapid growth, however, frequently does not allow compensatory changes in circulation or in binocular adjustment, so that the visual acuity change may be much more rapid (and diplopia more troublesome) than with the slower growing tumors.

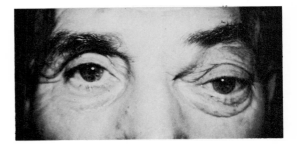

Fig 16-17. Orbital tumor displacing left eye.

Because of the close association of the orbital tissues with the openings into the cranial cavity, there may be a serious spread of neoplastic growth before the diagnosis is made and treatment undertaken.

Carcinoma and Adenocarcinoma

A great number of orbital carcinomas extend from the lids, conjunctiva, sinuses, and pharynx. Metastases from the breast and intestinal tract also occur.

Benign and malignant mixed tumors of the lacrimal gland—as well as adenocarcinomas (of the adenoid cystic type)—constitute the most common epithelial tumors of the orbit. Benign mixed tumors may recur in the orbit after excision if small areas of local direct extension through the pseudocapsule have occurred. Malignant transformation is common. Adenoid cystic carcinomas frequently invade orbital

bone. Distal metastases are common. They are radioresistant.

Sarcoma

Sarcomas comprise a group of tumors of mesodermal origin which are highly cellular in composition and are frequently poorly differentiated. In childhood, the most common primary orbital form is the rhabdomyosarcoma. Lymphomas and lymphosarcomas of the lacrimal gland constitute the most frequent adult tumor of this group. Angiosarcomas, chondrosarcomas, osteosarcomas, and fibrosarcomas rarely occur as primary orbital tumors, and most reported examples have been late manifestations of excessive orbital radiation in childhood—usually given for the treatment of intraocular retinoblastomas.

Many of the sarcomatous tumors are resistant to radiation therapy. Exenteration of the orbit is usually required.

•   •   •

Bibliography

Albert, D. M.: Microtubules on retinoblastoma. Am J Ophth **69**:296-9, 1970.

Albert, D. M.: Tissue culture study of human retinoblastoma. Invest Ophth **9**:64-72, 1970.

Ash, J. E.: Epibulbar tumors. Am J Ophth **33**:1203-19, 1950.

Aurora, A. L.: Reappraisal of basal cell carcinoma of the eyelids. Am J Ophth **70**:329-36, 1970.

Bedford, M. A., Bedotto, C., & P. A. Macfaul: Retinoblastoma. Brit J Ophth **55**:19-27, 1971.

Boniuk, M.: Ocular and Adnexal Tumors. Mosby, 1964.

Chopdar, A.: Malignant melanoma of the conjunctiva. Brit J Ophth **54**:631-3, 1970.

Davidorf, F. H.: Conservative management of malignant melanoma. II. Transscleral diathermy as a method of treatment for malignant melanomas of the choroid. Arch Ophth **83**:273-80, 1970.

Dykstra, P. C.: The cytologic diagnosis of carcinoma and related lesions of the ocular conjunctiva and cornea. Tr Am Acad Ophth **73**:979-95, 1969.

Hoyt, W. F.: Optic glioma of childhood. Natural history and rationale for conservative management. Brit J Ophth **53**:793-8, 1969.

Huber, A.: Eye Symptoms in Brain Tumors, 2nd ed. Mosby, 1971.

Lincoff, H., McLean, J., & R. Long: The cryosurgical treatment of intraocular tumors. Am J Ophth **63**:389-99, 1967.

Reeh, M. T.: Treatment of Lid and Epibulbar Tumors. Thomas, 1963.

Reese, A. B.: Tumors of the Eye, 2nd ed. Hoeber, 1963.

Reese, A. B., & R. M. Ellsworth: Evaluation and current concept of retinoblastoma therapy. Tr Am Acad Ophth **67**:164-72, 1963.

Smith, T. R.: Malignant tumors of the eye. CA **19**:360-3, 1969.

Spaeth, E. B.: Tumors of the lacrimal gland. Tr Am Acad Ophth **63**:739-51, 1959.

Zareth, M. M., & others: Laser photocoagulation of the eye. Arch Ophth **69**:97-104, 1963.

Zimmerman, L. E. (editor): Tumors of the Eye and Adnexa. Little, Brown, 1962.

17 . . .

Trauma

In spite of the protection afforded by the bony orbit, the cushioning effect of the retrobulbar fat, and the lids and lashes—and in spite of the great strides made in recent years in the development of protective devices, especially the use of safety goggles—the incidence of eye injuries remains high. Childhood eye injuries continue to occur as a result of air rifle, bow and arrow, catapult (slingshot), and throwing accidents.

Pain or photophobia caused by the injury may produce blepharospasm severe enough to prevent examination of the eye. If this happens, instill a sterile topical anesthetic. With the aid of a loupe and well-focused light, the anterior surface of the cornea is examined for foreign materials or wounds, regularity, and luster. The conjunctiva is inspected for hemorrhage, foreign material, or tears. The depth and clarity of the anterior chamber is noted. The size, shape, and light reaction of the pupil should be compared with those of the pupil of the uninjured eye. If the eyeball is intact, the lids are carefully inspected to the fornices, everting the upper lid. The lens, vitreous, and retina are examined with an ophthalmoscope for evidence of intraocular damage such as hemorrhage or retinal detachment.

If the patient complains of a foreign body sensation but none can be seen with oblique illumination, instill sterile fluorescein. This may demonstrate an irregularity of the corneal surface due to a minute abrasion, laceration, or foreign body.

A small child may be difficult to examine adequately. If a rupture or laceration of the eyeball is suspected, it is best not to struggle but to examine with the aid of a short-acting general anesthetic. If a severe injury is not suspected, the lids may be manually separated under topical anesthesia with the use of lid retracting forceps.

It is important to determine and record visual acuity (see p 17). Visual acuity should be tested again upon recovery from the injury, and a refraction performed if vision is below normal. This record may have legal significance.

In severe injuries it is important for the nonspecialist to bear in mind the possibility of causing further damage by unnecessary manipulation.

Caution: Topical anesthetics, dyes, and other medications placed in an injured eye **must be sterile.** Both tetracaine and fluorescein can be autoclaved repeatedly without impairment of their pharmacologic properties. Most ophthalmic solutions are now available in individual disposable sterile units.

NONPENETRATING INJURIES OF THE EYEBALL
(Abrasions, Contusions, Rupture, Superficial Foreign Bodies, Burns)

Abrasions

Abrasions of the lids, cornea, or conjunctiva do not require surgical treatment. The wound should be cleansed of imbedded foreign material. In order to facilitate the examination, the pain associated with abrasions of the cornea and conjunctiva can be relieved by instillation of a topical anesthetic such as 0.5% tetracaine (Pontocaine®) solution, but routine instillation of a topical anesthetic by the patient **must not be permitted** since it may delay the diagnosis of complications and is conducive to further injury. Antibiotic ointment, eg, polymyxin B–bacitracin (Polysporin®), helps prevent bacterial infection. An eye bandage applied with firm but gentle pressure lessens discomfort and promotes healing by preventing movement of the lids over the involved area. The dressing should be changed daily and the wound inspected for evidence of infection or ulcer formation.

Corneal abrasions cause severe pain and may lead to recurrent corneal erosion, but they rarely become infected.

Contusions

Contusions of the eyeball and its surrounding tissues are commonly produced by traumatic contact with a blunt object. The results

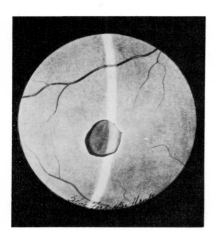

Fig 17-1. Hole in retina, macular area, posttraumatic.

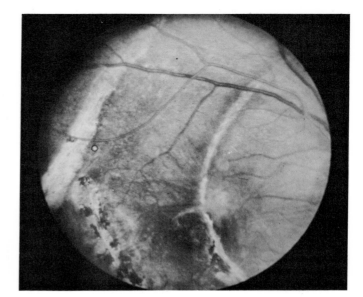

Fig 17-2. **Choroidal tears.**
(Photo by Diane Beeston.)

of such injury are variable and are often not obvious upon superficial examination. Careful study and adequate follow-up are indicated. The possible results of contusion injury are hemorrhage and swelling of the eyelids (ecchymosis, "black eye"), subconjunctival hemorrhages, edema or rupture of the cornea, hemorrhage into the anterior chamber (hyphema), rupture of the root of the iris (iridodialysis), traumatic paralysis of the pupil (mydriasis), paralysis or spasm of the muscles of accommodation, anterior chamber angle recession with subsequent secondary glaucoma (see p 206), traumatic cataract, dislocation of the lens (subluxation and luxation), vitreous hemorrhage, retinal hemorrhage and retinal edema (most common in the macular area, called commotio retinae, or Berlin's traumatic edema), detachment of the retina, rupture of the choroid posteriorly, and optic nerve injury.

Many of these injuries cannot be seen on casual external observation. Some, such as cataract, may not develop for many days or weeks following the injury.

Except for those involving rupture of the eyeball itself (see below), most of the immediate effects of contusion of the eye do not require immediate definitive treatment. However, any injury severe enough to cause intraocular hemorrhage involves the danger of delayed secondary hemorrhage from the broken vessel, which may cause intractable glaucoma and permanent damage to the eyeball. Patients who show evidence of intraocular hemorrhage should be put at absolute bed rest for 4 or 5

days with both eyes bandaged in order to minimize the chance of further bleeding. Secondary hemorrhage rarely occurs after 72 hours. A short-acting cycloplegic such as 5% homatropine may be used. Acetazolamide (Diamox®), mannitol, or other systemically administered agents to lower intraocular pressure may be necessary.

Rupture of the Eyeball

Rupture of the eyeball may occur due to penetrating trauma. It frequently occurs as a result of contusion which causes a sudden increase in ocular pressure, causing the wall of the eyeball to tear at one of the weaker points. The most common site of rupture is along the limbus; occasionally, rupture occurs around the optic nerve. Anterior ruptures can be repaired surgically by interrupted sutures of fine silk unless intraocular contents are so deranged that useful function of the eye is not possible, in which case evisceration or enucleation should be done. If either of these procedures is required, implantation of a plastic sphere is useful as a space-filler and to aid in movement of a prosthesis (artificial eye), which can be fitted much like a large contact lens 2 or 3 weeks later.

Corneal and Conjunctival Foreign Bodies

Foreign bodies are the most frequent cause of eye injury. Small metallic or nonmetallic foreign bodies are frequently blown into the eye and may become lodged under the upper lid or be embedded in corneal epithelium. In remov-

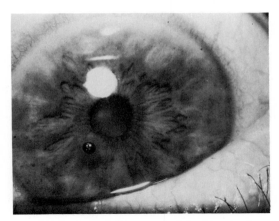

Fig 17-3. Metallic corneal foreign body.
(Courtesy of A. Rosenberg.)

ing corneal foreign bodies, a sterile topical anesthetic is essential. Minute corneal foreign bodies which are not readily visualized with the naked eye or loupe may be outlined with sterile fluorescein. If a foreign body containing iron has remained in the tissue for any length of time, rust penetrates the corneal tissue and must be removed to prevent further irritation.

Although foreign bodies may often be removed satisfactorily using a light and magnifying loupe, the most satisfactory method is under direct observation with the aid of the greater magnification and illumination of the slit lamp. Although the cornea is very tough, it is also thin (1 mm). Care must be taken not to penetrate the cornea in the process of removing a deeply imbedded foreign body. Many types of instruments are used for removing superficial corneal foreign bodies, including special ''hockey stick'' or ''golf club'' spuds, scalpel blades, and the points of hypodermic needles. A dental drill of the burr type is often useful for removing an imbedded rust ring.

Following removal of the foreign body, an antibiotic ointment such as polymyxin B–bacitracin (Polysporin®) should be instilled 3 times a day into the conjunctival sac to prevent contamination with bacteria such as Pseudomonas aeruginosa. If the wound is extensive, an eye bandage can be placed over the eye to minimize movement of the lid over the injured area. The wound should be inspected daily for evidence of infection until it is completely healed.

Burns

Thermal burns of the eye structures are treated as burns of skin structures elsewhere, as the tissues of the lids are most commonly involved. If the damage has been deep enough to cause sloughing of the corneal tissue, the eye is almost certainly lost by extensive scarring or perforation, necessitating enucleation.

Ultraviolet irradiation, even in moderate doses, often produces a superficial keratitis which is quite painful, although recovery occurs within 12-36 hours without complications. Pain often comes on 6-12 hours after exposure. This type of injury occurs following exposure to an electric welding arc without the protection of a filter. Many ''flash burns'' are caused by careless exposure in the mistaken belief that the eyes can be burned in this way only when looking directly at the arc. A short circuit in a high-voltage line may cause the same type of injury.

In severe cases of ''flash burn,'' instillation of a sterile topical anesthetic may be necessary for examination. A mydriatic (eg, homatropine hydrobromide, 2-5%) should be used. Systemic sedation or narcotics are preferable to topical anesthetics. Local corticosteroid therapy and cold compresses are indicated to relieve discomfort.

Infrared exposure rarely produces an ocular reaction. (''Glass-blower's cataract'' is rare today but once was common among workers who were required to watch the color changes in molten glass in furnaces without proper filters.) Viewing the sun or an eclipse of the sun without an adequate filter, however, may produce a serious burn of the macula resulting in permanent impairment of vision.

Excessive exposure to radiation (x-ray) has for many years been known to produce cataractous changes which may not appear for many months after the exposure. The same risk is inherent in exposure to nuclear devices.

PENETRATING INJURIES TO THE EYE
(Lacerations, Intraocular Foreign Bodies)

Note: Tetanus prophylaxis is indicated whenever penetrating eye injury occurs.

Lacerations

Lacerations are usually caused by sharp objects (knives, scissors, a projecting portion of the dashboard of an automobile, etc). Such injuries are treated in different ways depending upon whether there is prolapse of tissue or not.

A. Lacerations Without Prolapse of Tissue: If the eyeball has been penetrated anteriorly without evidence of prolapse of intraocular contents, and if the wound is clean and apparently free from contamination, it can

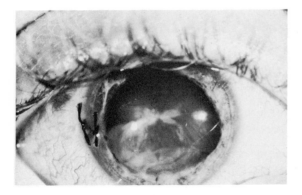

Fig 17-4. Corneal laceration with sutures in place. Note also traumatic cataract.

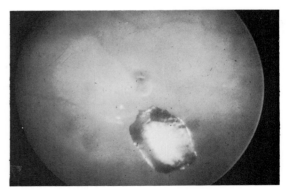

Fig 17-5. Ophthalmoscopic view of intraocular metallic (iron) foreign body in vitreous.

usually be repaired by direct interrupted sutures of fine silk or catgut. Blood clots can be gently removed from the anterior chamber by irrigation and the chamber re-formed after corneal repair by injection of normal saline solution or air. A mydriatic should be used and an antibiotic solution instilled in the conjunctival sac, and bilateral eye bandages applied. The patient should be placed at bed rest for a few days and systemic antibiotics given to minimize the chance of intraocular infection.

B. Lacerations With Prolapse: If only a small portion of the iris prolapses through the wound, this should be grasped with a forceps and excised at the level of the wound lip. Small amounts of uveal tissue can be removed in a similar way. The wound should then be closed in the same manner as a wound without prolapse, and the same follow-up care given. If uveal tissue has been injured, the possibility of sympathetic ophthalmia is always present.

If the wound has been extensive and loss of intraocular contents has been great enough that the prognosis for useful function is hopeless, evisceration or enucleation is indicated as the primary surgical procedure.

Intraocular Foreign Bodies

Foreign bodies which have become lodged within the eye should be identified and localized as soon as possible. Particles of iron or copper must be removed to prevent later disorganization of ocular tissues by degenerative changes (siderosis from iron and chalcosis from copper). Some of the newer alloys are more inert and may be tolerated. Other kinds of particles, such as glass or porcelain, may be tolerated indefinitely and are usually better left alone.

A complaint of discomfort in the eye with blurred vision and a history of striking steel upon steel should arouse a strong suspicion of an intraocular foreign body. The anterior portion of the eye, including the cornea, iris, lens, and sclera, should be inspected with a loupe or slit lamp in an attempt to localize the wound of entry. Direct ophthalmoscopic visualization of an intraocular foreign body may be possible. An orbital x-ray must be taken to verify the presence of a radiopaque foreign body as well as for medicolegal reasons.

Localizing x-rays can be obtained by several methods, usually by the method of Comberg, using a contact lens; or the method of Sweet, with a geometric calculation following accurate positioning of a guide post. By one of these special means the radiologist is able to plot the approximate position of the foreign body within the eye or orbit. The Berman metal locator (p 33) is an electronic instrument for detecting the presence of metals. It is useful in pinpointing an intraocular foreign body located near one of the accessible areas of the eyeball. The wand of the instrument can be sterilized and passed posteriorly over the exposed field at surgery.

If the foreign body is anterior to the lens zonules, it should be removed through an incision into the anterior chamber at the limbus. If it is located posteriorly, there are 2 schools of thought regarding its removal. Some believe that posterior intraocular foreign bodies should be removed through the area of the pars plana which is nearest to the foreign body because less retinal damage is caused in that manner. Others maintain that the damage has been done already and that the foreign body should be removed directly through that point on the wall of the eyeball which is nearest to it, unless that area is at the macula.

If the foreign body has magnetic properties, the sterilized tip of a hand magnet (or giant magnet) near the area of exit can be used to facilitate its removal. If it is nonmagnetic and removal is essential, small forceps have been devised for introduction into the posterior portion of the eye with minimal displacement and trauma. A special instrument has been devised to grasp a spherical air rifle or shotgun pellet.

Any damaged area of the retina must be treated with diathermy or photocoagulation to prevent retinal detachment.

INJURIES TO THE LIDS

Many lacerations of the lids do not involve the margins, and may be sutured in the same way as other lacerations of the skin. If the margin of the eyelid is involved, however, precautions must be taken in an attempt to prevent marginal notching. The most effective technic is to split the lid margin on both sides of the laceration in a frontal plane (anterior, posterior) through the gray line, forming 2 sheets of tissue. A small "V" of skin can then be removed from the anterior surface of one side of the laceration and a small "V" of tarsus removed from the other side, allowing the 2 flaps to overlap in 2 suture lines. This is called "halving the lid" and produces a smooth repair. Direct appositional closure utilizing a figure-of-eight suture is currently favored by many.

Rarely, extreme edema of the tissues prevents apposition of the wound for primary closure, and the repair must be delayed (secondary repair) until this has subsided. Local debridement and irrigation, with use of antibiotics, should be carried out until it is possible to approximate the edges of the wound.

Lacerations of the lids near the inner canthus frequently involve the canaliculi. If these are not repaired, permanent stricture with epiphora will result. In repair of a canaliculus, a small polyethylene tube or large piece of heavy stiff suture material is introduced through both portions of the severed canaliculus and maintained in place while the tissues are reapproximated. This procedure will often maintain a patent duct while the tissues are healing. The Viers canaliculus rod is an effective canaliculus splint for most cases. The pigtail probe is helpful in identifying the cut end of the canaliculus and serves as a guide for threading polyethlyene tubing. These should be left in place for several weeks, and subsequent dilatations performed if strictures tend to form.

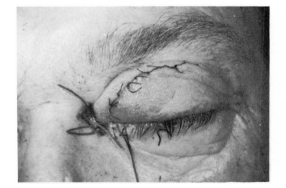

Fig 17-6. Complete laceration of upper lid and upper and lower canaliculi. Large sutures used in repair of severed canaliculi and medial canthal tendon.

Canaliculus repair should be performed immediately inasmuch as subsequent attempts at repair are much more difficult.

INJURIES INVOLVING THE ORBIT AND ITS CONTENTS

Bony Injury

Fractures of the walls of the orbit may be caused by direct blows or by extension of a fracture line from adjacent bones. The outer table of the frontal bone above the orbit may receive crushing injuries without damaging the orbital contents. Similarly, injuries of the zygomatic bone, nasal bone and accessory sinuses, and the medial wall of the orbit can be involved in depressed injuries to the face in automobile accidents. If a fracture involves the paranasal sinuses, emphysema may be noted by crepitation on palpation. Such an involvement frequently is followed by the development of chronic osteomyelitis.

Blowout Fracture

Isolated orbital floor or "blowout" fracture, without concurrent orbital rim fracture, usually follows blunt injury to the eye. Orbital contents herniate into the maxillary sinus, and the inferior rectus or inferior oblique muscle may become incarcerated at the fracture site.

Signs and symptoms are pain and nausea at the time of injury and diplopia on looking up or down. Diplopia may occur immediately or within a few days. Enophthalmos may not be present until the orbital reaction clears. The fracture site is best demonstrated by antral roof deformation on Waters' view x-rays or laminagrams. There is limited movement of the eye even with forced ductions.

If the fracture is large or muscle imbalance significant, prompt surgical reduction is imperative. If the vertical imbalance is small, surgery can be delayed a few days or weeks as long as steady improvement is noted.

Two effective means of surgical treatment are available. A Caldwell-Luc antrostomy can be used for antral packing after direct reduction from below. Packing is generally left in place 2 weeks. Traction on the extraocular muscles by forceps or sling sutures will verify reduction. The fracture site may be approached through the lower lid along the orbital floor. In this instance, the prolapsed tissue is reduced and the orbital floor defect is bridged with a graft of bone, cartilage, or plastic material.

Penetrating Injury

Penetrating injuries of the orbital tissue may be produced by flying missiles or sharp instruments. Radiopaque foreign bodies can be localized by x-ray methods similar to those used in locating foreign bodies within the eye. Most orbital foreign bodies are best left alone.

Contusions

Contusion injuries to the orbital contents may result in hemorrhage or subsequent atrophy of the tissue, with enophthalmos. Traumatic paresis of the extraocular muscles occasionally occurs in this way but is usually transient.

Pulsating Exophthalmos

Pulsating exophthalmos occasionally follows a penetrating or contusion injury to the orbital contents which has caused a shunt between the arterial and venous channels so that the pulse is transmitted into the orbital tissues. (This condition may develop spontaneously, but is more frequently traumatic in origin.) A common site of involvement is a fracture through the cavernous sinus.

Pulsating exophthalmos occasionally requires ligation of the carotid artery on the side of the aneurysm.

•　　•　　•

Bibliography

Byron, H. M.: Ocular trauma. Eye Ear Nose Throat Month 42:48-57, 1963.

Callahan, A.: Surgery of the Eye: Injuries. Thomas, 1950.

Cleasby, G. The orbit. Annual review. Arch Ophth 76:450-60, 1966.

Gregorson, E.: Traumatic hyphema: report of 200 consecutive cases. Acta Ophth 40:192-9, 1962.

Hoefle, F. B.: Initial treatment of eye injuries. Arch Ophth 79:33-6, 1968.

McDonald, P. R.: Penetrating wounds of the eye. Tr Am Acad Ophth 60:812-20, 1956.

Monahan, R. H., & C. W. Hill: Eye injuries. Journal-Lancet 86:257-61, 1966.

Oksala, A.: Treatment of traumatic hyphaema. Brit J Ophth 51:315-20, 1967.

Paton, D., & M. F. Goldberg: Injuries to the Eye, the Lids, and the Orbit. Saunders, 1970.

Pettit, T. H., & E. U. Keates: Traumatic cleavage of the anterior chamber angle. Arch Ophth 69:438-45, 1963.

Snow, J. B., Jr.: The management of orbital wall fractures. Tr Am Acad Ophth 74:1045-51, 1970.

18...

Ocular Disorders Associated With Systemic Diseases

IMPORTANT SYSTEMIC DISEASES WITH SIGNIFICANT RETINOPATHY

RETINOPATHY DUE TO ARTERIOSCLEROSIS

The central retinal artery branches within the eye into thin-walled arterioles with lumens larger than those of vessels of similar external size elsewhere. At arteriolar-venous crossings the walls of both vessels are intimately associated in a common sheath. With the thickening of the arteriolar vessel wall, the less resistant vein is deflected toward a right angle and compressed. This is known clinically as arteriovenous ("A-V") nicking.

If arteriolar sclerosis develops as a response to early hypertension, the prognosis for sight and life is much better than when little or no sclerosis develops. Sclerotic vessels tend to resist increased pressure, resulting in less damage to adjacent tissue. In general, the younger the patient at onset of hypertension (and the more acute the onset), the more generalized the damage that results. Mild arteriosclerotic changes normally occur in older individuals (late 50's). If the process occurs earlier, it may be associated with hypercholesterolemia or hyperlipidemia or compounded by the added insult of early persistent hypertension.

Appearance of Retinal Vessels

A. Blood Column: A normal arteriolar wall is transparent, so that what is actually seen is the column of blood within the vessel. A thin central light reflection in the center of the blood column appears as a yellow refractile line about $1/5$ the width of the column. Spasm of a vessel narrows the blood column, usually in an irregular fashion, and indicates hypertension. As the walls of the arterioles become infiltrated with lipids and cholesterol, the vessels become sclerotic. As this process continues, the vessel wall gradually loses its transparency and becomes visible; the blood column appears wider than normal, and the thin light reflex becomes broader. The grayish yellow fat products in the vessel wall blend with the red of the blood column to produce a typical "copper wire" appearance. This indicates moderate arteriosclerosis. As sclerosis proceeds, the blood column—vessel wall light reflection resembles "silver wire," which indicates severe arteriosclerosis; at times, even occlusion of an arteriolar branch may occur.

B. Arteriolar-Venous Crossings: (Fig 18-1.) The following changes indicative of arteriolarsclerosis are best evaluated 2-3 disk diameters from the optic disk (ophthalmoscopic examination).

1. Arteriolar-venous compression (concealment).

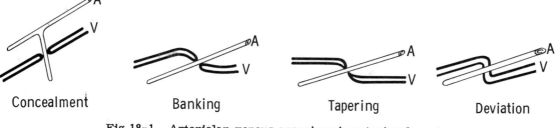

Concealment   Banking   Tapering   Deviation

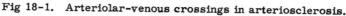

Fig 18-1. Arteriolar-venous crossings in arteriosclerosis.

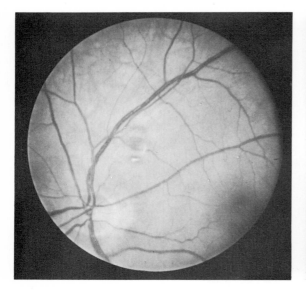

Fig 18-2. Keith-Wagener retinopathy stage I.
Minimal vascular changes; a nearly normal fundus.

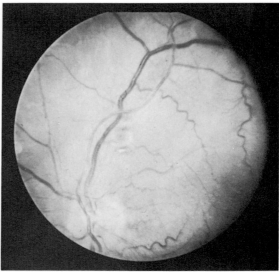

Fig 18-3. Keith-Wagener retinopathy stage II.
Tendency to right-angle crossing of the veins beneath the arterioles with compression of the veins; increased sclerosis of arterioles.

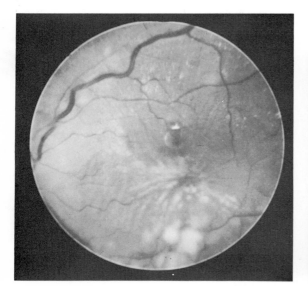

Fig 18-4. Keith-Wagener retinopathy stage III.
Retinal edema around the macular area (star figure) with "cotton-wool" patches.

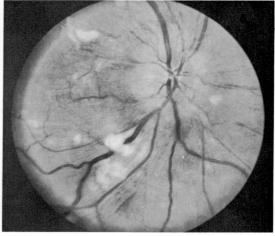

Fig 18-5. Keith-Wagener retinopathy stage IV.
Same changes as stage III plus papilledema. (Photo by Diane Beeston.)

2. Banking of the vein - Distal to its arteriolar crossing, the vein is more curved than normal.

3. Tapering of the vein - As the vein approaches the arteriolar-venous crossing, the blood column becomes gradually attenuated (narrowed).

4. Deviation of the vein - The wall of the vein is thinner than that of the arteriole and is deflected at the arteriolar-venous crossing toward a 90° angle.

C. Sheathing of Arterioles: In advanced sclerotic changes, the arteriolar wall may become distinguishable as a white line at the edges of the blood column. This is known as "sheathing of the arterioles."

Complications of Arteriosclerotic Changes

Narrowing of the lumen of an arteriole or vein causes partial or complete obstruction, with either "artery occlusion" or "venous thrombosis."

Symptoms of Arteriosclerotic Retinopathy

The visual impairment is dependent on the location of the vascular lesions and the nature of complications such as glaucoma, optic atrophy, thrombosis of a central retinal vessel, and, extremely rarely, transitory amblyopia due to arterial spasm.

RETINOPATHY DUE TO HYPERTENSION

Ophthalmoscopic Changes in Hypertension

In the early stages there may be minimal observable ocular evidence of hypertension: Keith-Wagener stage I (K-W I). Irregular narrowing of retinal arterioles occurs as a result of focal areas of spasm of the arteriole walls. Flame-shaped hemorrhages occur in nerve fiber layers. Small, round hemorrhages occur in the outer plexiform layer (K-W II).

Small, "hard-appearing" exudates (usually nonabsorbable) in the outer plexiform layer represent the nonabsorbable fraction of serum following retinal edema. Fluffy white areas ("cotton-wool patches," not true exudates) about $1/5$ as large as the disk appear in the nerve fiber layer. Pathologically, there are cytoid bodies, a collection of swollen glial cells resulting from an ischemic infarct of the terminal arteriole in the nerve fiber layer (K-W III).

Edema of the macula appears in severe hypertension and presents as a white star radiating from the fovea. This formation is due to edema in Henle's fiber layer (outer plexiform layer) of the retina. The star may be incomplete.

Papilledema is a serious finding in malignant hypertension (K-W IV). It may be associated with increased intracranial pressure due to altered cerebral circulation.

In general, the changes of hypertension, including vessel spasm, retinal edema, hemorrhages, cotton-wool patches, and papilledema, are reversible; whereas the changes in arteriosclerosis, including blood column reflex changes, sheathing, arteriovenous changes, exudates, and occlusion of large retinal vessels, are relatively irreversible.

In the classification below, hypertensive patients usually fall into either stages I and II or stages III and IV, ie, a patient does not as a rule advance from stage II to stage III. Persons in stages III and IV are generally younger individuals with severe hypertension and minimal arteriolar sclerotic changes.

Adequate antihypertensive therapy is of greatest value in stage III or IV but of questionable value in stage I or II. Controlled series have shown that such treatment prolongs life in stages III and IV. Prognosis varies greatly with the height of the diastolic blood pressure and the degree of cardiac, cerebral, or renal involvement. The younger the patient's age at onset, the poorer the prognosis. The changes of retinal vessels correlate well with vessel changes in the brain and kidney.

Table 18-1. A classification of hypertensive retinopathy (modified after Keith and Wagener).

Stage	Ophthalmoscopic Appearance	Clinical Classification
I	Minimal narrowing or sclerosis of arterioles.	"Essential" hypertension (chronic, benign, "arteriosclerotic").
II	Thickening and dulling of vessel reflection (copper-wire appearance). Localized and generalized narrowing of arterioles. Changes at arteriolar-venous crossings (A-V nicking). Scattered round or flame-shaped hemorrhages. Vascular occlusion may be present. Very small exudates.	
III	Sclerotic changes may not be marked. "Angiospastic retinopathy": Localized arteriolar spasm, hemorrhages, exudates, "cotton-wool patches," retinal edema.	Angiospastic hypertension (malignant).
IV	Same as III, plus papilledema (neuroretinopathy).	

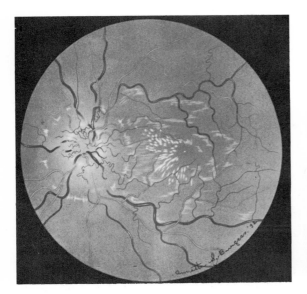

Fig 18-6. Keith-Wagener retinopathy stage IV. Severe hypertensive retinopathy showing papilledema, macular edema, A-V nicking, and narrow arterioles (drawing). (Reproduced, with permission, from Wilmer: Atlas Fundus Oculi. Macmillan, 1934.)

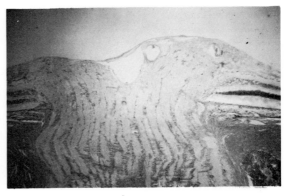

Fig 18-7. Photomicrograph showing pathologic changes in papilledema.

Symptoms of Hypertensive Retinopathy

On rare occasions, impaired vision may be the presenting symptom of hypertension. Unilateral or bilateral blurring of vision, scotomas, or partial amblyopia may occur, but complete blindness is extremely rare.

RENAL RETINOPATHY

A single attack of acute glomerulonephritis causes no permanent retinal damage. If the disease becomes subacute or chronic, retinopathy develops. In general, the process is indistinguishable from the "angiospastic retinitis" described in stage III and IV hypertensive retinopathy. The retinopathy is associated with the hypertension.

RETINOPATHY IN TOXEMIA OF PREGNANCY

Severe toxemia of pregnancy characteristically causes retinopathy of the "angiospastic" hypertensive type (stage III or IV). Generalized as well as localized constriction of the larger arterioles is the first sign of retinopathy. If the toxemia is not controlled, marked retinopathy occurs, including retinal edema with macular star formation, papilledema, cotton-wool patches, widespread hemorrhages, and serous retinal detachment. Nearly all cases show the advanced retinopathy at or near term. Marked retinopathy is an indication for termination of pregnancy, and the prognosis is good for life and vision if pregnancy is terminated before irreversible vascular changes have occurred.

SUBACUTE BACTERIAL ENDOCARDITIS

Multiple petechial conjunctival hemorrhages may occur in subacute bacterial endocarditis. Retinopathy is present in 40% of cases at some point during the course of the disease. This consists of hemorrhages, either deep or flame-shaped, and Roth spots— small white spots often surrounded by hemorrhages—believed to be collections of lymphocytes and edema fluid. It is thought that the bacteria cause a local toxic effect on the capillary walls which causes the hemorrhage. The spots may be localized lymphocytic accumulations or structureless deposits. Papilledema is present in one-third of cases. Occlusion of the central retinal artery by emboli is an occasional complication.

CYANOSIS RETINAE

Cyanosis of the retina may occur with those diseases that cause generalized cyanosis (eg, congestive failure, congenital heart disease). The conjunctivas are congested and cyanotic. Retinal veins are dark, tortuous, and dilated. Retinal arteries are dark but normal in size. The retina in general is dark and often edematous, with scattered hemorrhages.

BLOOD DYSCRASIAS AND LYMPHATIC DISEASES

Pernicious Anemia (Fig 18-8)

Early in the disease the fundus is pale and the veins somewhat tortuous and dilated. The arteries are normal. Later (when the red blood count drops below 2.5 million/cu mm), flame-shaped retinal hemorrhages appear near the vessels and choroidal hemorrhage is often seen. The hemorrhages become more numerous and may break through the retina to become preretinal. The visual acuity is affected only if hemorrhage occurs in the macula. The conjunctivas often have a suggestive pale appearance.

Retrobulbar neuritis is present in 5% of cases and leads to optic atrophy.

Chronic Anemia

Ocular changes in all chronic anemias are the same as early changes in pernicious anemia. In severe chronic anemias, the later changes of pernicious anemia (except for retrobulbar neuritis) may occur.

Acute Massive Hemorrhage

Complete and sudden, permanent blindness occurs rarely following acute massive hemorrhage, most commonly if bleeding is from the gastrointestinal tract or uterus. This occurs as a result of severe spasm of central retinal artery (reversible) or occlusion of the central retinal artery (irreversible). More often, generalized edema and a pale fundus with constricted arteries and dilated veins occur which clear as the red blood count returns to normal.

Hemorrhagic Disorders

Retinal and choroidal hemorrhage may occur in many types of hemorrhagic disorders; it is commonly associated with recurrent systemic hemorrhage (eg, thrombocytopenic purpura). Retinal edema, especially about the optic disk, may also be present. Following recovery or during remissions, the fundus is normal.

Leukemia (Fig 18-9)

There may be retinal pallor due to increased number of white blood cells. The various types of leukemia do not present characteristic fundus pictures. Retinopathy due to secondary anemia occurs as described above. Leukocytic infiltration of the conjunctiva and orbit may be present.

Polycythemia Vera (Fig 18-10)

Retinal veins are dark, tortuous, and dilated. Retinal arteries are normal. Scattered retinal hemorrhages are often present. Retinal edema and papilledema are occasionally present.

Lymphoma

Orbital involvement with lymphosarcoma or Hodgkin's disease is not uncommon. A tumor so placed may be the only manifestation of the lymphoma. It is usually present beneath the conjunctiva of the upper cul-de-sac and will readily respond to local radiation therapy. Characteristically, no retinopathy is present in these diseases.

DIABETES MELLITUS

Diabetes mellitus is a complex metabolic disorder that also involves the small blood vessels, often causing widespread damage to many body tissues, including the eyes.

The ocular complications of diabetes are dependent not only upon impaired carbohydrate metabolism but also upon as yet undefined complexes of factors, and these may occur before the characteristic findings of glycosuria, hyperglycemia, polyuria, and polyphagia become manifest. The ocular complications occur approximately 20 years after onset despite apparently adequate diabetic control. Improved treatment measures (eg, improved insulins, antibiotics) which have lengthened the life span of diabetics have actually resulted in a marked increase in incidence of retinopathy and other ocular complications. Diabetes has rapidly become the second largest cause of blindness in the USA and may soon lead the list. The outlook for adult (maturity onset) diabetes is considerably better than for juvenile diabetes.

The possibility of diabetes should be considered in all patients with unexplained retinopathy, cataract, extraocular muscle palsy, optic neuritis, or sudden changes in refractive error. Absence of glycosuria or a normal fasting blood glucose level does not exclude a diagnosis of diabetes. Postprandial blood glucose determinations and glucose tolerance

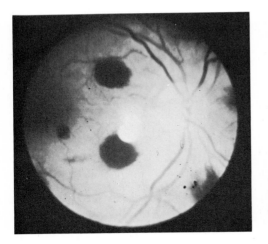

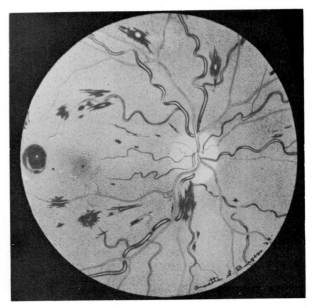

Fig 18-8. Retinal hemorrhages associated with severe pernicious anemia. (Woman, age 54.) Hemoglobin, 17%. RBC, 900,000/cu mm.

Fig 18-9. Retinal hemorrhages associated with chronic lymphatic leukemia. (Reproduced, with permission, from Wilmer: Atlas Fundus Oculi. Macmillan, 1934.)

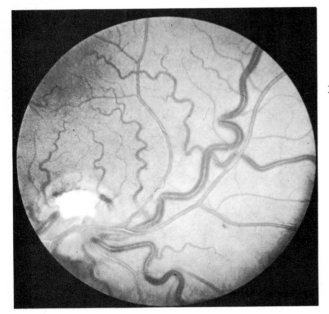

Fig 18-10. Engorged and markedly tortuous veins of polycythemia vera. Note that arteries are relatively unaffected. (Photo by L. Arlinghaus.)

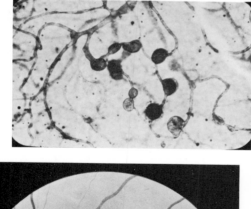

Fig 18-11. Diabetic retinopathy stage I.
Microscopic section showing microaneurysms of the retinal capillaries.

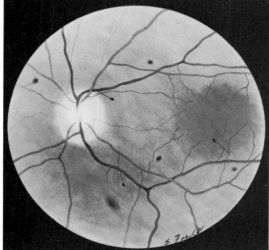

Fig 18-12. Diabetic retinopathy stage I.
Punctate hemorrhages and capillary aneurysms. All hemorrhages are essentially
round in form.

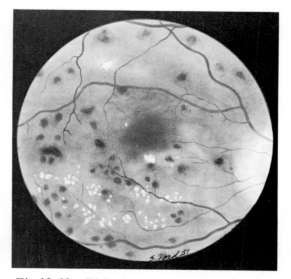

Fig 18-13. Diabetic retinopathy stage II.
Round hemorrhages are more prominent,
and some small waxy exudates are present.

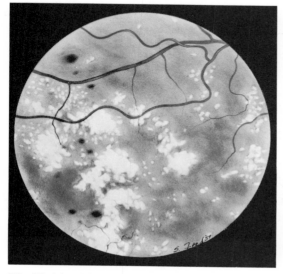

Fig 18-14. Diabetic retinopathy, late stage II.
Exudates coalesced into larger masses.

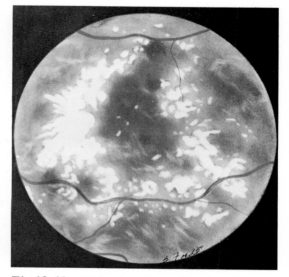

Fig 18-15. Diabetic retinopathy stage II.
Circinate distribution of coalesced exudates
around the macula.

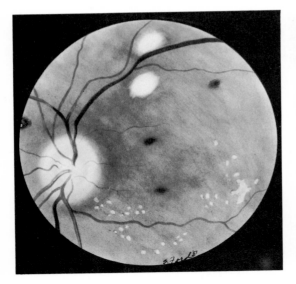

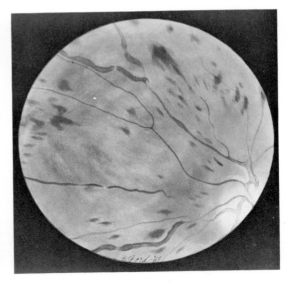

Fig 18-16. Diabetic retinopathy stage III.
Cotton-wool patches have been added to
hemorrhages and exudates.

Fig 18-17. Diabetic retinopathy stage IV.
Hemorrhages with marked disease of the
veins (link sausage appearance of veins).

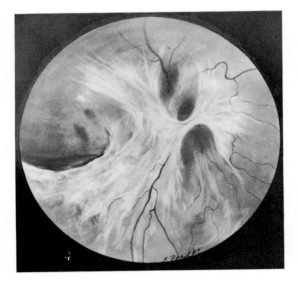

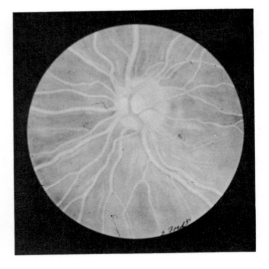

Fig 18-18. Diabetic retinopathy stage V.
Preretinal hemorrhage and retinitis proliferans.

**Fig 18-19. Lipemia retinalis in advanced
diabetes.**

(Figs 18-12 to 18-19 courtesy of F. Cordes.)

tests may be required. Rarely, the diabetic ocular change may become evident before there is demonstrable evidence of impaired glucose tolerance.

Careful control of diabetes in an attempt to retard or minimize retinopathy would seem prudent at the present time even though evidence supporting the value of rigid control remains controversial.

Hypophysectomy, or pituitary ablation by freezing probe or irradiation, has been employed in patients with advanced diabetic retinopathy with some encouraging results in highly selected patients with no renal dysfunction. Significant improvement of visual acuity and actual regression of retinal changes for over 6 years has been reported. Pituitary ablation carries the risk of blindness and hormonal problems caused by the operation.

Sealing off of retinal vessels involved in proliferative retinopathy with a Zeiss photocoagulator or by one of several types of laser photocoagulators shows promise of slowing down or stopping retinopathy in its more advanced stages.

Because of the highly variable course of diabetic retinopathy, it is difficult to evaluate the results of the above treatment methods. The retinopathy may be relatively stable, slowly progressive, or rapidly progressive. Spontaneous arrest or improvement may occur in as many as 10% of patients with progressive proliferative retinopathy who have received no photocoagulation or suppression of pituitary function.

Although most diabetic patients with severe retinopathy have a relatively short life expectancy (5-6 years), they may live 10-20 years or longer.

Retinopathy

The ophthalmoscopic appearance in diabetic retinopathy may be divided into 5 stages: (Figs 18-11 to 18-18.)

Stage I: Microaneurysms resembling small round hemorrhages appear near the optic disk and macula. Slight dilatation of veins may be present. The arterioles are normal. Histologically, microaneurysms occur on the venous side of capillaries in the inner nuclear layer.

Stage II: The veins are dilated, and scattered, small, waxy-yellowish, hard-appearing exudates are seen. Exudates in the outer plexiform layer are visible on histologic section.

Stage III: In addition to stage II findings there are cotton-wool patches (fluffy white areas in the nerve fiber layer, usually much smaller than the optic disk). These occur mainly when hypertensive retinopathy is also present. The cytoid body may be seen on his-

tologic section. This is the result of ischemic infarction of a terminal arteriole and appears as an eosinophilic, granular, disk-shaped area in the nerve fiber layer representing swollen glial cells.

Stage IV: Marked venous changes are present. Venules are dilated and appear cyanotic, with sheathing and a link-sausage appearance of vessels. Large and small hemorrhages are prominent, and may occur within any layer of the retina or become preretinal. Histologically, hemorrhages may be seen in any layer of the retina.

Stage V: Large retinal and preretinal hemorrhages, and hemorrhages into the vitreous. The latter gradually absorb, leaving fibrous scar tissue with new vessel formation. This gives the picture of retinitis proliferans. These fibrous strands are attached to the retina, and subsequent contraction of the scar tissue may detach the retina, leading to ultimate total loss of vision.

Lipemia retinalis: (Fig 18-19) This is a rare but spectacular ophthalmoscopic finding in young, severely involved diabetics who are out of control. The fundus is quite pale, and the vessels appear filled with milk because of the high fat content of the blood. Vision may be unaffected. Lipemia retinalis is seen in diabetic coma, or is an indication of impending coma. This condition is also observed in type I hyperlipoproteinemia (Fredrickson).

The presence and degree of retinopathy seem to be more closely related to the duration of the disease than to its severity. Control plays only a minor role (if any) in the onset of retinopathy, and once the process is well under way no amount of control seems to affect its progress.

The juvenile diabetic develops a severe form of retinopathy within 20 years in 60-75% of cases, even if under good control. The retinopathy often begins in stage IV and progresses to stage V. In older diabetic patients, retinopathy usually begins in stage I and seldom progresses beyond stage III. Macular degeneration may reduce the central visual acuity markedly in the later stages.

Lens Changes

A. True Diabetic Cataract (Rare): Bilateral cataracts occasionally occur with a rapid onset in severe juvenile diabetes. The lens may become completely opaque in several weeks. The process starts as snow-white areas in the cortex—posterior subcapsular and some anterior subcapsular opacities which progressively involve more and more cortex—and finally become confluent to make the entire lens opaque.

B. Senile Cataract in the Diabetic (Common): Typical senile nuclear sclerosis, posterior subcapsular changes, and cortical opacities occur earlier and more frequently in diabetics.

C. Sudden Changes in the Refraction of the Lens: Especially when diabetes is not well controlled, changes in blood glucose levels cause changes in sugar alcohols of the lens which in turn cause changes in refractive power by as much as 3 or 4 diopters. This results in blurred vision. Such changes do not occur when the disease is well controlled.

Iris Changes

Glycogen infiltration of the pigmented epithelium and sphincter and dilator muscles of the iris may cause diminished pupillary responses.

Rubeosis iridis is common in severe juvenile diabetes. Numerous small intertwining blood vessels develop on the anterior surface of the iris. Spontaneous hyphema may occur. The formation of peripheral anterior synechias is aided by the vascularization of anterior chamber structures, eventually blocking aqueous outflow sufficiently to cause secondary glaucoma.

Extraocular Muscle Palsy

This common occurrence in diabetes is manifested by a sudden onset of diplopia due to paresis of an extraocular muscle. The tendency is toward complete recovery within 4-6 weeks. An extraocular muscle palsy may be the clinical sign that leads to the diagnosis of diabetes.

Optic Atrophy

This complication of diabetes is being reported with increasing frequency.

Iridocyclitis

This is particularly common in juvenile diabetes and nearly always responds well to standard nonspecific treatment of topical corticosteroids and cycloplegics.

Optic Neuritis

Retrobulbar neuritis and papillitis are seen more commonly in diabetics than in nondiabetics, but they are much less common than optic atrophy. Isolated cases of papilledema have also been reported. The diabetic is also more susceptible to tobacco and other toxic amblyopias.

GOUT

An insidious nongranulomatous uveitis is the most common of the numerous ocular abnormalities associated with gout. At times the uveitis is quite severe, associated with increased intraocular tension, corneal edema, marked aqueous flare and cells, and numerous small keratic precipitates. These attacks usually clear promptly in response to mydriatic and local corticosteroid therapy.

Episcleritis, scleritis, eyelid eczema, and conjunctivitis are associated with gout less commonly and usually are easily controlled by topical corticosteroid therapy.

ENDOCRINE DISEASES

Disturbances of the endocrine glands have a number of important ocular manifestations. By far the most important of these are due to disturbances of the thyroid gland, although parathyroid and pituitary abnormalities also produce significant ocular changes.

THYROTOXICOSIS

The principal ocular sign of thyrotoxicosis is exophthalmos, which is seldom greater than 3 mm and most often is about 1.5 mm. The exophthalmos is usually unassociated with conjunctival hyperemia or chemosis. Retraction of the upper lid due to stimulation of Müller's muscle is common, and accentuates the appearance of exophthalmos. Lid lag (Graefe's sign) occurs in about 80% of cases. The upper lid lags above its normal position in downward rotation of the eyes, so that several mm of sclera are visible above the exposed superior limbus. Infrequent blinking (Stellwag's sign) may occur, as well as other less important lid signs.

Mild to moderate external ophthalmoplegia is often present (40% of cases), eg, impaired elevation due to weakness of the superior rectus muscle. Horizontal and downward movements are less commonly affected.

The BMR, PBI, T_4, radioactive T_3 red cell uptake, and radioiodine (^{131}I) uptake are all elevated. The radioiodine uptake cannot be suppressed by T_3 administration.

The exophthalmometer reading may show asymmetry. Orbital tonometry is usually normal.

Examination of tissues in cases of thyrotoxic exophthalmos reveals normal orbital contents with no edema or round cell infiltration. Some atrophy of the extraocular muscles is usually present.

Subtotal thyroidectomy (preceded by appropriate medical preparation) probably remains the most widely accepted treatment method available. Treatment with radioactive iodine appears to be an excellent alternative in older patients. Propylthiouracil, 100-250 mg 3 times daily for 6-18 months, is an acceptable form of therapy also, with a reported cure rate of about 60%

The results of adequate surgical or medical treatment are very good (95% cure) except for the ocular changes, which do not respond nearly as well as other signs and symptoms. Lid retraction and other lid signs often disappear, but exophthalmos is rarely favorably influenced and occasionally becomes progressive.

Untreated thyrotoxicosis can eventually cause marked general debility, including extreme weight loss, weakness, and cardiac failure. The exophthalmos remains stationary, but lid signs and external ophthalmoplegia tend to be progressive without adequate therapy. The lid signs may be diminished by the administration of topical 0.1% guanethidine given 2 or 3 times daily.

MALIGNANT EXOPHTHALMOS

An uncommon progressive type of exophthalmos which occurs most frequently in middle age may develop following thyroidectomy, but occasionally occurs during mild thyrotoxicosis, during thiouracil treatment, or in the absence

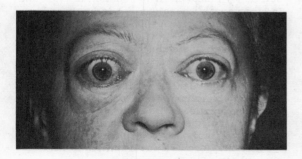

Fig 18-20. Thyrotoxic exophthalmos associated with hyperthyroidism. (Photo by Diane Beeston.)

of previously identified hyperthyroid disease. The cause of this so-called "malignant exophthalmos" is not completely understood, but overaction of the thyroid gland does not seem to be a factor. There is clinical and experimental evidence that excessive production of thyrotropic hormone by the pituitary gland or excessive secretion of a specific hormone, EPS (exophthalmos-producing substance), causes progressive exophthalmos. Experimentally, male sex hormones have intensified the exophthalmos; this finding is in accord with the observation that men are more frequently affected than women.

Pathologic findings include marked edema and round cell infiltration of the orbital fat, and marked enlargement (sometimes 5 times normal diameter) and lymphocytic infiltration of the extraocular muscles. Many individual muscle fibers degenerate and are replaced by fibrosis.

Clinical Findings

Symptoms consist of lacrimation, photophobia, foreign body sensation, diplopia, pain on eye movements, and a subjective feeling that the eyes are bulging. Proptosis can become extreme. Conjunctival injection may progress to massive chemosis. Other signs include bulging of the lids, external ophthalmoplegia, and increased orbital resistance, which can be estimated with an orbitometer. The process often starts unilaterally and may reach massive proportions before the fellow eye is involved. Sooner or later, however, the fellow eye is usually involved to some degree. Urinary excretion of thyrotropic hormone is increased. Basal metabolic rate, blood cholesterol, protein-bound iodine, and ^{131}I uptake are usually normal.

Complications and Sequelae

With increasing exophthalmos, the lids are no longer able to protect the cornea adequately and exposure keratitis occurs which can lead to secondary corneal ulcerations, perforation, panophthalmitis, and loss of all visual function. Papilledema and retinal hemorrhages occur. Optic atrophy supervenes if pressure on the optic nerve is not relieved in time.

Treatment

Malignant exophthalmos presents a difficult therapeutic problem. Medical means have met with little success. Large doses of corticosteroids systemically (up to 120 mg of prednisolone daily) may reverse the process. Corticosteroids by retrobulbar and subconjunctival injection may also reduce chemosis and proptosis. Thyroid hormone, although not always effective, should be given following thyroid surgery or propylthiouracil therapy to maintain the PBI at about 7-9 μg/100 ml whenever there is a progression of exophthalmos. Estrogens, thiouracil drugs, and irradiation of the pituitary gland have had a few reported successes but far more failures.

Local care of the eye is very important. Protective ointments, transparent shields, and prompt attention to secondary infection to prevent corneal ulceration are important. Lateral tarsorrhaphy will occasionally help protect the cornea.

Frequent measurements with an exophthalmometer are necessary. If patients can be tided over the active phase and the disease appears to be self-limited, radical surgery can be avoided. However, if corneal or optic nerve changes are resulting in visual loss, surgical decompression is mandatory. This can be accomplished transcranially by the Naffziger approach through the orbital roof. A slightly safer but possibly less effective method is the Krönlein approach, where the orbital contents are allowed to overflow through a bony opening into the temporal fossa. Decompression can also be accomplished by opening the antrum to orbital contents. In severe cases, more than one decompression procedure may be necessary to protect visual function.

Course and Prognosis

Without decompression, vision in both eyes may be totally lost. With surgical decompression there is usually some return of visual function, or the preoperative visual acuity is maintained. A residual prominence of the eyes, sometimes with extraocular muscle abnormalities, often remains, but the patient is able to resume normal activity. Tarsorrhaphy or resection of redundant conjunctiva following successful orbital decompression may enhance the cosmetic result.

MYXEDEMA

Significant ocular signs are not common in myxedema. Thin superficial corneal opacities and small, flaky, white opacities in the lens cortex, neither of which seriously interferes with vision, may be present. Optic neuritis, with eventual optic atrophy and serious visual disability, occurs very rarely. Orbital pseudotumor has been reported.

HYPOPARATHYROIDISM

Occasionally at thyroidectomy the parathyroid glands are removed inadvertently, causing hypoparathyroidism. Spontaneous cases, although rare, should be suspected in young patients with cataracts. The blood calcium decreases, and serum phosphates are increased. Tetany may ensue and can be severe enough to cause generalized convulsions. The ocular manifestations consist of blepharospasm and twitching eyelids. Small, discrete, punctate opacities of the lens cortex develop which may eventually require lens extraction. Treatment with calcium salts, calciferol, and dihydrotachysterol usually prevents further development of lens opacities, but any that have occurred prior to treatment remain.

HYPERPARATHYROIDISM

In hyperparathyroidism, deposition of calcium may rarely occur in soft tissue. "Metastatic" calcification of the cornea and conjunctiva may be an early sign of the hypercalcemia encountered in this disorder.

DISEASES DUE TO NUTRITIONAL DISTURBANCES

XEROPHTHALMIA
(Avitaminosis A)

Xerophthalmia is the general term applied to the ocular manifestations of pure vitamin A deficiency disease. It is common in India and in other areas where the diet is likely to be deficient in vitamin A. It is seldom seen in the USA.

At onset, the conjunctival and corneal epithelial linings lose their normal luster and become dry and thickened. Microscopically, there is keratinization of the corneal and conjunctival epithelium. In the cornea there is also degeneration of Bowman's membrane and infiltration of the corneal stroma with cells and edema fluid. Corneal ulceration and perforation may occur if the condition is not properly treated.

Clinical Findings

Night blindness is the earliest symptom. Irritation and blurred vision occur if the process continues. Xerosis of the conjunctiva is characterized by the formation of Bitot's spot, a white, foamy, wedge-shaped, lusterless area in the palpebral fissure with its base at the limbus and its apex directed toward the outer canthus. It contains many wrinkles, which are concentric with the limbus. Xerosis of the corneal epithelium occurs in 2 stages: pre-xerosis, a loss of corneal luster and a reduction in corneal sensitivity; and true xerosis, an extension to the cornea of the conjunctival xerosis. Keratomalacia is a late and severe stage of xerophthalmia in which the cornea becomes cloudy, soft, and ulcerative. Perforation, with subsequent panophthalmitis, becomes a serious threat.

Microscopic study of the scrapings from Bitot's spot shows large, keratinized epithelial cells with pale, indistinct cytoplasms and fragmented nuclei. The normal columnar conjunctival epithelium is keratinized and squamous. Xerosis bacilli (nonpathogenic diphtheroids originally thought to be the cause of xerosis) are numerous.

There is a close relationship between retinal function and vitamin A. The regeneration of visual purple is slowed in vitamin A deficiency. Slight night blindness is an early sign of vitamin A deficiency, and mild degrees occur fairly often during pregnancy. Night blindness quickly disappears following vitamin A therapy. Severe cases of night blindness due to vitamin A deficiency are rare.

Complications and Sequelae

In severe cases, perforation of the cornea and subsequent loss of the eye can occur. Bilateral corneal scarring is common.

Treatment

Vitamin A, 50,000 units IM, is given every day until the process is reversed. Broad-

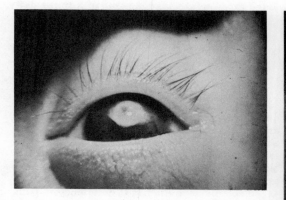

Fig 18-21. Keratomalacia. Case of xerophthalmia in a 5-month-old child.

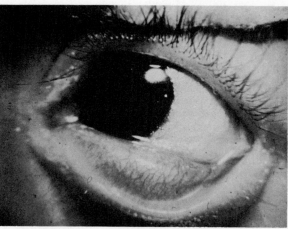

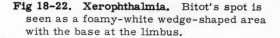

Fig 18-22. Xerophthalmia. Bitot's spot is seen as a foamy-white wedge-shaped area with the base at the limbus.

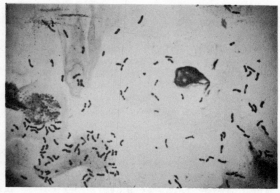

Fig 18-23. Hyperkeratinized conjunctival epithelial cells and xerosis bacilli from a patient with xerophthalmia.

spectrum antibiotic eye ointment (to prevent secondary infection) and vitamin A and D ointment are applied locally 4 times a day. A well balanced diet is necessary to prevent recurrences of deficiency disorders.

Course and Prognosis

Parenteral vitamin A is curative in all cases when given in the early stages. If the process is moderately advanced before treatment, corneal scarring is common. Without treatment, sight can be totally lost through corneal perforation and secondary infection.

HYPERVITAMINOSIS A

Chronic vitamin A intoxication is a cause of pseudotumor cerebri, manifested by bilateral papilledema. The skin and scleras may also appear to be yellowish. The papilledema may not disappear for as long as 4-6 months after the vitamin is discontinued.

HYPERVITAMINOSIS D

Calcium deposits in the cornea and conjunctiva are the most common ocular changes. Strabismus, epicanthal folds, osteosclerosis of orbital bones, nystagmus, papilledema, sluggish pupillary reaction, iritis, and cataract are less common ocular findings. The incidence of these changes has declined substantially since the content of vitamin D in milk and other foodstuffs has been subject to government regulation.

AVITAMINOSIS B$_1$
(Beriberi)

The principal effects of thiamine deficiency are polyneuritis and gastrointestinal disturbances. Up to 70% of patients have associated ocular abnormalities, particularly conjunctivitis and blepharitis. Optic atrophy and central scotoma have also been attributed to vitamin B$_1$ deficiency.

Wernicke's syndrome, previously attributed to alcoholism, is due to the accompanying thiamine deficiency (see Chapter 13).

Beriberi is treated with correction of dietary deficiency. Liver, whole wheat bread, cereals, eggs, and yeast are particularly good sources of vitamin B$_1$. Parenteral injection of thiamine hydrochloride, 50 mg twice daily for

one week, usually alleviates the ocular manifestations of beriberi.

AVITAMINOSIS B$_2$
(Pellagra)

Nicotinic acid and riboflavin make up most of the vitamin B$_2$ complex. A deficiency of nicotinic acid causes pellagra, which is characterized by dermatitis, diarrhea, and dementia. A few cases of optic atrophy causing central scotomas have been reported.

Riboflavin deficiency has been said to cause a number of ocular changes. Rosacea keratitis, vascularization of the limbal cornea, seborrheic blepharitis, and secondary conjunctivitis have all been attributed to riboflavin deficiency, but these conditions seldom respond to riboflavin therapy. Optic atrophy is at times caused by ariboflavinosis. Definite riboflavin-deficient conditions respond well to dried (brewer's) yeast, 25-30 gm 3 times daily.

AVITAMINOSIS C
(Scurvy)

Petechial or larger hemorrhages can occur in the orbit, lids, subconjunctival space, anterior chamber, or vitreous cavity. A striking picture of proptosis, sometimes bilateral, occurs in scorbutic infants who have had orbital hemorrhages. Orbital hemorrhages are rare in adults.

Treatment of vitamin C deficiency is with proper diet, particularly adequate amounts of citrus juice. Supplements of ascorbic acid, 200-300 mg/day orally, or sodium ascorbate injection, 0.5-1 gm IV or IM daily in divided doses, will help correct vitamin C deficiency rapidly.

CHRONIC GRANULOMATOUS INFECTIOUS DISEASES

Many of the so-called granulomatous infectious diseases, including tuberculosis, sarcoidosis, brucellosis, leprosy, and toxoplasmosis, undergo a chronic course with frequent exacerbations and remissions. The eye is often involved, particularly by anterior uveitis. The following paragraphs deal with other ocular complications of these systemic diseases.

TUBERCULOSIS

Ocular tuberculosis results from endogenous spread from systemic foci. The incidence of eye involvement is less than 1% in known cases of pulmonary tuberculosis.

Tuberculosis of the Uveal Tract
A. Iritis (Anterior Uveitis): Many cases of granulomatous uveitis are said to be tuberculous, although very few cases have been established. At times only the anterior segment of the eye is involved. Local treatment of iritis with mydriatics and corticosteroids is indicated. Systemic tuberculosis therapy is useful in the treatment of established cases of tuberculous uveitis.

B. Miliary Tuberculosis: In this usually fatal form of tuberculosis, many small discrete yellowish nodules are visible ophthalmoscopically in the posterior pole of the eye.

C. Solitary Tubercles: These occur as gray isolated masses about the size of the optic disk in the posterior fundus, and usually cause minimal functional disturbance. The tubercles may be the first sign of an impending generalized uveitis. Solitary tubercles are occasionally seen in the iris or ciliary body.

Occasionally, orbital periostitis due to a tubercle has occurred.

Tuberculosis of the Retina
Choroidal involvement usually causes associated retinitis as the pigmented epithelial layer is broken down. This process is spoken of as tuberculous chorioretinitis.

Eales' Disease
The cause of this syndrome of recurrent vitreous hemorrhages is not known. Young men are most commonly affected. When visible, the retina shows perivasculitis with sheathing of vessels and scattered hemorrhages and exudates. Over a period of time, the recurrent vitreous hemorrhages completely destroy vision. Occasional improvement has resulted from surface diathermy treatment (as described under treatment for retinal detachment) of localized periphlebitis, but treatment is usually not effective. The syndrome has not been proved to be tuberculous, and most patients with Eales' disease have no evidence of tuberculosis elsewhere. There is some evidence that the disease may be a peripheral vascular disorder. The patient may retain useful vision for many years, but at least half become blind eventually.

Other Structures
Corneal phlyctenulosis is often tuberculous. Interstitial keratitis is due to tuberculosis in fewer than 10% of cases. Deep scleritis (sclerosing keratitis) associated with interstitial keratitis is often due to tuberculosis. Optic neuritis as a result of tuberculous meningitis is not uncommon. Granuloma of the conjunctiva is rare.

SARCOIDOSIS

Although no organism has been isolated from the lesions of sarcoidosis, this disease is grouped with the granulomatous infectious diseases because of the similarities of the clinical and pathologic pictures.

Sarcoidosis is not rare. It is more common in Negroes than in people of other races. The lesions are widespread and spotty, including diffuse fibrosis about the hilar lung regions, nodular subcutaneous lesions over the body, rarefied long bones (especially the phalanges), and ocular changes. The course of the disease is usually benign and chronic, but serious localized damage, particularly to the eye, can result.

About 35% of cases have ocular involvement at some time during the course of the disease. A low-grade, usually bilateral granulomatous iritis is the most common eye finding. Choroiditis is less common. Typical skin lesions of sarcoidosis frequently involve the lids. Other structures, such as the lacrimal gland, retina, and episcleral tissue, may be involved. In about 25% of cases, conjunctival biopsy shows histologic evidence of sarcoidosis. The cranial nerves and the optic nerve (optic atrophy and papilledema) are occasionally involved.

Local treatment of the anterior uveitis with mydriatics and corticosteroids is indicated. Systemic steroids may be required in anterior uveitis and are usually necessary in posterior uveitis. Diagnosis and control of secondary glaucoma, frequently associated with the anterior uveitis of sarcoidosis, is important.

LEPROSY

Mycobacterium leprae causes chronic granulomatous disease. Leprosy is mildly contagious (more so in childhood), and causes skin and CNS lesions. Although rare in the USA, leprosy is still an important disease in some areas of the world. The eye is affected by endogenous spread during exacerbations of the generalized disease. In over 80% of cases there are eye complications, of which granulomatous uveitis is the most common. Interstitial keratitis, often superficial as well as deep, is also a common eye complication. Hypertrophy of the brows and lids and skin nodules on the lids—as well as ectropion—are common. Other eye structures are seldom affected. The uveitis requires local treatment. The generalized disease responds fairly well to sulfone therapy.

SYPHILIS

Congenital Syphilis

Manifestations of syphilis acquired in utero or at birth include mental deficiency, saddle nose, rhinitis, Hutchinson's teeth, alopecia, exanthemas, deafness, and bone lesions. The most common eye lesion is interstitial keratitis (see p 88). Chorioretinitis unassociated with interstitial keratitis occurs fairly often. There are many small yellow dots and pigment clumps in the peripheral fundus, giving the typical "salt and pepper" appearance. In other cases, the chorioretinitis occurs as larger isolated patches or may have the appearance of retinitis pigmentosa. Syphilitic conjunctivitis or dacryoadenitis is rare.

Congenital syphilis is treated with large doses of penicillin.

Acquired Syphilis

Ocular chancre (primary lesion) occurs rarely on the lid margins and follows the same course as a genital chancre.

Iritis and iridocyclitis occur in the secondary stage of syphilis along with the rash in about 5% of cases. The iritis is acute, with fibrous exudates in the anterior chamber. Posterior synechias are common if care is not taken to keep the pupil dilated.

Other less common ocular manifestations of acquired syphilis are interstitial keratitis and chorioretinitis, which occur much less frequently in acquired than in congenital syphilis; chorioretinitis usually is widespread and often destroys useful vision. Syphilitic chorioretinitis may resemble retinitis pigmentosa in clinical appearance; however, unlike the genetically determined disease, it can be unilateral.

Neuro-ophthalmologic Considerations

Argyll Robertson pupil is particularly common in tabes and paresis. Syphilis often causes complete internal ophthalmoplegia. Optic neuritis is usually due to basal meningi-

tis and may resemble retrobulbar neuritis. Visual fields show marked peripheral constriction. Optic atrophy follows severe chorioretinitis or optic neuritis. A gumma occasionally involves the optic nerve, causing optic atrophy. The third cranial nerve is most commonly involved, causing individual extraocular muscle palsies. The 6th nerve is less frequently involved; the 4th is rarely affected. Of the other cranial nerves, the 7th and 8th are most likely to be affected.

Seronegative Syphilis

Cases of late syphilis seronegative to the commonly used nontreponemal antigen tests (VDRL, Kahn, etc) have been suggested by ocular findings and identified by the much more reliable Treponema pallidum immobilization (TPI) and fluorescent treponemal antibody absorption (FTA-ABS) tests. These ocular signs include unexplained abnormal pupillary findings, optic atrophy, subluxated lens, chronic unresponsive uveitis, and fundi with retinitis pigmentosa-like lesions, especially if unilateral or asymmetrical. In a number of these patients, live Treponema pallidum organisms have been recovered from the eye by anterior chamber puncture. Antisyphilitic therapy is indicated to prevent other complications of late syphilis. Except for uveitis, the ocular changes are irreversible.

BRUCELLOSIS

During the chronic stage of this disease, ocular involvement by the endogenous route is fairly common. Iritis is the most frequent ocular complication. The uveitis is not always granulomatous; if nongranulomatous, the inflammation tends to subside in a short time. Less common complications include choroiditis, generalized uveitis, and nummular keratitis, which has the same clinical appearance as epidemic keratoconjunctivitis. These lesions usually heal well but occasionally ulcerate, and can develop into chronic keratitis with periodic exacerbations and remissions.

Other ocular complications of brucellosis, including scleritis, are rarely seen. Some cases of ocular brucellosis respond to systemic sulfadiazine and streptomycin, although the organism develops resistance easily. The iritis is treated locally by mydriatics. Corticosteroids are sometimes of value locally, but are contraindicated systemically.

TOXOPLASMOSIS

This disease is of great ocular importance. The organism is a protozoan parasite which infects a great number of animals and birds and has world-wide distribution. Although there have not been a great many proved human cases, toxoplasmosis is probably the most common cause of posterior chorioretinitis.

Congenital Toxoplasmosis

The fetus is infected in utero. The disease is recognized after birth by the typical posterior polar chorioretinitis, which is usually seen in the inactive stage. About 75% of cases also demonstrate cerebral or cerebellar calcification by x-ray, although only a minority of these show signs of CNS disease such as convulsions, mental deficiency, and hemiplegia or paraplegia. The congenital form is nearly always arrested by the time it can be diagnosed.

Acquired Toxoplasmosis

Adult toxoplasmosis is probably the most common cause of posterior uveitis. Associated CNS disease is much less common than in the congenital form. Uveal lesions are often seen in the active stage, and there may be evidence of an old healed lesion near the new uveal focus of activity. A positive Sabin-Feldman dye test titer, rising on repeated complement fixation tests, is diagnostic. The titer rises sharply for about the first 2 weeks of infection and then slowly falls to normal over the next several years. The toxoplasmin skin test is of value only for screening purposes. Treatment has been disappointing, although adult cases may seem to benefit from systemically administered tetracyclines, sulfonamides, and corticosteroids. The prognosis is good for life and peripheral vision, but poor for central vision since the uveitis involves the macular area in at least 50% of cases.

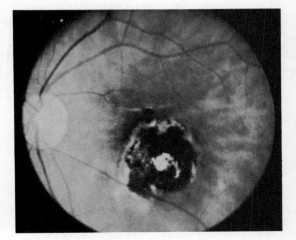

Fig 18-24. Healed toxoplasmic chorioretinitis. Note scarring in left macular area.

lids and lid margins. Herpes simplex may cause iridocyclitis, and may rarely cause severe encephalitis. Corticosteroids should not be employed.

HERPES ZOSTER
(Shingles)

When this neurotropic virus affects the first division of the 5th cranial nerve, many ocular complications can occur, including keratitis, iritis, scleritis, and optic neuritis. Involvement of the oculomotor nerve leads to incomplete or complete internal or external ophthalmoplegia. In about 25% of cases complete recovery within 3-6 weeks is the rule. Only local supportive and symptomatic treatment is of value.

SYSTEMIC VIRAL DISEASES

HERPES SIMPLEX

The most common manifestation of herpes simplex is fever blisters on the lips. The most common and serious eye lesion is herpes simplex (dendritic) keratitis (see p 78). Vesicular skin lesions can also appear on the skin of the

POLIOMYELITIS

Bulbar poliomyelitis severe enough to cause lesions of the 3rd, 4th, or 6th cranial nerves is usually fatal. Any type of internal or external ophthalmoplegia may result in survivors. Supranuclear abnormalities ("gaze" palsies, paralysis of convergence or divergence) are rare residual defects. Optic neuritis is rarely present. Treatment is purely symptomatic, although occasionally a residual extraocular muscle imbalance can be greatly improved by strabismus surgery.

GERMAN MEASLES
(Rubella)

Maternal rubella during the first trimester of pregnancy causes congenital anomalies, including serious heart disease, genitourinary disorders, and many serious ocular diseases in about 10% of infants. The most common eye complication is cataract, which is bilateral in 75% of cases. The embryonal and fetal nuclei of the lens are usually opaque, and visual acuity is often below 20/200. Other congenital ocular anomalies are frequently associated with the cataracts, eg, uveal colobomas, searching nystagmus, microphthalmos, strabismus, retinopathy, and infantile glaucoma. Congenital cataract, especially if bilateral, may require surgical removal, but the prognosis is always guarded since other ocular anomalies are often present which may not be recognized until the cataract is removed. Many physicians have felt that therapeutic abortion is advisable if rubella occurs during the first trimester of pregnancy since the rate of serious congenital anomalies is so high.

Cataract surgery should be delayed until at least age 2 since the live virus is present in ocular tissues for many months after birth. Earlier surgery results in a very high percentage of unsatisfactory results.

MEASLES
(Rubeola)

Acute conjunctivitis is common early in the course of measles. Koplik's spots can occur on the conjunctiva. There may also be an associated epithelial keratitis.

Optic neuritis and eventual optic atrophy occur rarely in measles meningitis or encephalitis.

The treatment of the eye complications of measles is symptomatic unless there is secondary infection, in which case local antibiotic ointment is used.

MUMPS

The most common ocular complication of mumps is dacryoadenitis. A diffuse keratitis with corneal edema resembling the disciform keratitis of herpes simplex occurs rarely. It usually clears completely within 2-3 weeks. Other less common eye complications of mumps include episcleritis, iridocyclitis, choroiditis, and optic neuritis, all of which tend to heal with little or no residual damage. Mumps encephalitis can cause a wide variety of neuro-ophthalmologic abnormalities which may be permanent, including internal and external ophthalmoplegia, pupillary abnormalities, and gaze palsies. Convalescent serum and gamma globulin may help to modify the disease; otherwise treatment is symptomatic.

SMALLPOX
(Variola)

Conjunctivitis appears fairly often on about the 5th day after the onset of smallpox. Less commonly, pustules occur on the conjunctiva. Central corneal ulceration with secondary infection and hypopyon has been known to occur. Smallpox encephalitis, with onset during the second week of the disease, occurs infrequently but has a mortality of at least 30%. Those who survive seldom have residual CNS damage.

VACCINIA

The vesicles of vaccinia may occur on the skin of the lids, when the patient inadvertently touches the vaccinated area and then rubs his lids. Such lesions may cause a violent local reaction but heal with little or no scarring and no damage to the eyeball.

A severe encephalitis occurs rarely about 10 days following vaccination. Mortality is up to 50%, but survivors seldom have residual CNS disease.

CHICKENPOX
(Varicella)

Swollen lids, conjunctivitis, and, rarely, vesicular conjunctival lesions may occur as part of the clinical picture of chickenpox.

PEMPHIGUS

This rare but serious disease is presumed to be of viral etiology and may be confined to the eye. It occurs most frequently as a chronic conjunctivitis associated with cutaneous lesions and inflammation of the mucous membranes of the nose and throat. Acute generalized pemphigus is usually fatal within weeks unless it responds to systemic corticotropin or corticosteroids. (See Chapter 6.)

VOGT-KOYANAGI AND HARADA'S SYNDROMES

Bilateral uveitis associated with alopecia, poliosis, vitiligo, and hearing defects, usually in young adults, has been termed Vogt-Koyanagi disease. When the choroiditis is more exudative, serous retinal detachment occurs and the complex is known as Harada's syndrome. Japanese and Italians are affected more commonly than other groups, but even among these the disease is rare. There is a tendency toward recovery of visual function, but this is not always complete. Corticosteroids have been reported to have a favorable effect upon the disease. Local corticosteroids and mydriatics are indicated. There have been a few reports of isolation of a virus from these cases, but viral etiology has not yet been definitely established.

BEHÇET'S SYNDROME

This is a rare disease whose most constant finding is recurrent hypopyon and uveitis. Aphthous lesions of the mucous membranes of the mouth and genitalia are often present. The attacks of uveitis may occur at any time during adult life and slowly destroy useful visual function in both eyes. The disease is believed to be caused by a virus. CNS signs are present in 10-20% of patients, with cranial nerve palsies occurring more frequently than papilledema. There is no effective treatment. Mydriatics are indicated during attacks of uveitis.

INFECTIOUS MONONUCLEOSIS

Although this fairly common disease is often looked upon as benign and self-limited, there is increasing evidence that significant complications are not rare. The disease process can affect the eye directly, causing nongranulomatous uveitis, scleritis, conjunctivitis, retinitis, or papillitis. Complete recovery is usual, but residual visual loss can result. The CNS may also be involved, causing infranuclear muscle palsies, nystagmus, and pupillary abnormalities. No specific therapy is available, although gamma globulin has been used with questionable benefit.

COLLAGEN DISEASES AND OTHER DISEASES OF UNKNOWN ETIOLOGY

This ill-defined group of diseases is characterized by widespread inflammatory damage of connective tissue with deposition of fibrinoid tissue in the ground substance. There is evidence that an auto-antibody reaction against normal tissue antigens produces tissue damage. Ocular involvement is frequent in most collagen diseases.

LUPUS ERYTHEMATOSUS

Discoid lupus erythematosus is localized to the skin area at the sides of the nose in "butterfly" pattern, and may produce patchy erythema and atrophy of the skin of the lids by contiguity. There is no generalized manifestation of the disease.

Systemic or acute disseminated lupus erythematosus is characterized by widespread systemic involvement, including butterfly cutaneous lesions, fever, leukopenia, splenomegaly, arthritis, and nephritis. The diagnosis can be confirmed by finding characteristic "LE cells" in the peripheral blood. The most common ocular complication is a severe retinopathy with cotton-wool patches, perivasculitis, and widespread retinal hemorrhages. Episcleritis and scleritis sometimes occur and usually are controlled by topical corticosteroids. Papillitis or occlusion of the central retinal artery may destroy all vision. The untreated disease is usually fatal. Adrenal corticosteroid treatment has greatly improved prognosis; 50% of patients now survive for 5 years.

DERMATOMYOSITIS

This rare disease occurs most frequently in children. It is similar to disseminated lupus erythematosus but has a better prognosis.

Characteristically there is a degenerative subacute inflammation of the muscles, sometimes
including the extraocular muscles. The lids
are commonly a part of the generalized dermal
involvement and may show marked swelling
and erythema. Retinopathy consisting of multiple white, irregular opacities appearing much
like cotton-wool patches as well as fine
shaped hemorrhages may occur. High doses
of systemic corticosteroids will frequently
effect a remission which continues even after
cessation of therapy. The ultimate prognosis
is poor, however.

SCLERODERMA

This rare chronic disease is characterized by widespread alterations in the collage-
nous tissues of the mucosa, bones, muscles,
skin, and internal organs. Men and women between 15 and 45 years of age are affected. The
skin in local areas becomes tense and "leath-
ery" and the process may spread to involve
large areas of the limbs, rendering them vir-
tually immobile. The skin of the eyelids is
often involved. Iritis and cataract occur less
frequently. Retinopathy similar to lupus erythematosus and dermatomyositis may be present. Systemic corticosteroid treatment has
improved the prognosis substantially, and
retinopathy usually improves or disappears.

PERIARTERITIS (POLYARTERITIS) NODOSA

This rare disease may occur at any age,
usually in men and boys (80%). The general
picture is that of subacute illness, with remissions and exacerbations of fever, weakness,
and acute, localized pain in areas of necrotiz-
ing arteritis. Skin manifestations are common
and vary from mild erythema to purpura. The
kidneys are often involved (80%), causing generalized vasoconstriction and hypertension.
About 20% of cases show angiospastic retinopathy which rarely causes widespread retinal
detachment. Other occasional ocular complications include iritis, central retinal artery
occlusion, keratitis, ring ulcer of the cornea,
scleritis, and extraocular muscle palsies.
Eosinophilia suggests that this disease may be
a hypersensitivity phenomenon, and cases
ascribed to drug sensitivity have been reported.
Systemic corticosteroids are of some value,
but the long-term prognosis is uniformly bad.

ERYTHEMA MULTIFORME
(Stevens-Johnson Syndrome)

Erythema multiforme is a serious mucocutaneous disease that occurs as a hypersensitivity reaction to drugs or food. Children
are most susceptible. The manifestations consist of generalized maculopapular rash, severe stomatitis, and purulent conjunctivitis,
sometimes leading to symblepharon and occlusion of the lacrimal gland ducts (**dry eye syndrome**). In severe cases corneal ulcers, per-
forations, and panophthalmitis can destroy all
visual function. Systemic corticosteroid treatment often favorably influences the course of
the disease and usually preserves useful visual
function. Secondary infection with Staphylococcus aureus is common and must be vigorously treated by local antibiotics instilled into
the conjunctival sac. Frequently there is
marked reduction of tear formation which can
be helped by instillation of artificial tears 3
or 4 times a day.

TEMPORAL (CRANIAL) ARTERITIS

This uncommon syndrome is one of many
ways the underlying disease, giant cell arteritis, can cause symptoms. It is usually seen
in elderly people. It is characterized by inflammation of a cranial artery, which ordinarily causes severe boring headache. In about
half of cases there are associated mild or severe ocular manifestations. Visual disturbances are common as a result of occlusion of
the central retinal artery or one of its major
branches or as a result of optic neuritis. Less
commonly, involvement of cranial nerves III,
IV, and VI causes ptosis and diplopia. A high
sedimentation rate is an excellent corrobora-
tive laboratory test.

High doses of systemic corticosteroids
may arrest visual function loss or prevent involvement of the second eye. Despite treatment, bilateral total blindness from central
retinal artery occlusion is not uncommon.
Death usually occurs within 5 years, often as
a result of cerebrovascular accident or coronary occlusion.

IDIOPATHIC ARTERITIS OF TAKAYASU
(Pulseless Disease)

This disease, found most frequently in
young women and occasionally in children, is

a polyarteritis of unknown etiology with increased predilection for the aorta and its branches. Manifestations may include evidence of cerebrovascular insufficiency, syncope, absence of pulsations in the upper extremities, and ophthalmologic changes compatible with chronic hypoxia of the ocular structures. Ophthalmodynamometry may be of value in diagnosis by demonstrating decreased carotid blood flow on one or both sides. The disease is sometimes associated with rheumatoid arthritis, which lends support to the idea that it is a collagen disease.

Thromboendarterectomy, prosthetic graft, and systemic corticosteroid therapy have been reported to be successful.

RHEUMATOID ARTHRITIS

Rheumatoid arthritis is a disease of middle and old age that is 3 times more common in women than in men. Uveitis occurs in only 3% of cases. Scleritis is much more common, and occasionally is severe enough to weaken the sclera and cause bulging or perforating staphylomas (scleromalacia perforans). Scleral grafts or reinforcement by fascia lata may prevent ocular rupture. Recurrent conjunctivitis may merge into episcleritis. Anterior uveitis and episcleritis will usually respond to topical corticosteroids. Keratoconjunctivitis sicca is present in 10-15% of cases (see Sjögren's syndrome, below).

JUVENILE RHEUMATOID ARTHRITIS
(Still's Disease)

Uveitis is quite common in this disorder (up to 50% in some series). A low-grade bilateral iridocyclitis may precede or follow joint involvement. Band keratitis occurs in about 10% of cases.

SJÖGREN'S SYNDROME

Sjögren's disease is currently thought of as being an auto-immune collagen disease with delayed damage to the lacrimal gland. The complete syndrome (arthritis, keratitis, and dry mouth) occurs almost exclusively in women over 40. The ocular involvement is termed

keratoconjunctivitis sicca (see Chapter 6). There is associated dryness of the mouth and other mucous·membranes and frequently polyarthritis. Up to half of these patients have rheumatoid arthritis, and others with no arthritis have circulating rheumatoid factor.

There is no effective systemic therapy, although many forms of endocrine therapy have been tried. Keratoconjunctivitis sicca can occur without other systemic abnormalities; the ocular dryness is treated symptomatically with artificial tear solutions.

ANKYLOSING SPONDYLITIS

Ankylosing spondylitis is predominantly a disease of men (90%). The sacro-iliac joint is typically involved. Iridocyclitis, frequently with hypopyon, is the most common ocular finding (33%).

INHERITED SKELETO-OCULAR DISEASES

ARACHNODACTYLY
(Marfan's Syndrome)

The most striking feature of this rare syndrome is increased length of the long bones, particularly of the fingers and toes. Other characteristics include scanty subcutaneous fat, relaxed ligaments, and, less commonly, other associated developmental anomalies, including congenital heart disease and deformities of the spine and joints. Ocular complications are often seen—in particular, dislocation of the lenses, usually superiorly and nasally. Less common ocular anomalies include severe refractive errors, megalocornea, cataract, uveal colobomas, and secondary glaucoma. There is a high infant mortality. Removal of a dislocated lens may be necessary. The disease is genetically determined, nearly always as an autosomal dominant, often with incomplete expression, so that mild, incomplete forms of the syndrome are seen. Several reports have correlated cytogenetic changes with Marfan's syndrome.

MARCHESANI'S SYNDROME

This is a rare hereditary disorder characterized by multiple skeletal and ocular abnormalities which is transmitted as an autosomal recessive trait. Patients are short and stocky, with well developed muscles. The hands and feet are characteristically spade-shaped; in childhood, x-rays show delayed carpal and tarsal ossification. Ocular complications include spherophakia and ectopia lentis, which gives rise to lenticular myopia, iridodonesis, and glaucoma. The prognosis for vision is usually poor because the glaucoma resists all forms of treatment.

OSTEOGENESIS IMPERFECTA
(Brittle Bones and Blue Scleras)

This rare autosomal dominant syndrome is characterized by multiple fractures, blue scleras, and, less commonly, deafness. The disease is usually manifest soon after birth. The long bones are very fragile, fracturing easily and often healing with fibrous bony union. The bones become more fragile with age. The very thin sclera allows the blue color imparted by the underlying uveal tract to show through. There is often no visual functional impairment. Occasionally, abnormalities such as keratoconus, megalocornea, and corneal or lenticular opacities are also present which do interfere with visual function.

Ophthalmologic treatment is seldom necessary.

DISEASES RESULTING FROM INBORN ERRORS OF METABOLISM WITH OCULAR SIGNS

GARGOYLISM
(Hurler's Syndrome)

Gargoylism is a rare autosomal recessive metabolic disorder associated with the accumulation of mucopolysaccharides in the tissues. It results in grotesque facies, mental deficiency, dwarfism, changes in bone shape, corneal opacities, and heart failure. The clinical features appear early in life, and are progressive. The corneal clouding consists of a uniform opalescence of the entire stroma,

appearing much like nonspecific corneal edema on slit lamp examination. Papilledema from hydrocephalus may occur.

There is no treatment.

Rare cases of corneal involvement alone have been described in which the cornea is the only body tissue storing excessive amounts of mucopolysaccharides.

HEPATOLENTICULAR DEGENERATION
(Wilson's Disease)

This rare autosomal recessive disease of young adults, characterized by abnormal copper metabolism, causes changes in the basal nuclei, cirrhosis of the liver, and a pathognomonic corneal pigmentation called the Kayser-Fleischer ring. The ring appears as a green or brown band peripherally and deep in the stroma near Descemet's membrane, and may only be visible with a slit lamp. The disease is progressive and often results in death by age 40.

Treatment with dimercaprol (BAL) and penicillamine (Cuprimine®) has resulted in sustained clinical improvement in some cases.

CYSTINOSIS

This rare autosomal recessive derangement of amino acid metabolism causes widespread deposition of cystine crystals throughout the body. Dwarfism, nephropathy, and death in childhood from renal failure is the rule. Cystine crystals can be readily seen in the conjunctiva and cornea, where fine particles are seen predominantly in the outer third of the corneal stroma.

There is no treatment.

ALBINISM

Generalized albinism is a disease affecting the metabolism of melanin and is inherited as an autosomal recessive. The skin and hair are white, and there is a generalized lack of pigment throughout the body which is apparent from birth. The eyebrows and lashes are white. The irides appear reddish, and the pupil appears red. The fundus is red, with a prominent choroidal vessel pattern since the pigmented epithelium of the retina is deficient. Photophobia is prominent. The macula is often poorly developed, greatly impairing visual function, and this often causes an associated searching nystagmus which reduces visual acuity to about 20/200.

Another variant, ocular albinism, is confined to the eye and characteristically follows a sex-linked recessive pattern of inheritance.

HOMOCYSTINURIA

Homocystinuria is a rare autosomal recessive disorder of amino acid metabolism characterized clinically by mental retardation, downward dislocation of the lenses of the eyes, and genu valgum evident by age 1. The plasma homocystine and methionine levels are elevated. Urinary excretion of homocystine is increased, and the nitroprusside test of the urine is positive. Thrombosis of medium-sized arteries is common, often resulting in early death from cerebrovascular, coronary, or renal vascular occlusions.

GALACTOSEMIA

Galactosemia is a rare autosomal recessive disorder of carbohydrate metabolism which becomes clinically manifest soon after birth by feeding problems, vomiting, diarrhea, abdominal distention, hepatomegaly, jaundice, ascites, cataracts, mental retardation, and elevated blood and urine galactose levels. Dietary exclusion of milk and all foods containing galactose and lactose for the first 3 years of life will prevent the clinical manifestations and will result in improvement of existing abnormalities. Even the cataract changes, which are characterized by vacuoles of the cortex, are reversible in the early stage.

Identification of the carrier state is possible by finding a 50% reduction of galactose-6-phosphatase.

MISCELLANEOUS SYSTEMIC DISEASES WITH OCULAR MANIFESTATIONS

WERNER'S SYNDROME

Werner's syndrome is a rare hereditary disorder characterized ocularly by juvenile cataracts, glaucoma, and corneal opacities.

It is probably transmitted as a recessive trait. The onset is usually between age 20 and 30, with graying and thinning of the hair of the scalp, genital region, and axillas. Atrophic skin changes may occur on the face, limbs, hands, and feet.

LAURENCE-MOON-BIEDL SYNDROME

Obesity, mental deficiency, polydactyly, hypogenitalism, and retinitis pigmentosa form the complete syndrome. The retinal changes are not always typical of retinitis pigmentosa and may be present soon after birth or develop during adolescence. This rare syndrome is genetically determined and follows an autosomal recessive pattern with a high rate of consanguinity. The heterozygous state may be identified by mild incomplete evidences of the disease. It is interesting that a single abnormal gene can account for such a multiplicity of clinical findings.

ROSACEA
(Acne Rosacea)

This disease of unknown etiology is primarily dermatologic, beginning as a hyperemia of the face associated with acneiform lesions and eventually causing hypertrophy of tissues (such as rhinophyma). Chronic blepharitis due to staphylococcal infection or seborrhea is often present. Rosacea keratitis develops in about 5% of cases. Episcleritis, scleritis, and nongranulomatous iridocyclitis are rare ocular complications.

Topical corticosteroids are helpful in controlling keratitis or iridocyclitis, but there is no specific therapy.

REITER'S SYNDROME

This disorder consists of conjunctivitis, urethritis, arthritis, and frequently diarrhea. It is often included among the rheumatoid syndromes. (See Chapter 6.)

ULCERATIVE COLITIS

Ulcerative colitis is frequently associated with Reiter's syndrome and spondylitis and sometimes a severe uveitis that is resistant to all forms of therapy.

LOWE'S SYNDROME

This rare syndrome consists of cerebral defects, mental retardation, and ocular anomalies associated with dwarfism due to renal dysfunction (a congenital defect of reabsorption in the renal tubules, causing aminoaciduria). The eye findings include congenital cataract, infantile glaucoma, and nystagmus. All cases reported to date have occurred in males, suggesting sex-linked inheritance. There is a high early mortality rate.

OCULAR COMPLICATIONS OF CERTAIN SYSTEMICALLY ADMINISTERED DRUGS

ANTICHOLINERGICS
(Atropine and Related Synthetic Drugs)

All of these drugs, when given preoperatively or for gastrointestinal disorders, may cause blurred near vision in presbyopic patients due to a direct action on accommodation. They also tend to dilate the pupils, so that in patients with narrow anterior chamber angles there is the added threat of angle-closure glaucoma. This is the cause of angle-closure glaucoma (frequently attributed to "nervousness") occasionally seen in patients hospitalized for general surgery.

CHLORAMPHENICOL

Chloramphenicol, in addition to the possibility of causing severe blood dyscrasias, hepatic and renal disease, and gastrointestinal disturbances, can sometimes cause optic neuritis. This latter is especially true in children. Bilateral blurred vision with central scotomas occurs. Discontinuance of treatment does not always restore vision.

Despite the possibility of toxic optic neuropathy, chloramphenicol may still be required for the treatment of bacterial endophthalmitis. The drug is generally not administered for more than 1 week.

CHLOROQUINE
(Aralen®)

Originally employed as an antimalarial drug, chloroquine has also been widely used in the treatment of many collagen diseases, especially systemic lupus erythematosus and rheumatoid arthritis, and skin diseases, including discoid lupus erythematosus and sarcoidosis. With high dosage—often 250-750 mg daily administered for months or years—serious ocular toxicity has occurred. Corneal changes were described first, and consisted of diffuse haziness of the epithelium and subepithelial area, occasionally sufficient to simulate an epithelial dystrophy. These changes cause only mild blurring of vision and are reversible upon drug withdrawal. Similar changes have been described in patients receiving quinacrine. Minimal corneal involvement is not necessarily an indication for discontinuance of chloroquine therapy. Corneal changes have been reported in about 30% of patients on long-term chloroquine treatment.

A less common but more serious ocular complication of long-term chloroquine therapy is retinal damage, causing loss of central vision as well as constriction of peripheral visual fields. Pigmentary changes and edema of the macula, marked alteration of the retinal vessels, and in some cases peripheral pigmentary changes can be seen ophthalmoscopically. Fluorescein fundus photography aids greatly in establishing early diagnosis or evaluating the extent of macular involvement. Visual field examination reveals central scotomas and peripheral field constriction. There are also changes of the electroretinogram, dark adaptation, and color vision. The damage is always bilateral and is usually equal in both eyes. The visual loss is irreversible, and may even progress after cessation of therapy. No treatment is of any value.

Long-term chloroquine therapy must be undertaken only upon urgent indications. These patients should be examined by an ophthalmologist every 3-4 months. Between examinations, the patient should make a rough test of his visual acuity once weekly.

CHLOROTHIAZIDE
(Diuril®)

Xanthopsia (yellow vision) has been reported in patients taking this oral diuretic.

CONTRACEPTIVES, ORAL

Although numerous reports suggest that in predisposed individuals oral contraceptives can provoke or precipitate ophthalmic vascular occlusive disease or optic nerve damage, it is difficult to establish a definite cause and effect relationship. Optic neuritis, retinal arterial or venous thrombosis, and pseudotumor cerebri have been described in patients taking oral contraceptives. Since there is some uncertainty regarding the possibility of such ocular complications, oral contraceptives should be used only by healthy women with no history of vascular, neurologic, or ocular disease.

CORTICOSTEROIDS

It has been clearly demonstrated that long-term systemic corticosteroid therapy can cause chronic open-angle glaucoma and cataracts and can provoke and worsen attacks of herpes simplex keratitis. Locally administered corticosteroids are much more potent in this respect and have the added disadvantage of causing fungal overgrowth if the corneal epithelium is not intact. Steroid-induced subcapsular lens opacities cause some impairment of visual function but usually do not progress to advanced cataract. Cessation of therapy will arrest progression of the lenticular opacities, but the changes are irreversible.
Systemic corticosteroids may also cause papilledema associated with pseudotumor cerebri, both during administration and shortly after withdrawal.

DIGITALIS

Blurred vision and disturbed color vision are said to be the most common ocular complications of digitalis toxicity, although the actual incidence of such symptoms in patients receiving digitalis is extremely low. The purified glycosides of digitalis probably produce fewer of the toxic ocular symptoms than the whole leaf.

Visual acuity may be decreased. Objects may appear yellow (xanthopsia) or, less commonly, green, brown, red, "snowy," or white. The patient may complain of photophobia and flashes of light. Scotomas and, very rarely, transient and permanent amblyopia have been described. The toxic effects of digitalis may be due to direct effects on the retinal reception cells or retrobulbar neuritis, or they may be of central origin.

OXYGEN

Any concentration of oxygen in excess of that in air may lead to retrolental fibroplasia in premature infants. Premature infants should receive only the amount of oxygen necessary for survival. The concentration should not exceed 40% for brief periods as indicated. In adults, administration of hyperbaric oxygen (3 atmospheres) can cause constriction of the retinal arterioles. In one reported case, a patient with an old inactive retrobulbar neuritis exposed to 100% oxygen at 2 atmospheres of pressure developed almost complete loss of visual field in 2 hours.

PHENOTHIAZINES

The phenothiazines usually exert an atropine-like effect on the eye so that the pupils may be dilated, especially with large dosages. Of greater clinical significance, however, are the pigmentary ocular changes, which include pigment deposits on the corneal endothelium and anterior lens capsule and pigmentary retinopathy. The corneal and lens pigmentation may cause blurring of vision, but the pigment deposits usually disappear several months after the drug is discontinued. In pigmentary retinopathy, there is a diminution of central vision, night blindness, diffuse narrowing of the retinal arteries, and occasionally severe blindness.
Chlorpromazine (Thorazine®) and thioridazine (Mellaril®) are the principal phenothiazines causing ocular complications. In the case of chlorpromazine these complications usually occur only after many months at high dosages (> 200 mg daily), whereas the pigmentary retinopathy has been reported as occurring in a period of only 3 weeks following high dosages of thioridazine.

Patients receiving large dosages or prolonged treatment with phenothiazines should be
questioned regarding visual disturbances and
should have periodic ophthalmoscopic examinations.

QUININE AND QUINACRINE

Quinine and quinacrine, when used in the
treatment of malaria, may cause bilateral
blurred vision, sometimes following a single
dose. There is constriction of the visual field
and, rarely, total blindness. The tendency is
toward partial recovery, although usually there
are permanent peripheral field defects. The
ganglion cells of the retina are affected first,
presumably as a result of vasoconstriction of
the retinal arterioles. Varying degrees of
retinal edema occur early. Optic atrophy is
a late finding.

SALICYLATES

Salicylic acid derivatives in very large
doses can cause ocular manifestations similar
to those caused by quinine and quinacrine.
Withdrawal of the drug usually results in improved visual function, but complete recovery
is rare.

SEDATIVE TRANQUILIZERS

When taken regularly, the so-called minor
tranquilizers can decrease tear production by
the lacrimal gland, thus resulting in ocular
irritation due to dry eyes. Tear production
returns to normal when the tranquilizers are
discontinued.

The principal drugs in this group are
meprobamate (Miltown®), chlordiazepoxide
(Librium®), and diazepoxide (Valium®).

VITAMIN A

When vitamin A is given in large doses
over a period of months, patients (particularly
children) can develop blurred vision due to
papilledema secondary to increased intracranial pressure. The papilledema disappears
several weeks after discontinuing the vitamin
A.

VITAMIN D

Band-shaped corneal calcification and
optic atrophy may result from excessive doses
of vitamin D. Children are more vulnerable
than adults.

•   •   •

Bibliography

Anderson, B., Sr.: Rheumatoid syndromes.
Am J Ophth **64**:35-50, 1967.

Can, R.E., & others: Ocular toxicity of
antimalarial drugs: Long-term follow-
up. Am J Ophth **66**:738-44, 1968.

Chizeck, D.J., & A.T. Franceschetti:
Oral contraceptives: Side-effects and
ophthalmological manifestations. Survey
Ophth **14**:90, 1969.

Cocke, J.G., Jr.: Chloramphenicol optic
neuritis. Am J Dis Child **114**:424, 1967.

Cogan, D.G.: Ocular correlates of inborn
metabolic defects. Canad MAJ **95**:1055-
65, 1966.

Cordes, F.C.: The diabetic: His visual
prognosis. Arch Ophth **48**:531-56, 1952.

Crick, R.P., Hoyle, C., & H. Smellie:
The eyes in sarcoidosis. Brit J Ophth
45:461-81, 1961.

Davis, M.D.: The natural course of diabetic retinopathy. Tr Am Acad Ophth
72:237, 1968.

Donaldson, D.D.: Atlas of External Dis-
eases of the Eye, Vol. I. Congenital
Anomalies and Systemic Diseases.
Mosby, 1966.

Ellsworth, R.J., & R.W. Zeller: Chloroquine (Aralen)-induced retinal damage.
Arch Ophth **66**:269-72, 1961.

Gamble, C.N., Aronson, S.B., & F.B.
Brescia: The pathogenesis of recurrent
(Auer) uveitis. Arch Ophth **84**:331-41,
1970.

Hardy, J., & I.S. Ciric: Anterior hypophysectomy in diabetic retinopathy.
JAMA **203**:73-9, 1968.

Hardy, J., & I.S. Ciric: Pituitary ablation
for diabetic retinopathy. I. Results of
hypophysectomy. JAMA **203**:79-85, 1968.

Hogan, M.J.: Ocular toxoplasmosis. Am J Ophth 46:467-94, 1958.

Hollenhorst, R.W.: Vascular status of patients who have cholesterol emboli in the retina. Am J Ophth 61:1159-65, 1966.

Irvine, A.R., & E.W.D. Norton: Photocoagulation for diabetic retinopathy. Am J Ophth 71:437-45, 1971.

Kimura, S.J., & others: Uveitis and joint diseases. Arch Ophth 77:309-16, 1967.

Krill, A.E., Potts, A.M., & C.E. Johanson: Chloroquine retinopathy. Investigation of discrepancy between dark adaptation and electroretinographic findings in advanced stages. Am J Ophth 71:530-43, 1971.

Leopold, I.H.: Diabetic retinopathy. Survey Ophth 6:483-612, 1961. [Entire journal devoted to diabetic retinopathy.]

Leopold, I.H.: Ocular complications of drugs. JAMA 205:631-3, 1968.

Macri, F.J.: Pharmacology and toxicology of ophthalmic drugs. Annual review. Arch Ophth 84:532-45, 1970.

Meyer-Schwickerath, G.R.E., & K. Schott: Diabetic retinopathy and photocoagulation. Am J Ophth 66:597, 1968.

Nowicki, N.J.: The ocular manifestations of collagen diseases. M Clin North America 49:131-9, 1965.

Nylander, U.: Ocular damage in chloroquine therapy. Acta ophth (Suppl 92), 1967.

Pearson, O.H.: Hypophysectomy for the treatment of diabetic retinopathy. JAMA 188:116-22, 1964.

Ray, B.S., & others: Pituitary ablation for diabetic retinopathy. II. Yttrium 90 implantation in the pituitary gland. JAMA 203:85-8, 1968.

Robertson, D.M., Hollenhorst, R.W., & J.A. Callahan: Ocular manifestations of digitalis toxicity. Arch Ophth 76:640-5, 1966.

Salmon, M.L., Winkelman, J.Z., & A.J. Gay: Neuro-ophthalmic sequelae in users of oral contraceptives. JAMA 206:85, 1968.

Schutz, S., Newhouse, R., & J.D. Russo: Alternate-day steroid regimen in the treatment of ocular disease. Brit J Ophth 52:461-3, 1968.

Sever, J.L., Nelson, K.B., & M.R. Gilkeson: Rubella epidemic, 1964. Effect on 6000 pregnancies. Am J Dis Child 110:395-407, 1965.

Shell, J.W., & S.P. Eriksen: Toxicity and ophthalmic drugs. Survey Ophth 13:215-8, 1969.

Smith, J.L., & others: Seronegative ocular and neurosyphilis. Am J Ophth 59:753-63, 1965.

Smith, J.L.: The current status of ocular syphilis. Survey Ophth 14:176-8, 1969.

Sorsby, A. (editor): Modern Ophthalmology, 4 Vols. Butterworth, 1963-1964.

Talal, N.: Sjögren's syndrome. Bull Rheum Dis 16, March, 1966.

Toussaint, D., Cogan, D.G., & J. Kubawara: Extravascular lesions of diabetic retinopathy. Arch Ophth 67:42-7, 1962.

Wagener, H.P., & N.M. Keith: Diffuse arteriolar disease with hypertension and the associated retinal lesions. Medicine 18:317-430, 1939.

Walsh, F.B., & W.F. Hoyt: Clinical Neuro-ophthalmology, 3rd ed. Williams & Wilkins, 1969.

Walsh, F.B., & others: Oral contraceptives and neuro-ophthalmologic interest. Arch Ophth 74:628-40, 1965.

Werner, S.C.: Prednisone in emergency treatment of malignant exophthalmos. Lancet 1:1004-7, 1966.

Willetts, G.S.: Ocular side-effects of drugs. Brit J Ophth 53:252-62, 1969.

19 . . .
Hereditary Aspects

As genetic factors are proved responsible for more and more diseases, it becomes increasingly important to understand the principles of genetic transmission. Much of the background work in clinical medical genetics has been done in ophthalmology, since the eye seems unusually prone to genetically determined disease. Mainly because the cornea is a convenient window through which the inner eye can be observed, accurate diagnosis of ocular disease is the rule.

It is now possible to estimate the chances for occurrence of many genetically determined diseases (usually the rare but severe ones), but the familial incidence of many other diseases also known to be genetically determined still cannot be accurately predicted.

The electron microscope has stimulated interest and progress in the science of genetics. It is now possible to study the structure of individual chromosomes in some detail. It has been definitely established that there are 23 pairs of chromosomes in the nucleus of the normal human somatic cell. Twenty-two of these pairs are somewhat similar, and therefore have been termed **autosomal**. Each pair is made up of 2 identical chromosomes. The twenty-third pair are sex chromosomes. With the electron microscope, it has been possible to classify the chromosomes. Cytogenetic studies have shown abnormal chromosomal numbers in several syndromes such as Turner's syndrome and Down's syndrome that include ocular anomalies.

The gametes (spermatozoon and ovum) are produced by a special type of cell division called reduction-division meiosis in which the 23 pairs of chromosomes dissociate; each chromosome of a pair separates and passes intact to a daughter cell to give it 23 unpaired chromosomes. At fertilization, each chromosome of the spermatozoon joins its corresponding chromosome of the ovum to produce a cell with 46 chromosomes. All cell divisions after fertilization (mitosis) involve a longitudinal splitting of all the chromosomes to produce cells with the constant number of 46 chromosomes.

Each chromosome is composed of many small units termed **genes**. Genes are arranged in pairs and determine bodily characteristics. Paired genes are either similar (homozygous) or dissimilar (heterozygous). If dissimilar, one determines the bodily characteristic and is termed **dominant** while the other gene is unexpressed and is termed **recessive**. At fertilization the reassortment of chromosomes is purely by chance, so that either chromosome of a pair from one parent has an equal chance to combine with either chromosome of the same pair from the other parent. Normal characteristics are inherited in the same way as genetically determined disease, which is discussed below under the headings of autosomal dominant, autosomal recessive, and sex-linked recessive inheritance.

AUTOSOMAL DOMINANT INHERITANCE

An abnormal dominant gene produces its specific abnormality even though its paired gene (allele) is normal. Males and females are affected alike and have a theoretical 50% chance of passing along the affected gene (and therefore the abnormality) to each of their offspring, even when mated to genotypically normal individuals. (See Fig 19-1.)

Given a particular group of pedigrees, autosomal dominant inheritance is established if the following conditions are met: (1) Males and females are about equally affected. (2) Direct transmission has occurred over 2 or more generations. (3) About 50% of individuals in the pedigrees must be affected.

Quite a large number of uncommon but serious diseases with ocular manifestations are transmitted in this way: Forms of juvenile glaucoma, Marfan's syndrome, congenital stationary night blindness (see Fig 19-2), osteogenesis imperfecta, and all the phakomatoses, which include neurofibromatosis, Lindau-Von Hippel disease, tuberous sclerosis, and Sturge-Weber syndrome. The process of

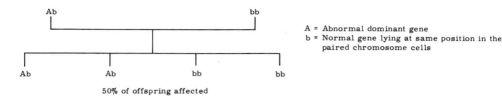

A = Abnormal dominant gene
b = Normal gene lying at same position in the
    paired chromosome cells

50% of offspring affected

Fig 19-1. Autosomal dominant inheritance.

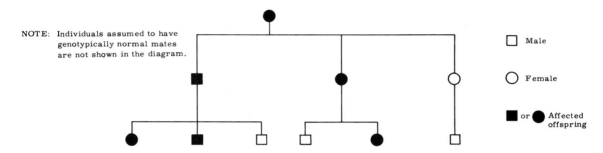

NOTE: Individuals assumed to have
       genotypically normal mates
       are not shown in the diagram.

☐ Male

○ Female

■ or ● Affected
         offspring

Fig 19-2. Pedigree of congenital stationary night blindness (abnormal dominant gene).

natural selection tends to keep most of these serious diseases at a low incidence in the general population since many of these people are unable to produce children even if they live to the age of reproduction.

Dominant disease may be more or less severe from generation to generation depending upon its **expression**; a disease with "variable expression" is one which can occur in a mild or severe form. An example is neurofibromatosis, in which genotypically affected individuals may have merely café au lait spots or may have many serious manifestations. One cannot predict if or when the disease will be more serious (with CNS tumors or optic nerve gliomas) in a succeeding generation. If the genetic pattern is present but there is no evidence of the disease, one says that its **penetrance** is reduced. It may be quite difficult to differentiate dominant inheritance with reduced penetrance from recessive inheritance (see below). To quote Duke-Elder, "It may well be said that dominance and recessiveness are not two distinct antitheses but represent the two extremes of a continuous series of variable types of hereditary transmission, all of which are fundamentally the same." Those pedigrees which demonstrate neither a definite autosomal dominant nor a definite recessive pattern are properly classified as irregular dominants (dominant inheritance with variable expression) or incomplete recessives (carrier state identifiable clinically).

AUTOSOMAL RECESSIVE INHERITANCE

Abnormal recessive genes must lie in pairs (duplex state) to produce manifest abnormality. Thus each parent must contribute one recessive abnormal gene. Each parent is clinically unaffected (genotypically affected but phenotypically normal), since a normal dominant gene makes the abnormal gene recessive. (See Fig 19-3.)

It is difficult to establish that a given disease results from autosomal recessive inheritance. Some of the criteria used to establish recessive inheritance are the following:

(1) Occurrence of the same disease in collateral branches of the family.

(2) History of consanguinity. The higher the rate of consanguinity in the pedigrees of a given disease, the more likely the disease is to be recessive and the rarer the occurrence of the disease in the general population. Consanguinity creates greater opportunities for the genes to lie in the duplex state, inasmuch as an individual with 2 related parents can receive the same affected gene from each, a common ancestor having originally passed on the affected gene.

(3) The occurrence of the disease in about 25% of siblings. This only holds for groups of pedigrees. There is a 25% chance that the 2 abnormal genes will be passed on to one individual. There is a 50% chance that a normal gene will modify the affected gene. In this case the individual is a carrier of the disease (just like the parents) but is not affected with the disease (ie, genotypically affected but

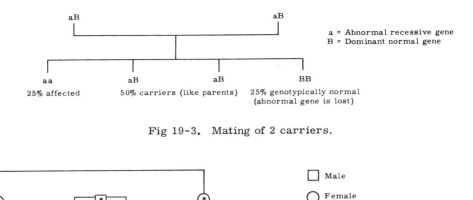

Fig 19-3. Mating of 2 carriers.

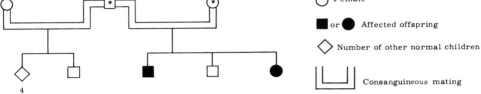
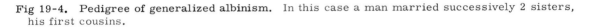

*These individuals must be carriers, although there may be no clinical method of detection.

Fig 19-4. **Pedigree of generalized albinism.** In this case a man married successively 2 sisters, his first cousins.

phenotypically normal). In the remaining 25% of siblings, 2 normal genes lie together and the abnormal gene is completely lost (ie, the individual is genotypically normal). Although a number of pedigrees are required to definitely establish recessive inheritance, even a single pedigree is suggestive if more than one sibling is similarly affected without antecedent history.

Many disease processes have been definitely established as resulting from autosomal recessive inheritance, and many others are suspected of having such a genetic background. Included among the definite cases are some forms of albinism (see Fig 19-4), juvenile amaurotic idiocy, megalocornea, infantile glaucoma, keratoconus, and the Laurence-Moon-Biedl syndrome.

RECESSIVE INHERITANCE OF A VERY COMMON RECESSIVE GENE (Pseudo-Dominant Inheritance)

An attractive hypothesis has been put forward to explain the genetic basis of several common disease entities. Diabetes mellitus and open-angle glaucoma undoubtedly have a genetic background and, because of their high incidence (at least 2% of the adult population),

have often been thought to be governed by autosomal dominant inheritance. However, groups of pedigrees of diabetes and glaucoma do not fit all the criteria necessary to establish dominant inheritance. The pedigrees fit much better into a pattern of recessive inheritance of a very common gene.

For example, there is evidence that the gene for diabetes is carried by as many as 35% of the population (heterozygote carriers), whereas about 3% will manifest clinical diabetes (homozygotes). Therefore, approximately one-third of matings by diabetics will be with carriers of the disease. One can see in Fig 19-5 that 50% of these offspring are affected, just as in dominant inheritance. Because of this confusion, the term pseudo-dominant has been used. Open-angle glaucoma and many common degenerative diseases probably fall into this category. It has been suggested that the carrier state of open-angle glaucoma is detectable when an increase of 8 mm Hg intraocular pressure is noted after 2 weeks of topical administration of steroid drops (1 drop 4 times daily). About one-third of patients so tested give this positive response, which correlates well with the suspected rate of diabetic carriers, showing the similarity of inheritance of these 2 entities.

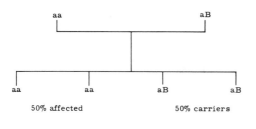

a = Abnormal recessive gene
B = Normal dominant gene

Fig 19-5. Pedigree of diabetes mellitus.
Example of inheritance of a common recessive gene (pseudo-dominant inheritance).

SEX-LINKED RECESSIVE INHERITANCE

One of the 23 pairs of human chromosomes is called the sex chromosomes. Identical chromosomes appear in females; these have been labeled the X chromosome. One such chromosome appears with a dissimilar mate in the male; this smaller chromosome has been labeled the Y chromosome. Therefore, XX is female and XY is male. Many of the genes of the X chromosome are unopposed by a gene of the Y chromosome, which is much smaller. Abnormalities of these genes cause disease in the male, whereas in the female an abnormal recessive gene of the sex chromosome is neutralized by its normal allele. Therefore, nearly all of the sex-linked diseases are manifested in males, whereas the disease is passed through the female. A male and his maternal grandfather are affected, and the intervening female is the carrier. Several important eye diseases have a sex-linked genetic pattern, such as color blindness (see Fig 19-6) and a type of retinitis pigmentosa. Other rarer eye diseases also have this mode of inheritance.

CYTOGENETIC ABNORMALITIES

Electron microscopy allows visualization of chromosomes during mitosis from small pieces of tissue cultured in vitro. When mitosis is interrupted in metaphase, the chromosomes can be spread on a slide, counted, and photographed. These cytogenetic studies have made possible the classification of chromosomes into 7 groups. The classification is based upon characteristics such as size and the position of the centromere. The groups contain as few as 2 or as many as 7 chromosomes, with the chromosomes of any group being indistinguishable from each other. Cytogenetics has also established that some clinical states can be correlated with an abnormal number of chromosomes, most frequently one more (trisomy) or occasionally one less (monosomy) than the normal number of 46. A few of the more common syndromes are summarized briefly below. Since the addition or subtraction of an entire gene is obviously a major genetic abnormality, these syndromes are characterized by many and extensive deformities. Undoubtedly, many such abnormal fertilizations result in many early abortions and stillbirths.

SYNDROMES ASSOCIATED WITH AN ABNORMAL NUMBER OF CHROMOSOMES

13-15 Trisomy
Anophthalmos, microphthalmos, retinal dysplasia, optic atrophy, coloboma of the uvea, and cataracts are the major eye anomalies; cerebral defects, cleft palate, heart lesions, polydactyly, and hemangiomas are the more severe nonophthalmic changes. Cytogenetically there is an extra chromosome indistinguishable from the group 13-15. Death by age 6 months is the rule. Only a few such cases have been reported to date.

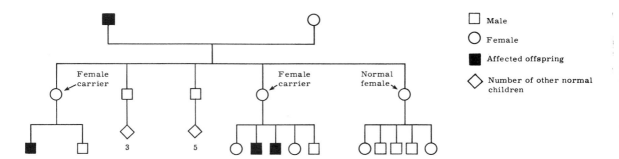

Fig 19-6. Pedigree of red-green color blindness.

16-18 Trisomy

The main features of this rare syndrome are mental and physical retardation. Corneal opacities and unilateral ptosis have been described.

21 Trisomy (Mongolism, Down's Syndrome)

Although Down's syndrome is a fairly common and well known entity, the hereditary pattern was ill defined until cytogenetic studies revealed an extra chromosome indistinguishable from chromosome 21. The principal manifestations are small stature, a flattened, round, mongoloid facies, saddle nose, thick lower lip, large tongue, soft, seborrheic skin, thick, smooth hair, obesity, small genitalia, short fingers, a simian fold, congenital heart anomalies, mental retardation, and frequent psychic disturbances. The ocular signs include hyperplasia of the iris, narrow palpebral fissures with Oriental slant, frequent strabismus, epicanthus, frequent cataract, high myopia (33%), and Brushfield (silver-gray) spots on the iris.

The incidence of Down's syndrome is significantly increased in children born to older women, particularly past age 40. Not all cytogenetically studied cases have demonstrated the same chromosomal anomaly, but a high percentage have shown the 21 trisomy (47 total chromosomes).

ABNORMALITIES INVOLVING SEX CHROMOSOMES

Turner's syndrome is a monosomy (45 chromosomes). For some reason, the affected female receives only one X chromosome. Clinically, there is growth retardation, rudimentary ovaries and female genitalia, amenorrhea, pterygium colli, epicanthus, and cubitus valgus. Of particular ophthalmic interest is the high incidence of color blindness (8%). This is the same frequency as for males (female incidence, 0.4%), and is readily explained by the fact that the normally recessive gene is unopposed and is expressed just as in the male.

Klinefelter's syndrome is a trisomy involving the X chromosomes. These phenotypical males have 47 chromosomes: the normal 44 autosomes and 3 sex chromosomes, XXY. These individuals are sterile, with small testes, frequently gynecomastia, and a eunuchoid physique. The ocular finding of interest is the very rare occurrence of color blindness, since the recessive X chromosome is masked by a normal dominant (as in the normal female).

There are other scattered reports of syndromes being correlated with an abnormal chromosomal pattern. Marfan's syndrome and Sturge-Weber syndrome are examples of syndromes which may need to be reclassified into the trisomy group. Despite these advances, one must not lose sight of the fact that while it is quite possible to identify an extra chromosome, there is no indication that an individual abnormal gene will ever be detected under the microscope.

OTHER GENETIC CONSIDERATIONS

Genetic Counseling

Valuable advice can often be given to families or engaged couples concerned with the possibilities of transmitting serious disease to future generations. This entails a working knowledge of basic genetic principles. A careful history of the pedigree in question is very important, as a single disease may have more than one mode of transmission (eg, retinitis pigmentosa has 3 or more basic patterns). On the other hand, careful inquiries about maternal health during pregnancy may suggest that the anomaly is developmental and therefore unrelated to the genes. The recognition of the genetic carrier state may enable the physician to give intelligent advice.

Advice against consanguineous marriage is certainly essential, since it is estimated that the average individual carries 5-10 undesirable recessive genes.

Genetic Carrier State

Recognition of the genetic carrier state is most important. Detection is possible in many diseases. There are 3 types:

A. Autosomal dominant diseases in which the disease appears in a mild or subclinical form (low expression). Because the offspring of such individuals still have the theoretical 50% chance of passing on the disease process, the recognition of this carrier state is important in genetic counseling.

B. Autosomal recessive diseases with heterozygous manifestations. Affected genes which are normally balanced by a normal allele may cause minor subclinical abnormalities which disclose the presence of the abnormal gene. One can predict the 25% possibility of occurrence of some autosomal recessive diseases if the carrier state can be recognized in both potential mates. Critical provocative tests for such common diseases as open-angle glaucoma (cortisone test) and diabetes mellitus (glucose tolerance test) may allow the detection of the heterozygous state as well as early detection of the disease (homozygous state).

C. Female carrier in sex-linked recessive disease. Subclinical evidence of the disease in daughters of affected fathers differentiates carriers from noncarriers in a number of sex-linked recessive diseases (often quite obvious in tapetoretinal degenerative conditions).

Mutation

Mutation occurs when a gene undergoes alteration in the germ cell due to spontaneous chemical change within the gene and is manifested by a new characteristic. The causes of the change are not entirely understood, but such extrinsic environmental factors as heat, x-rays, and exposure to radioactive materials may induce it. Most often the new characteristic is unfavorable (ie, disease producing), but some mutations are favorable and account for the evolution of species (Darwin).

Certain mutations occur repeatedly in specific genes and cause specific disease. Hemophilia, which follows a sex-linked pattern, and retinoblastoma, which follows an autosomal dominant pattern, are examples of disease occurring as a result of mutation. Very few individuals with severe abnormalities reproduce, so that the incidence of such diseases is dependent almost entirely upon mutation. Mutations causing less severe disease are inherited as dominant, recessive, or sex-linked traits depending upon the type of mutated gene.

GLOSSARY OF GENETIC TERMS*

Abiotrophic disease: Genetically determined disease which is not evident at birth but which becomes manifest later in life.

Acquired: Not hereditary; contracted after birth or in utero.

Alleles: See Allelic genes.

Allelic genes: Paired genes or partner genes; genes occupying the same locus on homologous (paired) chromosomes and which, therefore, normally segregate from each other during the reduction-division of mitosis.

Autosomes: The chromosomes (22 pairs of autosomes in man) other than the sex chromosomes.

---

*Modified from Krupp, Sweet, Jawetz, & Biglieri: Physician's Handbook, 16th ed. Lange, 1970.

Chromosome: A small thread-like or rod-like structure into which the nuclear chromatin divides during mitosis. The number of chromosomes is constant for any given species (23 pairs in man: 22 pairs of autosomes and one pair of sex chromosomes). Each chromosome is composed of a linear arrangement of small bodies called genes, each of which occupies a specific locus on its chromosome.

Congenital: Existing at or before birth; not necessarily hereditary.

Dominant: Designating a gene whose phenotypic effect largely or entirely obscures that of its allele.

Familial: Pertaining to traits, either hereditary or acquired, which tend to occur in families.

Gamete (germ cell): A cell which is capable of uniting with another cell in sexual reproduction (ie, the ovum and spermatozoon).

Gene: A unit of heredity which occupies a specific locus in the chromosome which, either alone or in combination, produces a single characteristic. It is usually a single molecule which is capable of self-duplication or mutation.

Genetic carrier state: A condition wherein a given hereditary characteristic is not manifest in one individual but may be genetically transmitted to the offspring of that individual.

Genotype: The hereditary constitution, or combination of genes, which characterizes a given individual or a group of genetically identical organisms.

Germ cells (gametes): Cells capable of uniting with other cells sexually in reproducing the organism, spermatozoa in the male and ova in the female.

Hereditary: Transmitted from ancestor to offspring through the germ plasm.

Heterozygous: Having 2 members of a given hereditary factor pair which are dissimilar, ie, the 2 genes of an allelic pair are not the same.

Homozygous: Having 2 members of a given hereditary factor pair which are similar, ie, the 2 genes of an allelic pair are identical.

Meiosis: A special type of cell division occurring during the maturation of sex cells, by which the normal diploid set of chromosomes is reduced to a single (haploid) set, 2 successive nuclear divisions occurring, while the chromosomes divide only once.

Mutation: A transformation of a gene, often sudden and dramatic, with or without known cause, into a different gene occupying the same locus as the original gene on a particular chromosome; the new gene is allelic to the normal gene from which it has arisen.

Penetrance: The likelihood or probability that a gene will become morphologically (phenotypically) expressed. The degree of penetrance may depend upon acquired as well as genetic factors.

Phenotype: The visible characteristics of an individual or those which are common to a group of apparently identical individuals.

Recessive: Designating a gene whose phenotypic effect is largely or entirely obscured by the effect of its allele.

Sex chromosome: The chromosome or pair of chromosomes which determines the sex of the individual. (In the human female, the sex chromosome pair is homologous, XX; in the male, nonhomologous, XY.)

Sex linkage: The influence of sex on transmission of hereditary traits. There are 2 main types of sex-linked inheritance depending upon whether the sex-linked genes are located in the X or the Y chromosome. Sex linkage may be absolute or incomplete.

Somatic cells: Cells incapable of reproducing the organism.

Trisomy: The existence of 3 chromosomes of one variety, rather than the normal pair of chromosomes.

Zygote: The cell formed by the union of 2 gametes in sexual reproduction.

•   •   •

Bibliography

Crow, J. F., & others: Symposium: Genetics in the practice of ophthalmology and otolaryngology. Tr Am Acad Ophth **69**:17-51, 1965.

Duke-Elder, S.: System of Ophthalmology. Vol. VII, pp. 3-113. Mosby, 1962.

Francois, J.: Heredity in Ophthalmology. Mosby, 1961.

Francois, J., & M. T. Matton-Van Leven: Chromosome abnormalities and ophthalmology. J Pediat Ophth **1**:5-18, 1964.

Sorsby, A.: Genetics in Ophthalmology. Mosby, 1951.

Waardenburg, P. J., Franceschetti, A., & D. Klein: Genetics and Ophthalmology. Thomas, Vol. I, 1961, Vol. II, 1963.

20...

Optics and Refraction

The sense of sight depends upon an external stimulus which is received by the eye in the form of light rays that pass to the retina through the cornea, aqueous, lens, and vitreous. The varying optical densities (or refractive indices) of these structures cause the light rays to change direction as they pass through. If the image does not focus on the fovea, the object will appear to be blurred. The science of optics forms the basis of the diagnosis and correction of refractive errors of the eyes.

Light is that form of radiant energy which gives objects visibility. When light strikes a substance it may be reflected from its surface, may be absorbed by the substance, or may pass through it. The visibility of objects depends upon the light reflected from their surfaces. Substances such as air, clear glass, or clear water through which light passes and through which objects can be easily seen are said to be **transparent.** Substances which transmit light poorly, such as opal, frosted glass, or thin paper, are called **translucent.** Substances which do not transmit light are called **opaque.** It is with the properties of reflection and transparency that we are particularly concerned in relationship to the eye.

Light travels in the form of **rays.** When the source is close, the rays are divergent when they reach the viewer's eye. When the light source is distant (eg, sunlight), the rays are parallel. Because of the relatively small aperture of the eye (pupil), it is the custom in ophthalmology to consider rays of light farther than 20 feet away to be parallel.

A collection of parallel light rays is called a **beam**; a collection of rays from a light source is called a **pencil**; and a convergent or divergent collection of rays meeting at a point is called a **focus.** The power of a pencil of light is expressed in diopters (D). At a distance (d) of one meter from the point of focus, the power of a pencil of light would be 1 diopter, since $1/d = D$, where d is expressed in meters. In optics, the diopter* is used to express (1) the

*The symbol D is used for diopter in optics; the symbol Δ is used for diopter in power of a prism.

power of a lens, (2) the power of a pencil of light, and (3) the power of a prism.

OPTICS OF PLANE SURFACES

When light strikes a transparent substance at an oblique angle while passing from one medium to another of different density, it is deflected or bent at the interface; this is known as **refraction.** If the ray travels perpendicular to the surface it goes through in a straight line. The constant relationship for the bending of light between any 2 media is expressed in the law of refraction: "The relationship of the angles of incidence to the angles of refraction for any 2 transparent media is such that the ratio of their sines is constant." This trigonometric concept is used as a basis for

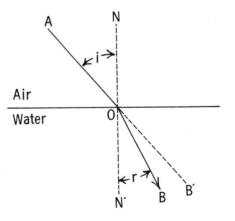

Fig 20-1. Refraction at a plane surface. NN´ is the perpendicular to the surface at O, where the incident ray strikes. A ray coming from A is bent toward the perpendicular (AB) in a denser medium. The apparent image is at B´, as if it were on a plane with A. i = angle of incidence; r = angle of refraction.

computing refractive powers of materials and lenses.

Prisms

A prism is an optical medium with 2 plane surfaces inclined toward each other. A ray of light incident to one of the inclined surfaces is bent toward the base of the prism and emerges at the second surface with further bending. However, the apparent displacement of an object viewed through the prism is toward the apex, or away from the base.

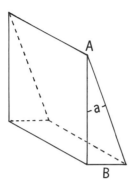

Fig 20-2. Prism sketched in perspective. A is the apex, B is the base, and a is the apex angle of the prism.

Convex Lenses (Fig 20-5)

Parallel rays of light converge to a focus (F), the principal focus of the lens. The distance LF in Fig 20-5 is the principal focal distance or focal length of the lens.

Concave Lenses (Fig 20-6)

Parallel rays of light diverge, but produce a **virtual image** which is focused at (F), the principal focus of the lens.

Prismatic Power of a Convex Lens (Fig 20-7)

Light entering a convex lens behaves as if the thicker central portion of the lens were the base of a prism. The central rays are little deflected, but the more peripheral rays deviate more, as if there were succeeding prisms of greater strength toward the edge of the lens.

Cylindric Lenses (Fig 20-8)

If a curved refracting surface is not perfectly spherical in all meridians, there will be one principal meridian with a greater curvature than the others. This cylindric effect is commonly found in the human eye, which is seldom perfect. The difference in curvature produces **astigmatism,** and prevents a point focus of the objects viewed through that lens system.

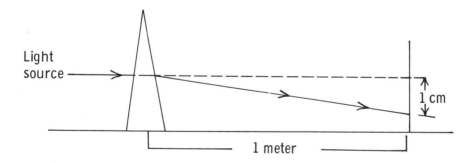

Fig 20-3. Prism deviation. A prism of 1 prism diopter strength will deviate a ray of light 1 cm in a distance of 1 M.

OPTICS OF SPHERICAL SURFACES

Refraction by a Spherical Surface (Fig 20-4)

Nonparallel rays of light entering a spherical refracting surface are bent toward the principal axis (OO´). The more peripheral rays are bent at a steeper angle, and the result is a "focal line" (U´R´).

Aberrations of Lenses

Ophthalmic lenses have many faults or aberrations according to their strengths and the materials from which they are made.

A. Spherical Aberration: When a beam of light passes through a convex lens, the rays closest to the axis are focused at the greatest distance from the lens, and each circle of rays farther from the axis is focused at areas farther in front of the more axial rays. This spherical aberration constitutes a longitudinal

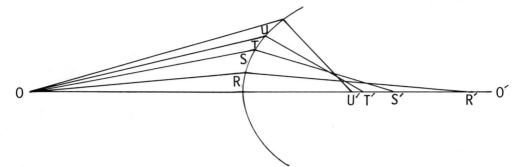

Fig 20-4. Refraction by a spherical surface.

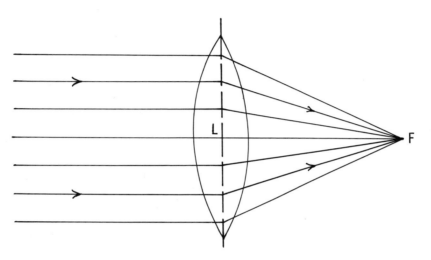

Fig 20-5. Refraction by a convex lens.

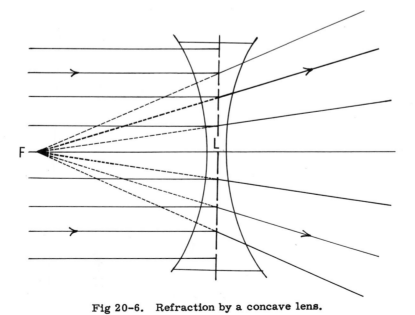

Fig 20-6. Refraction by a concave lens.

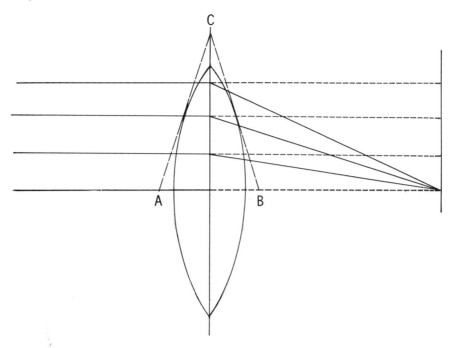

Fig 20-7. Prismatic power of a convex lens.

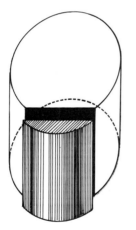

Fig 20-8. Cylindric lens. A cylindric lens is illustrated as being formed as a segment of a cylinder. It has an axis (vertical) along the plane surface, with no refracting power (axis of the cylinder), and an opposite meridian of greatest curvature (horizontal).

aberration which becomes greater as the lens aperture becomes larger. Between the focus of the axial rays and the more peripheral rays, a 3-dimensional conical figure called a "caustic" is produced. Spherical aberration has little importance as regards the eye because

the size of the pupil restricts the rays to the more axial ones.

B. Chromatic Aberration: (Fig 20-9) This is caused by the dispersion of white light into its component colors. Red is bent the least and has the longest focal distance; violet is bent the most and has the shortest focal distance. Blue, green, yellow, and orange lie between the violet and the red. Color correction is necessary in camera lenses but not in spectacle lenses because of the relatively low power and the low dispersive index of the glass used.

C. Curvature of Image: If a flat object at a great distance is focused through a lens of short focal length, the relatively shortened image distance from the center of the lens will produce a curved image instead of a flat one. This is not important in the eye since it is compensated by the curvature of the retina.

D. Distortion: Increasing magnification as the rays approach the edge of a lens causes a peripheral distortion which produces an apparent inward curvature of the sides of a square seen through a convex lens. Seen through a concave lens the sides appear to bulge outward.

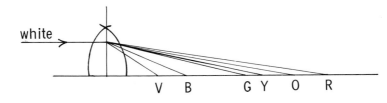

Fig 20-9. Chromatic aberration.

PHYSIOLOGIC ASPECTS OF OPTICS

Emmetropia, Hyperopia, Myopia

The **emmetropic** (normal) eye is one in which parallel rays of light are brought to a focus on the fovea without the use of accommodation. A **hyperopic** (farsighted) eye is smaller than normal and fails to converge the rays of light enough to focus upon the fovea without the use of accommodation. The act of accommodation or the placing of a convex ("plus") lens in front of the eye helps converge the light to a focus on the fovea. A **myopic** (nearsighted) eye is larger than normal and tends to focus the light in front of the fovea. A concave ("minus") lens in front of the eye helps to diverge the light rays to focus on the fovea.

Since the size of the eyeball governs the focus to such a large extent, and the eyeball continues to grow until about age 25, it is easy to see how a farsighted eye of a 10-year-old child becomes less farsighted or even nearsighted by age 20, and a normal or nearsighted eye becomes more nearsighted. This is a normal growth phenomenon, tempered by an inherited tendency toward nearsightedness, and explains why "exercises" or visual training have no influence on a condition due primarily to the size of an organ. (Rarer causes of myopia and hyperopia due to abnormal refractive changes in the optical media are not considered here.)

Accommodation

Accommodation is the mechanism by which the focusing apparatus of the eye adjusts to objects at different distances. Contraction of the ciliary muscle, which is supplied by the parasympathetic third nerve, results in increased curvature and gives the eye greater dioptric power, so that divergent rays of light coming from within infinity are now focused on the retina. The mechanism is largely reflex and so well adjusted that normal individuals are not aware of the process.

Just how contraction of the ciliary muscle increases the curvature of the lens is still disputed. Young and Helmholtz assumed that

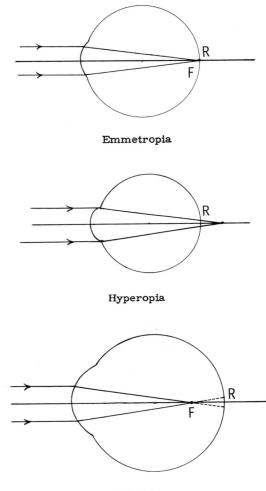

Emmetropia

Hyperopia

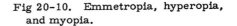

Myopia

Fig 20-10. Emmetropia, hyperopia, and myopia.

the lens was elastic and that contraction of the ciliary muscle, particularly the circular fibers of the ciliary muscle (fibers of Muller), drew the ciliary processes together so that the zonule of Zinn was relaxed. The zonule is a sheet of tissue made up of numerous fibers that support the lens in its capsule.

The lens itself is actually not elastic, but the lens capsule is. When the lens is taken out of the eye in its capsule, it is more circular than when it is in the eye during the non-accommodated state. When the zonule relaxes, the elastic lens capsule forces the lens to assume a more spherical form and hence its anterior surface becomes more convex.

Contraction of the ciliary muscle causes a change in refractive power of the crystalline lens from the earliest age at which accommodation can be measured up to about age 45 or 50.

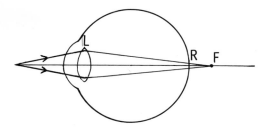

Fig 20-11. Unaccommodated eye.

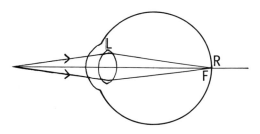

Fig 20-12. Accommodated eye.
Note lens shape more convex.

Table 20-1. Table of accommodation.*

Age (Years)	Mean Accommodation (Diopters)
8	13.8
25	9.9
35	7.3
40	5.8
45	3.6
50	1.9
55	1.3

*Modified after Duane.

Visual Acuity

Many subjective tests have been proposed for the determination of visual acuity using pictures of different objects, circles and dots, and letters and numerals. Snellen was the first to construct a system of test objects so arranged that acuity could be expressed by a number. In his test chart, the characters consist of letters or numerals, each stroke or space of which occupies an angle of 1 minute of arc, with the whole character occupying 5 minutes of arc at the stated distance.

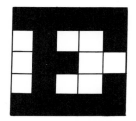

Fig 20-13. Snellen block E.

Many expressions of relative acuity have been devised to attempt to record the value as a fraction, but the majority in common use compare the patient's acuity with the average normal for that distance. (''20/20'' indicates the line read by average normal people at 20 feet.)

Snellen tests for near vision are constructed on the same principle as those for distance. A common near card is the Jaeger test type.

Visual acuity test results vary greatly with the illumination of the test cards; some increase in acuity is noted with increase in illumination up to a certain point of brightness. It has been suggested that a diffuse illumination of about 80-100 foot candles on the chart is best.

REFRACTIVE ERRORS

Optical System of the Eye

A ray of light entering the eye passes through the cornea, the aqueous, the anterior and posterior surfaces of the lens, and the vitreous to focus upon the fovea. Because of its greater curvature, the refractive power of the cornea is greater than that of the lens. However, the cornea has no powers of accommodation; its optical function is to refract light and to be clear and uniformly curved.

Because the aqueous has the same refractive index as the cornea (1.33), these 2 optical media are considered as one.

The variable refractive medium of the eye is the **crystalline lens** (in recent literature called simply the **lens**). The lens is an elastic structure situated in the anterior portion of the eye behind the iris (see p 3). In shape it resembles a biconvex glass lens ("magnifying glass"). In young people the lens is capable of precise instantaneous adjustments in its shape in order to bring into focus objects at varying distances from the eye within a range of 20 feet. This is known as **accommodation** (see above). Light rays entering the eye from objects farther away than 20 feet are considered to be parallel, and so accommodation is not necessary. In this case the eye is said to be **unaccommodated.**

The vitreous has no optical function other than light transmission. It is a clear gelatinous medium between the lens and the retina through which light rays pass unrefracted.

Emmetropia

In the absence of neural and retinal disorders and opacities of the cornea, lens, and vitreous, and assuming that the eyeball is of normal size, the unaccommodated eye will receive and focus parallel rays of light from a distant light source into a sharp image upon the fovea. This condition is called **emmetropia** ("sight in proper measure"). Emmetropia is best thought of as an ideal rather than a normal condition since almost all adults have some degree of refractive error. The emmetropic eye is diagrammed on p 269.

Ametropia

Variations from the emmetropic state not due to opacities or disease are collectively referred to as **ametropia** ("sight not in proper measure"). The principal forms of ametropia are **hyperopia** (hypermetropia, "far sight"), **myopia** ("near sight"), **astigmatism** ("not at a point"), and **presbyopia** ("old sight"). Less important variations are **anisometropia** (variation in refractive errors in the two eyes) and **aniseikonia** (difference in image size in the two eyes).

Nonvisual Symptoms and Signs

In addition to the visual disturbances caused by refractive errors, a great many associated symptoms may occur. These are especially important in the diagnosis of refractive errors in children. Common signs and symptoms include blinking, frowning, rubbing the eyes, head tilting, closing one eye, clumsiness, photophobia, injection, and tearing. Adults may complain of "eyestrain" caused by the effort of accommodation. Headache, dizziness, and occasionally nausea may have their origin in refractive errors.

Inheritance of Refractive Errors

Refractive errors of all kinds tend to be inherited but in no definitely predictable way. An important reason for this is the number of variables which influence refraction such as corneal curvature, depth of anterior chamber, length of the eye, and shape of the lens.

HYPEROPIA
(Hypermetropia, Farsightedness)

In hyperopia, parallel rays of light are brought to a focus behind the retina when accommodative powers are relaxed. The result is indistinct vision at all distances. Accommodative efforts bring objects into focus up to the limits of the powers of accommodation.

Hyperopia may be caused by shortness of the eyeball or weakness of the refractive power of the cornea or lens. "Physiologic" hyperopia is present at birth in about 80% of children. This is due to the shortness of the eye, partially compensated for by the fact that the infant lens is more convex than the adult lens. About 5% of children are born myopic, and about 15% emmetropic. During the years from about age 2 to about age 25, there is a slight gradual decrease in hyperopia. Most persons remain slightly hyperopic during adulthood.

Clinical Findings (See Fig 20-14)

Except in severe degrees of hyperopia, vision is normal beyond a range of 20 feet. If the effort required for accommodation is not too great, near vision may likewise be unimpaired (latent hyperopia). If greater accommodative effort is required, the patient complains of "eyestrain," sometimes accompanied by eye pain, headache, and nausea. In severe degrees of hyperopia ("high hyperopia"), distant vision can be maintained only by accommodative effort and near vision is blurred even with maximum accommodative effort. Hyperopia may be confused with myopia when a child holds a book close to his eyes in order to have an enlarged image when the print blurs.

In children such nonvisual symptoms as headache and disinterest in reading are occasionally associated with hyperopia of moderate to severe degree.

Convergent strabismus in children is frequently associated with hyperopia (accommodative esotropia; see p 184).

The lens required in the ophthalmoscope to focus on the retina is a rough index of the degree of hyperopia (or myopia). The space between the retinal vessels is smaller than normal, the optic disk is smaller than normal, and the retinal veins may be tortuous. Precise diagnosis depends upon the trial lens examination. Because children have strong accommodative powers, a cycloplegic drug is required. Because the accommodative powers decrease in adults, this is not necessary after about age 40.

Treatment

Hyperopia may be corrected with the use of convex lenses to increase the angle of incidence of the light rays entering the cornea and lens (Fig 20-5). Correction of a moderate degree of hyperopia in children without symptoms or strabismus is rarely necessary.

Course and Prognosis

Most children with hyperopia do not need corrective lenses unless esotropia is present (see Accommodative Esotropia, p 184). As accommodative ability fails (late in the 4th decade), a partial strength correction may be needed for reading. Bifocals (or 2 pairs of glasses) are usually required by age 45.

SIMPLE MYOPIA
(Nearsightedness)

In myopia, parallel rays of light are brought to a focus in front of the retina. Thus the "far point" of the eye, which is at infinity in emmetropia and hyperopia, is at a definite finite distance somewhere short of 20 feet, according to the degree of myopia. With myopia of 1 D, for example, the far point of clear focus is 1 meter from the eye; as the myopia increases, the far point decreases (inverse ratio).

Myopia may be caused by largeness of the eyeball (axial myopia) or by an increase in the strength of the refractive power of the media (refractive myopia). Most cases are axial in type. Heredity plays a large role in myopia. Myopia usually increases during the teen ages and levels off at about age 25 regardless of external factors such as amount of close work, lighting, rest, vitamins, endocrine balance, exercise, etc.

Clinical Findings (Fig 20-14)

The most common symptom is the inability to distinguish objects clearly in the distance, such as the blackboard in school or road signs. Many myopic children, however, never having experienced sharp distance vision, are not aware of what is missing and are usually only discovered to be myopic by routine visual screening tests in school.

Frowning (squinting) in an effort to see is common, as the acuity is sharpened by making a tiny lid aperture similar to the "pinhole camera"; this achieves a lens-like focus by eliminating peripheral rays of light entering the eye, allowing only the more axial rays to reach the retina for a clearer image. (This increases the depth of focus and is similar to "stopping down" the aperture of a camera.) This frowning sometimes results in fatigue headaches and lid irritation, and is often interpreted as photophobia.

Myopic children may hold their reading material quite close to the eyes if the degree of myopia is sufficient to bring the far point closer than the normal reading distance.

Treatment

Concave (minus) lenses to diverge the rays of light so that they will focus on the retina will afford the myopic individual "normal vision," and should not be looked upon as a crutch which will be habit-forming or which should be limited in use. Corrective lenses neither "strengthen" nor "weaken" eyes but allow the patient to see more clearly or more comfortably.

Corrective lenses for mild degrees of myopia (less than 1 or 1.5 D) in children in the first few grades of school are not indicated, as the demands for sharp distance vision are not great during this time.

Course and Prognosis

Myopia tends to increase during the teens and levels off by about age 25. Presbyopic symptoms in the 40's necessitate bifocals or removing the corrective lenses for reading.

Contrary to popular belief, the degree and progress of myopia are not affected either by wearing or refusing to wear corrective lenses. "Eye exercises" likewise have no effect since the size of the eyeball or the refractive power of the media cannot be altered in this way.

PSEUDOMYOPIA

Pseudomyopia is a rare disorder that is usually due to a spasm of the ciliary muscles (spasm of accommodation), which causes parallel rays of light to converge to a focus in front of the retina, as in true myopia. This may occur with excessive accommodative effort in uncorrected hyperopia, or it may be a hysterical phenomenon.

The diagnosis of pseudomyopia is confirmed upon relaxation of the spasm (and the correction of the myopia) by the instillation of a cycloplegic drug. Refraction without the use of a cycloplegic drug and the prescription of concave lenses only necessitate greater accommodative effort, which increases spasm and therefore the degree of pseudomyopia.

DEGENERATIVE MYOPIA
(Malignant Myopia, Progressive Myopia)

Since myopia is frequently progressive, the term "progressive myopia" is a poor one for this special condition, which may be more aptly called degenerative myopia, since the diagnosis is based upon the changes which are observed in the retina and choroid upon ophthalmoscopic examination.

Degenerative myopia is much less common than simple myopia. It has been reported to have a higher incidence in females and in certain races and ethnic groups, eg, the Chinese, Arabs, and Jews, and is undoubtedly genetically determined—usually as a recessive. It is more common in Southern Europe than in Northern Europe and the USA. Two types have been described: congenital and developmental. The pathology is the same in either case.

Clinical Findings
The manifestations of degenerative myopia are the same as those of simple myopia except that with severe degenerative changes the visual acuity may not be corrected to normal with any lenses. The degenerative changes may have no direct relationship to the degree of myopia. Thus a myopia of mild degree may show marked degenerative changes, while a "high" myopia of 6-20 D may show no degenerative changes. The diagnosis, therefore, depends upon ophthalmoscopic examination. The main characteristics are as follows:

A. Changes at the Optic Disk: A temporal crescent is seen ophthalmoscopically where the choroid pulls away from the edge of the disk, baring the white sclera. Outside of this area there may be a second choroidal crescent of disturbed pigmentation. In nasal supertraction of the vessels on the disk the retinal tissue seems to have been pulled over the nasal edge of the disk, distorting the course of the vessels.

B. Changes in the Choroid and Retina: The choroid is stretched and thinned, with areas of atrophy and pigment change. These changes may result in bare white patches of sclera showing through, or in pigment clumping resembling the changes seen in chorioretinitis. Rarely, there may be a proliferation of an unusual amount of pigment in the region of the macula to form the Forster-Fuchs black spot.

C. Changes in the Sclera: There may be a localized stretching of the sclera to form a staphyloma. The most common site is the posterior pole of the eye. The staphyloma increases the axial length of the eye and thus makes that area more myopic than the surrounding retina.

D. Changes in the Vitreous: Fibrillary degeneration and posterior vitreous detachment are common.

Pathology
Pathologic changes are degenerative in nature, with a generalized thinning and atrophy of the coats of the eye.

Treatment
As long as the visual acuity can be corrected with concave lenses, these should be used. Surgical shortening or reinforcing of the posterior sclera is still largely experimental. Complications (eg, retinal detachment) have to be specifically dealt with.

Course and Prognosis
The degenerative changes may gravely affect visual function. Thinning and atrophy of the choroid is almost always accompanied by loss of retinal function in the involved area. Choroidal hemorrhages may occur. Changes in the macula will markedly reduce central vision. Retinal detachment is a frequent complication, and vitreous degenerative opacities reduce vision. There is also a higher incidence of cataracts and secondary glaucoma among these patients.

ACQUIRED MYOPIA

A few instances of myopia do not fall into the above categories. If there is a history of fairly rapid blurring of distant vision and if a myopic change in refractive error has been demonstrated, several conditions should be investigated. They must be differentiated from true refractive errors.

Diabetes Mellitus
Uncontrolled diabetes mellitus tends to produce refractive error, either myopia or hyperopia, probably as a result of a change in

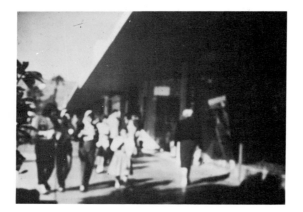

Slightly blurred figures seen from a distance (about 50 feet) through the eyes of a moderately myopic or significantly hyperopic person.

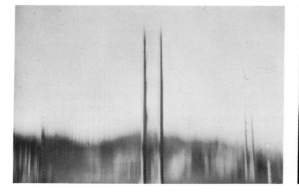

Severe astigmatism with the rule. Note vertical lines in focus.

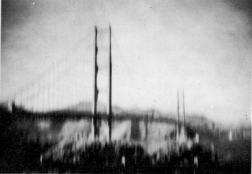

Moderate astigmatism with the rule.

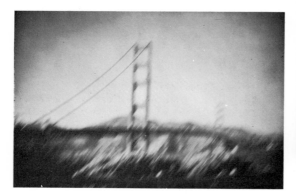

Moderate oblique astigmatism (axis 45°). Note cable at 45° in focus.

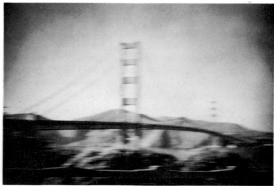

Moderate hyperopic astigmatism against the rule (axis 180°; can be corrected by proper convex cylindrical lens with axis at 180°). Note transverse structures in focus, vertical structures blurred.

Fig 20-14. Photographic interpretation of uncorrected refractive errors of various types. (Courtesy of E. Goodner.) The photographs on this page were taken with trial lenses in front of the camera to approximate the refractive error.

tissue fluids in the lens substance. Control of the diabetes by appropriate medical means usually reverses this state. The authors have examined several such cases where routine urine examination for sugar and even fasting blood glucose values were normal, but where glucose tolerance tests confirmed the suspected diabetes.

Cataract

In the incipient stage of cataract development the change in the substance of the lens may be merely a fluid change, producing myopia without noticeably affecting the transparency of the lens.

ASTIGMATISM

Astigmatism is distorted vision caused by a variation in refractive power along different meridians of the eye. Astigmatism may be "regular" or "irregular." "Regular" astigmatism may be "with the rule" or "against the rule." Most cases are due to irregularities in the shape of the cornea, but the lens may also cause astigmatism (eg, in old age, due to cataractous change). Heredity plays a role in astigmatism as well as in myopia and hyperopia.

In **regular astigmatism** the varying refractive powers in different meridians can be reduced to 2 principal meridians at right angles to each other. In astigmatism **with the rule** the vertical meridian has the greater curvature. This is usually the case with astigmatism in young people, since most such cases are caused by the shape of the cornea. Later in life the cornea tends to flatten, so that small amounts of astigmatism with the rule may disappear, or astigmatism **against the rule** (with the greater curvature in the horizontal meridian) may appear. **Irregular astigmatism** is due to the uneven bulges of keratoconus, corneal scarring, lens irregularities, and the pressure on the cornea of small tumors in the lids.

Astigmatism is identified as to the type of cylindric lens needed to correct it: a concave cylinder would be used for myopic astigmatism, and a convex cylindric lens for hyperopic astigmatism.

Astigmatism may be simple (no hyperopia or myopia) or combined with hyperopia (compound hyperopic astigmatism), or with myopia (compound myopic astigmatism), or mixed (myopic combined with hyperopic astigmatism or hyperopic combined with myopic astigmatism).

Clinical Findings (Fig 20-14)

With mild degrees of astigmatism there may be no symptoms, or merely asthenopia with prolonged use of the eyes. The person with astigmatism tries to achieve a clearer image by rapidly changing focus (accommodation), with resultant fatigue. With greater degrees of astigmatism, clear visual acuity may not be possible at any distance. Astigmatism may be discovered through routine screening tests in school or through comparison of visual abilities with normal associates.

The child with astigmatism tends to hold reading material close. There is also a tendency to frown, to obtain the "pinhole" effect, as in myopia. Headaches due to the frowning and accommodative effort are common.

Because of the difference in refractive powers of the 2 principal meridians, the retinal blood vessels coursing in one direction may be out of focus upon ophthalmoscopic examination while those in the opposite meridian are clear, and a different lens must be rotated into the ophthalmoscope to obtain a clear image. The disk is elongated. The retina itself is normal. The precise determination of the amount and axis of astigmatism depends upon a careful refraction with trial lenses.

Treatment

The refractive error is treated with a cylindric concave or convex lens oriented in the proper meridian (axis) to restore a spherical effect, with a combination lens incorporating concave or convex spheres for the resultant myopia or hyperopia. Small degrees of astigmatism are physiologic, and need no correction.

Mild degrees of irregular astigmatism due to keratoconus or corneal astigmatism which cannot be corrected with simple lenses are often benefited by corneal contact lenses, which tend to restore the spherical refracting surface over the cornea.

Course and Prognosis

Aside from the changes described above which tend to alter small amounts of regular astigmatism during the growth period, most moderate astigmatic errors are fairly constant throughout life. Irregular astigmatism due to keratoconus usually progresses to an uncorrectable degree; corneal transplants are eventually necessary.

PRESBYOPIA
(Old Sight)

At birth the lens substance is soft and pliable, and is easily altered in shape by the action of the ciliary muscles (accommodation). Throughout life there is a gradual hardening of this substance, beginning with the nucleus, so that it becomes more resistant to changes in shape until by the mid 40's the average person with normal vision has difficulty in focusing on near objects and reading fine print. This is presbyopia, and does not imply an increase in hyperopia but merely a lessening of the effective powers of accommodation.

Statistical studies similar to those of Duane (see p 270) have correlated the power of accommodation with age, so that if this power of accommodation is measured a fairly accurate estimation of the person's age may be made.

Clinical Findings

The symptoms occur with close work. There is blurring of near objects, or discomfort or fatigue with attempted near work. Persons with normal vision may complain of a blurring of distant objects for a few moments after looking up, due to the lag of relaxation of accommodation after excessive effort at near focusing. Usually the person has noticed that he must hold his reading material farther from his eyes to see the print, and a frequent statement is to the effect that his "arms are too short."

Treatment

Following refraction, a lens is prescribed which corrects the basic refractive error, together with the proper convex reading addition ("add") which brings the near point within suitable range for the individual's requirements. Since this lens will blur the distance vision, these requirements may necessitate a bifocal or multifocal lens for convenience in use. Some persons are content with the use of only the reading lens, whereas others prefer 2 pairs of glasses.

Course and Prognosis

The average person requires his first reading glasses between the ages of 42 and 45. This first prescription merely makes up the deficiency of the accommodative powers at that time. A new prescription is required about every 2 years. As these powers fail in the following years several changes in strength of reading additions may be required until the early 50's, at which time the glasses accomplish most of the change in focus required for close work. Little change may be necessary thereafter unless there is some alteration in the refractive state of the eye caused by developing lens opacities, glaucoma, degenerative myopia, or other pathologic changes.

PRINCIPLES OF REFRACTION OF THE EYE

The term "refraction" is an accepted clinical term commonly used by ophthalmologists to designate the examination for determining the refractive state of the eye. The term also refers to the bending of light passing through the optical structures of the eye itself.

METHODS OF REFRACTION

A detailed discussion of the technics of refraction is beyond the scope of this book. In general, the procedures fall into 2 main classes: cycloplegic and noncycloplegic.

Cycloplegic Refraction

By the use of certain solutions (scopolamine, atropine, homatropine) instilled in the conjunctival sac, the ciliary muscle is weakened and accommodative power lowered (cycloplegia). Dilation of the pupil (mydriasis) is coincidental but facilitates ophthalmoscopy. In this way the refractive state of the eye at rest can be determined. This can be done by objective retinoscopy or by subjective trial of lenses to obtain the best visual sharpness.

Retinoscopy is performed by directing a beam of light from a retinoscope into the pupil of the eye, and neutralizing the movement of a light "shadow" in the fundus by placing appropriate lenses in front of the eye.

Noncycloplegic Refraction

Without the use of the cycloplegic drugs, allowances are made for the action of accommodation, which is very active in youth and diminishes with age (presbyopia). As in cycloplegic refraction, objective or subjective methods can be used.

PRESCRIPTION OF LENSES

The 2 principal reasons for wearing corrective lenses are to improve visual acuity and to help relieve symptoms caused by refractive errors.

A visual acuity rating of 20/20 is not essential for everyone. Preschool children and even children in the first few grades are able to carry on their visual tasks effectively with much less than 20/20 visual acuity. In the absence of symptoms, therefore, a delay in the prescription of lenses often is possible. Even in older persons who are not driving motor vehicles, diminished visual acuity is often ignored, and correction may even be refused by the patient.

In cases of anisometropia, however, especially in children, where there is danger that amblyopia will develop due to lack of use of one eye (amblyopia ex anopsia), the prescription of lenses and even an occlusive patch to force the use of the amblyopic eye is frequently in order. In other instances, corrective lenses will influence muscle balance and may even help to prevent strabismus.

Partial or total relief of symptoms is a strong incentive for wearing corrective lenses. Experience, integrity, and insight will tell the examiner to refuse prescriptions for a small refractive error in the presence of unrelated symptoms. Many a patient has been made an "eye cripple" for life by corrective lenses prescribed with insufficient justification.

After a history of the presenting complaints is evaluated and the refraction is performed, the prescription of the proper lenses for that patient still embodies some of the "art of medicine," as it is impossible to write rules governing each case. The comfort of the patient is the final goal of the examiner.

CONTACT LENSES

Lenses which fit on the eyeball itself first became practicable in the early 1930's. They were first hand-blown, of glass, and later individually molded out of plastic. In 1947 the first of the plastic **corneal contact lenses** made their appearance. They are much smaller than the scleral lenses and very thin. The flow of tears over all surfaces provides the necessary lubricating fluid and plays an important role in refraction also.

In recent years corneal contact lenses have enjoyed a great increase in popularity since they now can be worn with comfort for longer periods. They must still be worn only intermittently, and should not be worn when infection or marked inflammation is present.

Corneal lenses are most often fitted at the patient's request for cosmetic purposes or because his activities (athletics, working in steamy or rainy atmospheres) make them convenient. The ophthalmologic indications are as follows: (1) corneal diseases in which correction of refractive error by spectacle lenses is unsatisfactory (eg, keratoconus) and (2) unilateral aphakia, where the greater discrepancy in image size which occurs with spectacle lenses interferes with binocular vision. The patient who elects to wear contact lenses should be intelligent, cooperative, and responsible, as more and more damaged eyes are being reported as a result of careless contact lens wear, usually in the presence of inflammation or infection.

"Soft" Contact Lens

The "soft" contact lens is a very porous plastic contact lens which is shaped much like the conventional "hard" contact lens but is more pliable and somewhat larger, measuring about 13 mm in diameter. Developed originally in Czechoslovakia in the early 1960's, it was available only for experimental purposes in the United States until early 1971. Primarily because of the danger of contamination and resultant corneal infection and because the lens has therapeutic value in some types of corneal disease, the lens has been declared a drug (and therefore subject to regulation by the FDA) rather than a device (as are the commonly used "hard" contact lenses, which are therefore not subject to FDA regulation).

The soft lens absorbs up to 40% of its dry weight when placed in normal saline solution. In its hydrated state, the lens is soft and pliable and acts as a refracting medium. The FDA has granted approval only for limited distribution of soft lenses, but wider distribution is anticipated soon. Early reports of the results of the use of soft lenses in the treatment of some cases of corneal disease, particularly bullous keratopathy, are quite favorable. Much more work is needed to determine how important the lenses may be in the treatment of a wide variety of corneal diseases.

For persons with normal corneas but significant refractive errors, the main advantage of the soft lens is comfort. One major concern has been the possibility of causing corneal infection, since no sterilizing solution has received FDA approval and the soft lenses must be boiled daily to assure sterility. Early reports indicate that many wearers have some "blur," especially if they have significant astigmatism. The durability of the lens under normal wearing conditions remains to be evaluated, but with anticipated technical improvements the soft contact lens will surely be of value optically as well as in corneal therapy.

Much research work is being done on the use of the soft lens as a means of delivering topical medications to the eye. Solutions such as pilocarpine and antibiotics can be placed in the lens at the time of hydration. Sustained release of the medication for many hours occurs when the lens is placed upon the eye.

• o •

Bibliography

Blair, H. L. , & T. G. Martens: Refraction and visual physiology. Annual review. Arch Ophth **71**:889-916, 1964.

Cowan, A.: Refraction of the Eye. Lea & Febiger, 1948.

Curtin, B. J.: Myopia: A review of its etiology, pathogenesis and treatment. Survey Ophth **15**:1-17, 1970.

Duke-Elder, S. , & D. Abrams: Ophthalmic Optics and Refraction. Mosby, 1970.

Raiford, M. B. (editor): Contact Lens Management. Internat Ophth Clinics. Little, Brown, 1961.

Rubin, M. L.: Optics and visual physiology. Annual review. Arch Ophth **75**:836-79, 1966.

Siegel, I. M.: Optics and visual physiology. Annual review. Arch Ophth **86**:100-12, 1971.

Sloane, A. E.: Manual of Refraction. Little, Brown, 1961.

21...
Preventive Ophthalmology

The most productive area of health care is that of prevention. Prevention of ocular disorders includes both elimination of hazards to the eyes (eg, accident prevention, sterility of ophthalmic solutions) and recognition of disease states at a time when improvement, containment, or cure can be achieved with proper management (eg, glaucoma).

The responsibility for effective prevention often rests with nonspecialists. If all practicing physicians were alert to the special problems of preventive ophthalmology, many cases of visual impairment due to injury, glaucoma, strabismus, infection, etc could be prevented. It is indeed a tragedy to find hitherto undetected advanced ocular disease in a patient who has been receiving regular medical treatment for another illness. Every physician should be aware of the disorders potentially leading to blindness so that he may take advantage of the opportunities for prevention by detection, proper management, and education of the patient.

GLAUCOMA

Approximately 2% of all persons over 35 have glaucoma. In the USA alone it is estimated that there are 1 million people with undetected glaucoma. About 90% of these people have chronic open-angle glaucoma, which does not cause symptoms in the early stages but can ultimately lead to blindness. Patients do not seek treatment until late in the disease because there is no pain and the visual acuity (central vision) remains good as the peripheral field is constricting.

The best means of detecting glaucoma is routine tonometric examination every 3 years on all persons over 20 (or every year if there is a family history of glaucoma). The next most important diagnostic steps are the visual field examination and the ophthalmoscopic examination for pathologic cupping of the optic disk. The visual field examination is normally done on the tangent screen. A confrontation field testing using the examiner's fingers as a target will pick up only gross visual field defects.

In recent years many glaucoma surveys have been carried out in various parts of the world. Their chief value is case-finding. Tonometry should be a part of every physical examination in the age group over 20. This can be accomplished by teaching tonometry to medical students, general practitioners, internists, and other interested physicians. It would also be worthwhile to establish permanent glaucoma detection centers. These could be established as single units or as parts of multiphasic disease detection centers.

AMBLYOPIA EX ANOPSIA
("Lazy Eye")

Amblyopia ex anopsia can be defined for the purposes of this discussion as decreased visual acuity in one eye in the absence of organic eye disease. The function of vision develops from birth to age 7. If vision has not developed by age 7, there is no chance that it will develop later.

In the absence of eye disease the 2 main abnormalities that will prevent a child from learning to see are strabismus and anisometropia.

Strabismus: If a young child develops esotropia or exotropia, he will have double vision. He quickly learns to suppress the image in the deviating eye and therefore uses only the straight eye, and learns to see normally with this eye. Unfortunately, vision does not develop in an unused eye; unless the good eye is patched, thus forcing the child to use the deviating eye, sight never will develop in that eye and the child will grow up with one perfectly normal eye which is essentially blind since it has never developed a functional connection with the visual centers in the brain. This is more likely to occur with esotropia than with exotropia.

Anisometropia: Young children are more concerned with perception of near objects than with distance vision. If one eye is nearsighted (myopic) and the other farsighted (hyperopic), the child will favor the nearsighted eye. Small children are concerned primarily with near objects, and it takes no effort to focus the nearsighted eye whereas it does take effort to focus with the farsighted eye. Hence the farsighted eye will not be used even though it is straight. The result will be the same as in untreated strabismus, ie, monocular blindness due to failure of visual development in an unused eye. The incidence of anisometropia is about 0.75-1%.

The best way to prevent amblyopia is visual acuity testing of all preschool children. By the time a child reaches school, it is usually too late for occlusion therapy. The test can be done by the parents at home using the illiterate "E" chart. Pediatricians and others responsible for the care of small children should test visual acuity at age 4.

CORNEAL OR INTRAOCULAR INFECTION

The invasion of the cornea by microorganisms is barred effectively by the intact corneal epithelium. Once this barrier is broken, however, there is no defense and organisms may enter the cornea freely and cause infection. One very dangerous and opportunistic organism, which actually grows in the cornea better than in any other known medium, is Pseudomonas aeruginosa. This organism may be a contaminant of many commonly used eye solutions.

Any ophthalmic solution placed in an injured eye must be sterile. If a contaminated solution has been instilled into the eye, a serious infection will probably result and may destroy the cornea and ultimately the eye. For this reason physicians, nurses, and manufacturing or prescription pharmacists should exercise at least the same degree of care in compounding ophthalmic solutions for use in injured eyes as in preparing solutions for intravenous administration or for use in a surgical field.

In this discussion, "intact eye" will be used to mean one in which the corneal epithelium has not been damaged and "injured eye" one in which the corneal epithelium has been damaged. The use of sterile eye drops is desirable in the care of an intact eye, but in the case of an injured eye it is an absolute neces-

sity. Fortunately, the vast majority of liquid eye medications are used at home and in the physician's office in eyes whose corneal epithelium is intact. If contaminated drops are instilled into an intact eye, a conjunctivitis may result which can usually be brought under control; if they are instilled into an injured eye, serious infection can develop and the eye may even be lost. Therefore, 2 standards are recommended for the preparation and use of ophthalmic solutions: (1) For the intact eye, sterile solutions which may be packaged in multiple-dose containers. (2) For the injured eye, small single disposable units containing sterile solutions for single patient use.

Two procedures that will ensure sterility of multiple-dose containers are autoclaving and sterile filtration.

OPHTHALMIA NEONATORUM

In many parts of the world it is customary for an antimicrobial agent to be placed in the eyes of newborn babies. This procedure was originally designed for the prevention and treatment of gonococcal conjunctivitis, which, if allowed to progress, can cause corneal ulceration and blindness. For many years silver nitrate (1%) was the only solution used, and this is still the only method of prophylaxis approved by the FDA. If inadvertently used in strong solution (5-10%), silver nitrate can cause permanent corneal scarring and possibly blindness.

Penicillin and other antibiotics have been used in many hospitals. Penicillin is effective against Neisseria gonorrhoeae, does not cause sensitization in newborns (who have weak antibody responses), and does not cause a chemical conjunctivitis as silver nitrate often does. Most states have laws requiring the use of silver nitrate.

INTRAOCULAR FOREIGN BODIES

Intraocular foreign bodies still occur as industrial accidents. They usually happen when a worker is striking steel on steel and a piece of the hammer flies off at high speed and passes through the sclera or cornea into the eye. Prevention consists of properly fitted safety glasses.

SOLAR RETINITIS
(Eclipse Retinopathy)

Following each solar eclipse there are many instances of ocular injury resulting from direct observation of the sun without an adequate filter. The optical system of the eye behaves as a strong magnifying lens in focusing the light onto a small spot on the macula, usually in one eye only, producing a thermal burn. The localized edema of the retinal tissue which results may clear with minimal loss of function or may cause significant atrophy of the tissue and produce a defect which is visible ophthalmoscopically as a macular hole. In the latter case a permanent central scotoma will result.

Eclipse retinopathy is easily preventable if adequate filters are used in observing eclipses, but the safest way to do so is on television.

A similar type of self-inflicted macular defect has recently been reported as a result of sungazing by US Army recruits.

The damage which results from a focus of intense light upon the retina has been put to practical use in the photocoagulation treatment of minimal degrees of retinal detachment and in the prevention of retinal detachment.

XEROPHTHALMIA

Occasional cases of xerophthalmia still occur even in the USA, and the disease is quite common in areas where nutrition is apt to be poor (eg, India). Vitamin A deficiency disease may be due to deficient diet resulting from poor economic circumstances, chronic alcoholism, deprivation weight-reducing diets, dietary therapy of an allergic condition; or failure of absorption of vitamin A in the gastrointestinal tract (as in obstruction of bile ducts or the common duct, or in severe diarrhea). In prescribing dietary therapy for any disorder the physician must be careful to include vitamin A among the vitamin supplementation. The estimated daily requirement of vitamin A is 1500 to 5000 IU daily for infants and children and 5000 IU daily for adults. Large parenteral doses are used for treatment of the established process. Early recognition and treatment of vitamin A deficiency disease can prevent loss of sight due to corneal perforation or secondary infection.

VISUAL LOSS DUE TO DRUGS
AND OTHER IATROGENIC FACTORS

Differential Diagnosis of "Red Eye" (See inside front cover.)

In the local treatment of eye disease the patient with the "red eye" presents the most common diagnostic challenge. The majority of cases of ocular inflammation are due to conjunctivitis, which is usually self-limited; but if a diagnosis of conjunctivitis is not clear-cut one must consider iritis, glaucoma, and corneal ulcer—all of which are far more severe and a greater threat to vision than conjunctivitis. If the patient has iritis, the pupil must be dilated with a cycloplegic such as atropine or scopolamine. If the patient has glaucoma, cycloplegic agents may cause permanent blindness. Corneal ulcer must be treated promptly with specific antibiotics in order to prevent scarring.

Hazards of Prolonged Corticosteroid Therapy

It has been clearly demonstrated that long-term systemic corticosteroid therapy can cause chronic open-angle glaucoma and cataracts and can both provoke and worsen attacks of herpes simplex keratitis. Locally administered corticosteroids are much more potent in this respect and have the added disadvantage of causing fungal overgrowth if the corneal epithelium is not intact. For these reasons, corticosteroids in any form must be administered with discretion.

Hazards of Chloroquine

Chloroquine (Aralen®) given over a prolonged period, as in the treatment of discoid lupus erythematosus, involves an approximately 10% risk of partial visual loss. The corneal opacities caused by chloroquine disappear when the drug is discontinued, but macular edema and pigmentation are often irreversible. Patients requiring chloroquine on a chronic basis should be examined by an ophthalmologist every 4-6 months. Between examinations the patient should make a rough test of his own visual acuity once a week.

Hazards of Mydriatics

In dilating the pupils to facilitate observation of the lens and retina, the physician should estimate the depth of the anterior chamber. If the iris appears to be quite close to the cornea, it is best to leave the decision to dilate in the hands of the ophthalmologist. Acute angle-closure glaucoma can be produced in less than 30 minutes, and surgery is almost always required to relieve it. Surgery is usually but not always successful, and permanent and complete blindness may be the result.

22...
The Eye Examination
in Infants and Children

The immediate examination of the newborn infant consists of a brief observation of color, responses, extremities, and digits, and a quick inspection of body surfaces. The more complete examination is done in the nursery.

Because the development of the eye often reflects organ and tissue development of the body as a whole, many congenital somatic defects are mirrored in the eye. A careful eye examination soon after birth may suggest the need for further investigative procedures. Subjective response is limited to the following response to a moving light. The only instruments required for the ocular examination of the newborn are a good hand light, an ophthalmoscope, and a loupe if necessary for magnification.

External Inspection

The eyelids are inspected for growths, deformities, lid notches, and symmetric movement with opening and closing of the eyes. The absolute and relative size of the eyeballs is noted, as well as position and alignment. The size and luster of the corneas are noted, and the anterior chambers are examined for clarity and iris configuration. The size, position, and light reaction of the pupils are also noted.

Ophthalmoscopic Examination

With undilated pupils, some information can be obtained by use of the ophthalmoscope in a dimly lighted room. Ideally, however, all newborns should be examined with an ophthalmoscope through dilated pupils. Ophthalmoscopic examination will demonstrate any corneal, lens, or vitreous opacities as well as abnormalities in the fundus. Neonatal retinal hemorrhages are not uncommon, usually clearing completely within a few weeks and leaving no permanent visual dysfunction.

Pediatric Eye Examination Schedule

Hospital Nursery

External eye examination and ophthalmoscopic examination through dilated pupils as outlined in the text. Two drops of sterile 5% homatropine and 2.5% phenylephrine in each eye are instilled one hour prior to examination. Special emphasis should be placed on the optic disks and maculas; detailed examination of the peripheral retinas is not necessary.

Age 4

Visual acuity test with illiterate "E" chart to rule out amblyopia ex anopsia. Visual acuity is normal 20/20 to 20/30 by 4-5 years of age.

Ages 5-16

Test visual acuity at age 5. If normal, test visual acuity with the Snellen chart every 2 years until age 16. Color vision should be tested at age 8-12. No other routine eye examination (eg, ophthalmoscopy) is necessary if visual acuity is normal and the eyes appear normal upon inspection.

THE NORMAL EYE IN INFANTS AND CHILDREN

Eyeball

In the newborn, the eye is relatively larger in comparison with body size than in later life. However, the anteroposterior diameter, which determines the focusing of the eye, is relatively short (averaging about 17.3 mm). This would produce a marked hyperopia if it were not for the greater curvature of the lens at this time.

Cornea

The cornea of the newborn is also relatively large, and reaches adult size by about 2 years of age. It is flatter than the adult cornea, however, and the curvature is greater at the periphery than in the center, whereas the opposite is true in the adult.

Lens

At birth the lens is more globular than in adulthood, and its greater refractive power compensates for the shortness of the eye. The lens grows throughout life as new fibers are added to the periphery, and this causes it to flatten. The consistency of the lens material changes throughout life from a soft plastic-like material to the glassy consistency seen in old age. This accounts for the gradual loss in power of accommodation with advancing age.

Refractive State

About 80% of children are born hyperopic, 5% myopic, and 15% emmetropic. About 10% have refractive errors which require correction before age 7 or 8. Hyperopia remains relatively static or gradually diminishes until 19 or 20 years of age. After age 7-8, myopia often increases until about age 25, with the greatest change at the time of puberty. There is usually little change in refractive error during the 3rd and 4th decades. Much greater curvature of the lens is the rule in prematures, and leads to myopia (usually temporary).

Iris

At birth there is little or no pigment on the anterior surface of the iris. The posterior pigment layer shows through the translucent tissue, usually giving the effect of a bluish or slate-gray color. As the pigment begins to appear on the anterior surface, the iris assumes its definitive color. If considerable pigment is deposited, the eyes become brown. Less pigmentation results in blue, gray, hazel, or green eyes. It may take 1-2 years for the pigmentary deposits to occur; in the meantime it is impossible to ascertain the ultimate color of the eyes.

Pupil

In the newborn the pupil is situated slightly to the nasal side of and below the center of the cornea. Because of the refractive power of the cornea in the neonatal period, the pupil appears larger than it actually is. The apparent diameter varies between 2.5 and 5.5 mm and averages about 4 mm. In infancy the pupil is smaller than at birth. The pupillary reflexes appear at about the 5th fetal month and are active by the 6th month. At about age 1 the pupil begins to widen, and it reaches its greatest diameter during adolescence. It again becomes smaller in old age. Myopes have larger pupils than hyperopes.

Normal pupils are round and regular and their diameters are constantly changing. Anisocoria, a difference in the size of the 2 pupils, is often a normal finding; in the absence of neurologic abnormalities, it requires no further special diagnostic consideration.

Position

During the first 3 months of life, eye movements may be poorly coordinated and there may be some doubt about the straightness of the eyes. By 6 months of age, however, the binocular reflexes are well developed; any deviation noted after that time should be investigated.

Nasolacrimal System

The fetal development of the nasolacrimal passages begins as cords of cells which usually hollow out about the time of birth. Because there may normally be a few weeks' delay in duct formation, failure of tear production in the first few weeks does not necessarily indicate any difficulty; failure of the tear ducts to function by 3 months of age, however, demands attention.

Optic Nerve

The medullation of optic nerve fibers usually takes place soon after birth.

The Normal Ocular Fundus of Infants and Children

The ophthalmoscopic appearance of the normal fundus in an infant differs greatly from that of an adult. Most of the differences are due to the distribution of pigments.

In premature infants, remnants of the tunica vasculosa lentis are frequently visible with the ophthalmoscope, either in front of the lens, behind the lens, or in both positions. The remnants are usually absorbed by the time the infant has reached term, but rarely they remain permanently and appear as a complete or partial "cobweb" in the pupil. At other times remnants of the primitive hyaloid system fail to absorb completely, leaving a cone on the optic disk which projects into the vitreous and is called Bergmeister's papilla.

Physiologic cupping of the disk is usually not seen in premature infants and is rarely seen at term; if seen then, it is usually very slight. In such cases the optic disk will appear gray, resembling optic nerve atrophy. This relative pallor, however, gradually changes to the normal adult pink color at about 2 years of age.

The foveal light reflection is absent in infants. Instead, the macula has a bright "mother-of-pearl" appearance with a suggestion of elevation. This is more pronounced in Negro infants. At 3-4 months of age, the macula becomes slightly concave and the foveal light reflection appears.

The peripheral fundus in the infant is gray, in contrast to the orange-red fundus of the adult. In Caucasian infants the pigmentation is more pronounced near the posterior pole, and gradually fades to almost white at the periphery. In Negro infants there is more pigment in the fundus and a gray-blue sheen is seen throughout the periphery. In Caucasian infants a white periphery is normal and should not be confused with retinoblastoma. During the next several months pigment continues to be deposited in the retina, and usually at about 2 years of age the adult color is evident.

CONGENITAL EYE DEFECTS

Most congenital ocular defects are genetically determined. Examples include congenital ptosis, refractive errors, aniridia, strabismus, retinitis pigmentosa, and arachnodactyly (Marfan's syndrome). Absence of a positive family history is no proof that the defect is not in the germ plasm (see Chapter 19).

Other congenital defects may be caused by interference with the development of the embryo, such as the multiple defects associated with rubella infection of the mother during the first 3 months of pregnancy. In this instance the infant may suffer from any or all of the following: cataracts, heart disease, deafness, microcephaly, microphthalmos, and mental deficiency. Eye defects are common in cerebral palsy.

Anophthalmos

This is a rare condition in which one or both eyeballs are absent or rudimentary. There may be either a congenital absence of any ocular structure, or an arrest of development to the point where only histologic evidence is present. The eyelids are usually present. They are often adherent at the margins but can be separated. Anophthalmos is associated with a chromosomal variation (16-18 trisomy; see p 262).

Cyclopia

Cyclopia, which is a rare midline fusion of developing eye structures together with generalized anterior brain and skull defects, is usually not compatible with life since it is transmitted by a recessive lethal gene.

Microphthalmos

In microphthalmos, one or both eyes are markedly smaller than normal. Many other ocular abnormalities may be present also, eg, cataract, glaucoma, aniridia, and coloboma. Somatic abnormalities are also often present, eg, polydactyly, syndactyly, clubfoot, polycystic kidneys, cystic liver, cleft palate, and meningoencephalocele. Microphthalmos is nearly always genetically determined—most frequently as a recessive but occasionally as a dominant trait.

Corneal Defects

There may be partial or complete opacity of the corneas such as are found in congenital glaucoma, faulty development of the cornea with persistent corneal lens attachments, birth injuries, intrauterine inflammation, interstitial keratitis, and lipid infiltrations of the cornea as in lipochondrodystrophy (Hurler's syndrome). The most frequent cause of opaque corneas in infants and young children is congenital glaucoma. In most instances, the eye is larger than normal (macrophthalmos, hydrophthalmos, buphthalmos). Birth injuries may cause extensive corneal opacities with edema as a result of rupture of Descemet's membrane. These usually clear spontaneously.

Megalocornea is an enlarged cornea with normal function usually transmitted as a sex-linked recessive trait. It must be differentiated from infantile glaucoma. There are usually no associated defects.

Iris and Pupillary Defects

Misplaced or ectopic pupils are frequently observed. The usual displacement is upward and laterally (temporally) from the center of the cornea. Such displacement is occasionally associated with ectopic lens, congenital glaucoma, or microcornea. Multiple pupils are known as **polycoria**. A true pupil must constrict on exposure to light, indicating a sphincter muscle. Congenital miosis is due to a poorly developed dilator muscle. Little change in pupillary size is noted after instillation of a mydriatic. Congenital mydriasis is characterized by large and inactive pupils and underdeveloped sphincter muscles, and must be differentiated from mydriasis due to juvenile paresis and pineal tumor. **Coloboma of the iris** indicates incomplete closure of the fetal ocular cleft and usually occurs below and nasally. It may be associated with coloboma of the lens, choroid, and optic nerve. **Aniridia** (absence of the iris) is a rare abnormality, frequently associated with secondary glaucoma (see p 205), and due to an autosomal dominant hereditary pattern. Various abnormalities in the shape of the pupils have been described, but are not necessarily significant. Persistent mesodermal remnants usually appear as thread-like bands running across the central pupillary space and attached to the lesser circle of the iris. They rarely have clinical significance or interfere with visual acuity.

The color of the iris is determined largely by heredity. Abnormalities in color include **albinism** (see p 252), due to the absence of normal pigmentation of the ocular structures and frequently associated with poor visual acuity and nystagmus; and **heterochromia**, a difference in color in the 2 eyes which may be a primary developmental defect with no functional loss or may be secondary to an inflammatory process.

Lens Abnormalities

The lens abnormalities most frequently noted are cataracts, although there may be faulty development, forming colobomas, or subluxation, as seen in Marfan's syndrome.

Any lens opacity which is present at birth is a congenital cataract, regardless of whether or not it interferes with visual acuity. Congenital cataracts are often associated with other conditions. Maternal rubella during the first trimester of pregnancy is a common cause of congenital cataract. Other congenital cataracts have a hereditary background.

If the opacity is small enough so that it does not occlude the pupil, adequate visual acuity is attained by focusing around the opacity. If the pupillary opening is entirely occluded, however, normal sight does not develop, and the poor fixation may lead to nystagmus and amblyopia ex anopsia.

Choroid and Retina

Gross defects of the choroid and retina are visible with the ophthalmoscope. The choroidal structures may show congenital colobomas, usually in the lower nasal region, which may also include the iris and all or part of the optic nerve. Central posterior (macular) scarring is a pigmentary disturbance often caused by intrauterine toxoplasmosis. Other congenital lesions of the choroid and retina include drusen, aneurysms, optic nerve malformations, medullated nerve fibers, and hereditary macular degeneration.

DEVELOPMENTAL BODY DEFECTS ASSOCIATED WITH OCULAR DEFECTS

Albinism

Congenital deficiency of pigment may involve the entire body (complete albinism) or a part of the body (incomplete albinism). When incomplete albinism involves only the eye, the function may be normal or impaired. In complete ocular albinism, there is usually an abnormal development of the macula, a severe refractive error, nystagmus, and severe photophobia. The eyebrows and eyelashes are white, the conjunctivas are hyperemic, the irides are either gray or red, and the pupil appears red. Treatment consists of relieving photophobia by means of tinted glasses or opaque contact lenses in which only a small hole is left in the center.

Marfan's Syndrome

This is a congenital and familial disorder of mesodermal origin which is nearly always transmitted as an autosomal dominant trait. The major features are (1) long, thin, spiderlike fingers and toes (arachnodactyly), (2) generalized relaxation of ligaments, (3) generalized muscular underdevelopment, (4) bilateral dislocation of the lenses (ectopia lentis), (5) abnormalities of the heart and, occasionally, aortic aneurysm, (7) high-arched palate, and (8) other deformities of the sternum, thorax, and joints.

The lenses are usually dislocated and visual acuity suffers because the patient is not seeing through the center of his lenses. Dislocation is usually upward, and often is incomplete. Cataracts frequently develop in the subluxated lenses. Cataract surgery in these cases carries a guarded prognosis.

Osteogenesis Imperfecta

This rare affliction is characterized by increased fragility of the bones and laxity of the ligaments, with frequent fractures and dislocations; dental defects, deafness, and blue scleras. The blue color is darker in the anterior parts of the scleras over the ciliary bodies. It is thought to be due to abnormal thinness of the sclera, and remains unchanged throughout life. Cataracts, megalocornea, and keratoconus may also be present. It nearly always occurs as an autosomal dominant trait.

Lipochondrodystrophy (Gargoylism, Hurler's Syndrome)

This is a rare condition due to autosomal recessive inheritance in which there is infiltration of lipids into the tissues, especially the liver, spleen, lymph nodes, pituitary gland, and corneas. Other ocular signs include slight ptosis, larger thickened eyelids, and strabismus (esotropia). The corneas show a diffuse haziness, which progresses to a milk-white opacity. Glaucoma may eventually develop. There is no satisfactory treatment.

Oxycephaly (Acrocephaly, Tower Skull, Steeple Head)

This deformity is evident at birth, but is often attributed to normal distortion during delivery and is seldom diagnosed at the time of delivery. It is characterized by a high, dome-shaped or pointed skull, high forehead, bulging temporal fossae, flattened cheekbones, shallow orbits, a high, narrow palatal arch, and synostosis of the cranial sutures. Syndactyly may also be present. The ocular signs include exophthalmos (due to flatness of the orbits), wide separation of the eyes, and exotropia. Closure of the eyelids may be difficult or impossible. Loss of vision may follow increased intracranial pressure. Nystagmus is common. Various operative procedures have been devised for the relief of intracranial pressure. If vision is to be preserved, surgery must be performed before optic atrophy has progressed. The syndrome is due to an autosomal dominant gene of weak penetrance.

Acrobrachycephaly

In this abnormality the head is wide, whereas in oxycephaly it is narrow. Acrobrachycephaly is caused by premature closure of the coronal sutures. Growth occurs only laterally and vertically, and the anteroposterior diameter is short. The ocular signs are similar to those of oxycephaly.

Other abnormalities involving skull development are scaphocephaly (increased anteroposterior diameter due to premature closure of the sagittal suture) and plagiocephaly (asymmetric flattening, usually due to premature closure of a single coronal suture).

Craniofacial Dysostosis (Crouzon's Disease)

This rare hereditary deformity, due to an autosomal dominant gene, is characterized by exophthalmos, atrophy of the maxilla, enlargement of the nasal bones, abnormal increase in the space between the eyes (ocular hypertelorism), optic atrophy, and bony abnormalities of the region of the perilongitudinal sinus. The palpebral fissures slant downward (in contrast to the upward slant of mongolism). Strabismus and nystagmus are also present.

Laurence-Moon-Biedl Syndrome

This syndrome includes retinitis pigmentosa, polydactyly, obesity, hypogenitalism, and mental retardation.

POSTNATAL PROBLEMS

The commonest ocular disorders of children are external infections of the conjunctivas and eyelids (bacterial conjunctivitis, sties, blepharitis), strabismus, ocular foreign bodies, allergic reactions of the conjunctivas and the eyelids, refractive errors (particularly myopia), and, to a lesser extent, the congenital eye disorders. Since it is more difficult to elicit an accurate history of causative factors and subjective complaints in children, it is not uncommon to overlook significant ocular disorders (especially in very young children). Aside from the altered frequency of occurrence of the types of ocular disorders, the etiology, manifestations, and treatment of eye disorders are about the same for children as for adults. Certain special problems encountered more frequently in infants and children are discussed below.

Ophthalmia Neonatorum (Conjunctivitis of the Newborn)

Conjunctivitis in the newborn may be of chemical, bacterial, or viral origin. Differentiation is usually made according to time of onset and by appropriate smears and cultures. Chemical conjunctivitis caused by the silver nitrate drops instilled into the conjunctival sac at birth is the most common form. Inflammation is greatest during the first or second day of life. Bacterial conjunctivitis is usually of staphylococcal, pneumococcal, or gonococcal origin, the latter being the most serious because of potential corneal damage. The onset of bacterial conjunctivitis is between the 2nd and 5th days of life; the diagnosis is confirmed by bacteriologic smear and culture. Inclusion blennorrhea has its onset between the 5th and 10th days. The presence of typical inclusion bodies in the epithelial cells confirms this diagnosis.

Silver nitrate conjunctivitis is usually self-limited, but is improved by the use of topical steroids and antibacterials to prevent secondary infection. Bacterial conjunctivitis requires instillation of antibacterial agents such as sodium sulfacetamide, bacitracin, or tetracycline ointment for several days. Treatment should be instituted without waiting for the results of the culture. Inclusion blennorrhea is treated with sulfonamide drops or ointments or a broad-spectrum antibiotic.

Silver nitrate solution (1%) should be used in sealed, single use, disposable containers. Some institutions advocate the use of antibiotic ophthalmic preparations in place of silver nitrate. Prenatal diagnosis and treatment of maternal gonorrhea will prevent many cases of neonatal gonococcal conjunctivitis; however, prophylactic medication of the newborn must not be neglected. Prevention of inclusion blennorrhea is difficult since it is carried in the mother's genitourinary tract. Instillation of silver nitrate or an antibiotic (usually penicillin) is required by the law in most states.

Retrolental Fibroplasia

This condition, seen as a white retrolental membrane in the pupillary opening, was until quite recently a frequent cause of blindness in infants weighing less than 4 lb. It occurred as a result of high oxygen concentrations in incubators. Recently revised recommendations for the administration of oxygen to premature newborns are summarized on p 113.

Congenital Glaucoma

Congenital glaucoma may occur alone or in association with many other congenital lesions. It is important to recognize this disorder early, as untreated glaucoma results in permanent blindness. It is often bilateral. Early signs are corneal haze or opacity, increased corneal diameter, a deep anterior chamber, and ill-defined discomfort. Since the outer coats of the eyeball are not as rigid in the child, the increased intraocular pressure expands the corneal and scleral tissues. Useful vision may be preserved by early diagnosis and medical and surgical treatment by an ophthalmologist.

Pseudoglioma

Parents will occasionally see a white spot through the infant's pupil (pseudoglioma). Although retinoblastoma (a glioma) must be ruled out, the opacity is more often due to cataract, retrolental fibroplasia, persistence of the tunica vasculosa lentis, or corneal scarring.

Retinoblastoma (Glioma of the Retina)

This rare malignant tumor of childhood is fatal if untreated. Two-thirds of cases occur before the end of the third year; rarely, cases have been reported up to 7 and 10 years of age. In about 30% of cases, retinoblastoma is bilateral. The tumor results from mutation of an autosomal dominant gene which is passed with fairly high penetrance. Children of survivors therefore have a nearly 50% chance of having retinoblastoma. It is more apt to be bilateral in succeeding generations. Parents who have produced one child with retinoblastoma run a 4-7% risk of producing the disease in each subsequently born child. Retinoblastoma is usually not discovered until it has advanced far enough to produce an opaque pupil. Infants and children with presenting symptoms of strabismus should be examined carefully to rule out retinoblastoma, since a deviating eye may be the first sign of the tumor.

Enucleation is the treatment of choice in all unilateral cases. Recent advances in treatment for the second eye in bilateral cases are outlined on p 222.

Strabismus

Strabismus is present in about 5% of children. Its early recognition is the responsibility of the pediatrician or the family physician. Systemic factors causing strabismus such as physical exhaustion, neuromuscular disorders, and hypoglycemia should be considered. Treatment of strabismus is best started at the age of 6 months to ensure development of the best possible visual acuity and a good cosmetic and functional result (binocular vision). The idea that a child may outgrow crossed eyes should be discouraged. Neglect in the treatment of strabismus may lead to undesirable cosmetic effects, psychic trauma, and permanent impairment of vision (see below) in the deviating eye. Strabismus is covered in depth in Chapter 14.

Amblyopia ex Anopsia (Lazy Eye)

Amblyopia ex anopsia is decreased visual acuity of one eye (uncorrectable with lenses) in the absence of organic eye disease. The 2 most common causes are uncorrected strabismus and anisometropia.

In uncorrected strabismus, the image from the deviated eye is suppressed (in order to prevent diplopia). If treatment is not instituted well before cessation of the visual maturing process (ie, before age 5 or 6), good vision cannot develop in the deviating eye. A similar situation exists when there is a great difference in refractive power of the 2 eyes (anisometropia). Even though the eyes may be correctly aligned, they are unable to focus together and the image of one eye is suppressed. If corrective measures are not instituted before the age of 5 or 6, amblyopia ex anopsia will result.

Early suspicion and prompt referral for treatment of the underlying condition are important in preventing amblyopia ex anopsia.

•   •   •

TESTS FOR VISUAL ACUITY

In the early years, visual acuity should be appraised as part of each general "well child" examination. It is best not to wait until the child is old enough to respond to visual charts, since these may not furnish accurate information until school age. Estimations of vision should be made in the first few days by ascertaining the pupillary responses to light, which rules out complete dysfunction of the eyes. In later weeks, light fixation reflexes can be elicited—single and bilateral reflexes first, and then binocular following and converging reflexes. A good response consists of prompt fixation and following reflexes, equal in each eye, with the light reflex centered in the pupil when the source is near the examiner's eyes. During the growing years, the parents' observations of the child's clumsiness, his awareness of his surroundings, and his apparent sharpness of vision are valuable aids. From about age 4 on, it becomes possible to elicit subjective responses by use of the illiterate "E" chart. Usually, at the first or second grade level, the regular Snellen chart may be employed.

The number of cases of amblyopia ex anopsia due to strabismus or anisometropia can be greatly decreased by the alert pediatrician or general physician who tests visual acuity at age 4. The mother's help can be solicited; she can be given an ''E'' card and asked to do the test at home and phone or mail the results to the doctor's office. The mother can often do a better job of this test than a nurse or even a physician because she has more time and a paramount interest in the child's health.

Development of Visual Acuity (Approximate)

Age	Visual Acuity
2 months	20/400
6 months	20/200
1 year	20/100
2 years	20/60
3 years	20/30
4-5 years	20/20

Appendix

COMMONLY USED EYE MEDICATIONS

LOCAL ANESTHETICS

Proparacaine hydrochloride (Ophthaine®, Ophthetic®), 0.5%, and benoxinate hydrochloride (Dorsacaine®), 0.4%, are effective local topical anesthetics. They have a rapid onset and short duration of action.

Tetracaine hydrochloride (Pontocaine®), 0.5%, is as effective as proparacaine and benoxinate but causes more allergic reactions.

Cocaine hydrochloride, 2-10%, produces a more profound corneal anesthesia than tetracaine. Cocaine should be used sparingly; when administered in excessive amounts it may act as a CNS stimulant and may even cause cardiovascular collapse.

Procaine hydrochloride, 1 and 2%, is commonly used locally by injection for eye surgery, including removal of chalazions and pterygiums as well as cataracts. Its duration of action is about 45 minutes.

Lidocaine hydrochloride (Xylocaine®), 1 and 2%, has a more rapid onset than procaine and the effect lasts longer.

PARASYMPATHOMIMETIC DRUGS

The parasympathomimetic drugs are used as miotics for controlling the intraocular pressure in glaucoma. They are divided into 2 groups: (1) those acting directly on the myoneural junction, and (2) cholinesterase inhibitors.

Group I (Pilocarpine and Carbachol)
The action of these drugs can be reversed with sympathomimetic agents.

Pilocarpine hydrochloride, 0.5-6%, is the most commonly used miotic and is the drug of choice in most cases of glaucoma. Its duration of action is 4-6 hours.

Carbachol (Doryl®), 1.5-3%, is poorly absorbed through the cornea and so is used only if pilocarpine is ineffective. Its duration of action is 4-6 hours. If benzalkonium chloride is used as the vehicle, the penetration of carbachol is significantly increased.

Group II (Physostigmine and Isoflurophate)
The action of these drugs is difficult to reverse.

Physostigmine salicylate (eserine), 0.25 and 0.5%, has a duration of action of about 6-8 hours. Because of its allergenic nature, in-stability, and shorter duration of action, physostigmine is gradually being replaced by the longer acting anticholinesterase drugs.

Isoflurophate (Floropryl®), 0.1% solution, is a powerful, long-acting (24 hours), oil-soluble miotic which was developed for use as a poisonous gas. Echothiophate iodide (Phospholine Iodide®), 0.03-0.25% solution, is a long-acting drug similar to isoflurophate which has the advantages of being water-soluble and causing less local irritation.

PARASYMPATHOLYTIC DRUGS

The parasympatholytic drugs are used as mydriatics and cycloplegics to facilitate ophthalmoscopic examination and refraction in young people.

Cycloplegics
The dose in each case depends upon the disorder being treated.

Homatropine hydrobromide, 2 and 5%, is used for refraction. Its duration of action is about 36 hours. Allergic reactions are rare.

Scopolamine hydrobromide (hyoscine), 0.2%, is used in the treatment of uveitis and in refraction of children. Its duration of action is 48-72 hours. Because of the low incidence of allergic reactions to scopolamine, this drug is often used in preference to atropine. Scopolamine occasionally causes dizziness and disorientation, mainly in older people.

Atropine sulfate, 0.5, 1, and 2%, is the most powerful drug in this group and has a duration of action of 10-14 days. It is used mainly in the treatment of uveitis and as a cycloplegic in refraction of young children. About 5% of the population are sensitive to atropine.

Cyclopentolate hydrochloride (Cyclogyl®), 0.5 and 1%, produces cycloplegia almost as profound as can be achieved with homatropine. Its shorter duration of action (less than 24 hours) is an advantage in cycloplegic refractions. Tropicamide (Mydriacyl®) is a short-acting (6 hours) cycloplegic whose action is similar to that of cyclopentolate.

SYMPATHOMIMETIC DRUGS

The sympathomimetic drugs are used primarily for mydriasis and as vasoconstrictors. Epinephrine is used as an anti-glaucoma agent. These drugs do not cause cycloplegia.

Phenylephrine hydrochloride (Neo-Synephrine®), 2.5 and 10%, acts for about 3 hours.

Hydroxyamphetamine hydrobromide ophthalmic solution (Paredrine®), 1%, has the same action and use as phenylephrine.

Epinephrine is widely used to lower intraocular pressure in open-angle glaucoma. It acts primarily by inhibiting aqueous production and secondarily by increasing aqueous outflow. It is also added to injectable local anesthetics because its vasoconstrictor effect decreases absorption of the anesthetic into the blood stream and so prolongs the action of the anesthetic.

DYES

Dyes are used for corneal staining to detect superficial corneal disorders.

Fluorescein sodium ophthalmic solution: Because Pseudomonas aeruginosa, a dangerous organism highly pathogenic for corneal tissues, grows well in fluorescein solutions, this dye is best used in the form of **sterile** fluorescein papers or **sterile** fluorescein solution (2%).

Merbromin (Mercurochrome®), 2%, does not stain the cornea as well as fluorescein but is less likely to become contaminated.

Rose bengal, 1%, is more effective than fluorescein in staining the mucous shreds seen in keratoconjunctivitis sicca.

IRRIGATING SOLUTIONS

An irrigating solution used in an injured eye must be sterile and for single patient use. It is permissible to use a sterile, nonirritating irrigating solution on more than one patient if the corneal epithelium and sclera are intact.

ANTIBIOTICS

Those antibiotics commonly used locally in the eye are discussed below. Systemic use may sometimes be necessary, eg, methicillin (Staphcillin®) for the treatment of infection by penicillinase-producing staphylococci or other antibiotics for intraocular infections. Of the antibiotics used systemically for intraocular infections, **chloramphenicol** (Chloromycetin®) affords the highest concentration in ocular tissues.

Neomycin sulfate (Mycifradin®) is effective against gram-negative or gram-positive organisms. A distinct advantage of neomycin over many antibiotics is that its severe nephrotoxic and neurotoxic properties have limited its systemic use; there is therefore little chance that the "priming dose" which may result from topical administration in the eye will form the basis of a sensitivity reaction upon subsequent systemic administration. Neomycin is usually combined with some other drug to widen its spectrum of activity. It is best known ophthalmologically as Neosporin®, both in ointment and solution form, in which it is combined with polymyxin and bacitracin. The frequency of application depends upon the severity of the infection. Its allergenic nature is a distinct disadvantage.

Chloramphenicol (Chloromycetin®) also has a wide range of activity against both gram-negative and gram-positive organisms. Its only disadvantage lies in the danger that local ocular use may sensitize the patient so that later systemic use would be dangerous. When used systemically this drug is said to penetrate the eye to a greater degree than most other antibiotics; for this reason it is used in high doses in intraocular infections. The rare chance of its producing aplastic anemia must be kept in mind, and frequent blood studies, including reticulocyte counts, are indicated as long as the patient is taking the drug.

Polymyxin B sulfate (Aerosporin®) is primarily effective against gram-negative microorganisms; it is not effective against gram-positive organisms. (The colicins [Coly-Mycin®] are an almost identical group of drugs.) Because polymyxin is clearly the most effective agent available against Pseudomonas aeruginosa, it is usually reserved for use in infections caused by this organism. It is applied topically in both the ointment and solution form and subconjunctivally in solution form. Polymyxin is also marketed as polymyxin E, but the 2 forms are similar enough in structure and clinical action to be considered identical. Because of its nephrotoxic effect it is rarely used systemically.

Gentamicin sulfate (Garamycin®), 0-3%, is also effective against both gram-negative and gram-positive organisms and so is a welcome new ocular antibiotic. It penetrates the cornea poorly and so will be most useful in the treatment of conjunctivitis and corneal ulceration.

Penicillin: In ophthalmology, local penicillin is sometimes used in newborns for prevention of ophthalmia neonatroum (but see p 280). It is used in ointment form, 100,000 units/gm once only at birth. Penicillin is used systemically in high doses (20 million units or more per 24 hours) in cases of intraocular infection, often in combination with chloramphenicol or gentamicin. Potassium penicillin G is usually used. For penicillinase producing organisms, sodium methicillin (Staphcillin®) or one of the other penicillinase resistant penicillins is recommended.

Bacitracin has a nephrotoxic factor when used systemically and is a good penicillin substitute for local use in the eye against gram-positive organisms. It is supplied as an ointment, 1000 units/gm, and in solutions containing 250 units/ml.

Erythromycin, 1%, is an effective penicillin substitute which finds its most important use against resistant staphylococcal organisms.

Streptomycin sulfate, 2.5-5%, is still used locally and systemically in gram-negative infections. In treating Pseudomonas infections, streptomycin is often combined with polymyxin.

Tetracycline (many brand names), **oxytetracycline** (Terramycin®), and **chlortetracycline** (Aureomycin®) have limited uses in ophthalmology because their effectiveness is so often impaired by the development of resistant strains. Solutions of these compounds are unstable with the exception of Achromycin® in sesame oil, widely used in the treatment of trachoma.

Nystatin (Mycostatin®), 100,000 units/gm, is not available in ophthalmic ointment form, but the dermatologic preparation is not irritating to ocular tissues and can be used with good results in the treatment of fungal infection of the eye. **Amphotericin B** (Fungizone®) is more effective than nystatin but is not available in ophthalmic ointment form and the dermatologic preparation is highly irritating. A solution (0.015%) must be made up in the pharmacy from the powdered drug.

SULFONAMIDES

The sulfonamides are the most commonly used drugs in the treatment of conjunctivitis. Their advantages include (1) activity against both gram-positive and gram-negative organisms, (2) relatively low cost, (3) low allergenicity, (4) minimal systemic use, and (5) the fact that they are not complicated by secondary fungus infections, as antibiotics sometimes are following prolonged use.

The commonest sulfonamides employed are **sulfisoxazole** (Gantrisin®), 4% ointment and solution, and **sulfacetamide sodium** (Sodium Sulamyd®), 10% ointment and solution.

ADRENAL CORTICOSTEROIDS

The adrenal corticosteroids are effective in treating inflammatory conditions of the eye, particularly those caused by uveitis, episcleritis, pingueculitis, and chemical burns. They are also valuable in decreasing vascularization and scarring following chemical burns, trauma, and severe inflammation. They are usually used 4-5 times daily in the affected eye in the form of a suspension or ointment.

Caution: The steroids enhance the activity of the herpes simplex virus, as shown by the fact that perforation of the cornea occasionally occurs when they are used in the eye for treatment of herpes simplex keratitis. Corneal perforation was an extremely rare complication of herpes simplex keratitis before the steroids came into general use. Other side effects of local steroid therapy are fungal overgrowth, cataract formation (unusual), and open-angle glaucoma (common). These effects are produced to a lesser degree with systemic steroid therapy. Any patient receiving local ocular corticosteroid therapy or long-term systemic corticosteroid therapy should be under the care of an ophthalmologist.

Cortisone acetate, 0.5-2.5% suspension and 1.5% ointment, is the least expensive of the corticosteroids and has sufficient clinical effectiveness in the great majority of cases.

Hydrocortisone, 0.5-2.5% suspension and 1.5% ointment, can be used in a lower concentration than cortisone because of its greater potency.

Prednisone, prednisolone, dexamethasone, and **betamethasone** are much more potent than hydrocortisone.

Fludrocortisone acetate (Florinef®, Alflorone®, F-Cortef®), 0.1%, has at least as much anti-inflammatory effect as hydrocortisone, prednisone, and prednisolone.

Medrysone®, 1%, is a new synthetic corticosteroid which gives promise of causing fewer side effects than other agents.

CARBONIC ANHYDRASE INHIBITORS

Acetazolamide (Diamox®) is a sulfonamide that was developed as a diuretic but is now used mainly to decrease the production of aqueous by the ciliary body in open-angle glaucoma. Carbonic anhydrase is an enzyme which is present in many body tissues. In the ciliary body it is directly concerned with the production of aqueous. When carbonic anhydrase is inhibited (eg, by acetazolamide), the amount of aqueous produced is decreased and the intraocular pressure is thus lowered.

Acetazolamide is used in selected cases of chronic and secondary glaucoma (and for preoperative preparation in primary acute glaucoma) which cannot be controlled by miotics alone. The dose is 5-10 mg/kg body weight every 4-6 hours. Acetazolamide is an extremely valuable drug but it does have many undesirable side effects. These include gastric distress, diarrhea, exfoliative dermatitis, kidney stones, shortness of breath, fatigue, acidosis, and tingling of the extremities. For this reason acetazolamide must be prescribed cautiously and used only in selected cases.

Other carbonic anhydrase inhibitors are dichlorphenamide (Daranide®, Oratrol®), ethoxzolamide (Cardrase®, Ethamide®), and methazolamide (Neptazane®)(has not been reported to cause kidney stones).

OPHTHALMIC PREPARATIONS AND EQUIPMENT

For the Physician's Bag
(1) Sterile topical anesthetic solution.
(2) Sterile fluorescein papers.
(3) Sulfacetamide sodium (Sodium Sulamyd®), 10% ointment or solution, or sulfisoxazole (Gantrisin®), 4% ointment, for treatment of bacterial conjunctivitis.
(4) Hand flashlight.
(5) Ophthalmoscope.
(6) Sterile irrigating solution.
(7) Sterile cotton applicators.
(8) Sterile spud for removal of corneal foreign bodies.
(9) Loupe or magnifying glasses.
(10) Tonometer.

For the Physician's Office
(1) All the above.
(2) Phenylephrine (Neo-Synephrine®), 2.5% solution, for mydriasis.
(3) Pilocarpine, 1%, for constricting pupils after mydriasis with phenylephrine.

VISUAL STANDARDS

INDUSTRIAL VISUAL EVALUATION*

The following mathematical calculation of loss of visual efficiency is used for legal and

*Modified and reproduced, with permission, from Arch Indust H **12**:439-49, 1955. For further explanation of the reasons behind the statistics and a legal discussion, see Spaeth, E.B., in Tr Am Acad Ophth **61**:592-601, 1957.

industrial cases, particularly in determination of compensation for injury.

Calculation of total visual efficiency is based on 3 factors of equal importance: percentage loss of central visual acuity, percentage loss of visual field, and percentage loss of coordinated ocular movements. Percentage loss of visual acuity in one eye does not represent the individual's total disability; even a total loss of one eye would not represent a 50% disability if the remaining eye were normal. Many people lead normal lives with one eye.

For evaluation of industrial visual efficiency, therefore, 3 visual functions are measured and mathematically coordinated: (1) visual acuity, (2) visual field, and (3) ocular motility (diplopia field, binocular field).

Visual Acuity
Distance and near vision are weighted evenly.

AMA Method of Estimation of Percentage Visual Loss (Using Best Correcting Spectacle Lens)

Distance (Snellen)	
Distance Visual Acuity	% Loss
20/20	0
20/25	5
20/40	15
20/50	25
20/80	40
20/100	50
20/160	70
20/200	80
20/400	90

Near	
Jaeger Test Type	% Loss
1	0
2	0
3	10
6	50
7	60
11	85
14	95

For purposes of calculating total visual acuity loss, near visual acuity is equally as important as distance acuity.

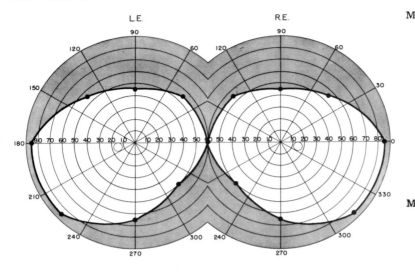

Minimal Normal Field:
Temporally	– 85°
Down and temporally	– 85°
Down	– 65°
Down and nasally	– 50°
Nasally	– 60°
Up and nasally	– 55°
Up	– 45°
Up and temporally	– 55°
Full field =	500°

Minimum Legal Visual Field

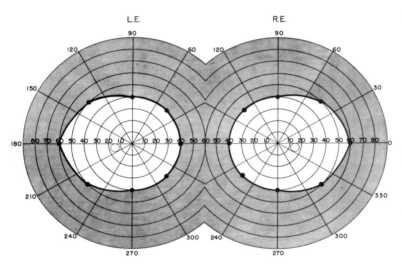

Moderate Loss of Field:
Temporally	– 60°
Down and temporally	– 50°
Down	– 40°
Down and nasally	– 40°
Nasally	– 40°
Up and nasally	– 40°
Up	– 40°
Up and temporally	– 50°
	360°

$$\frac{360 \times 100}{500} = 72\% \text{ field re-}$$
maining, or
28% field loss

Twenty-eight Percent Loss

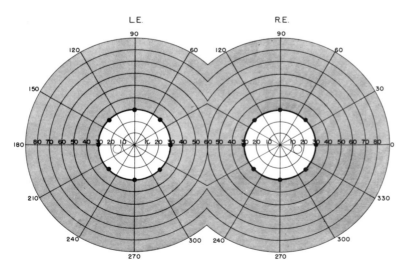

Severe Loss of Field:
Temporally	– 30°
Down and temporally	– 30°
Down	– 30°
Down and nasally	– 30°
Nasally	– 30°
Up and nasally	– 30°
Up	– 30°
Up and temporally	– 30°
	240°

$$\frac{240 \times 100}{500} = 48\% \text{ field re-}$$
maining, or
52% field loss

Fifty-two Percent Loss

Example: If the distance acuity is 20/80 and the subject can read Jaeger 6—

$$\frac{40 + 50}{2} = 45\% \text{ visual acuity loss, or } 55\%$$

visual acuity efficiency.

Visual Field

A white test object, 0.5°, is used in 8 meridians as diagrammed on p 294. This can be done with a 3 mm object at $1/3$ meter, using a perimeter. A full field represents 100% function. (Illumination should be at least 7 foot-candles.)

Ocular Motility

The extent of diplopia in the various directions of gaze is best determined using a tangent screen at 1 meter. A small test light is used and diplopia plotted along the 3 meridians above the horizontal 10, 20, and 30° from fixation. Diplopia fields are also plotted on the horizontal meridians and the 3 meridians below, 10, 20, 30, and 40° from the straight-ahead position. Diplopia within the central 20° represents 100% loss of motility efficiency of one eye since this condition usually requires patching one eye. If diplopia is not present in the central 20°, loss of ocular motility is calculated from a field diagram showing percentage loss. This value is then subtracted from 100 and expressed as ''80% motility efficiency,'' etc.

The inferior fields are weighted heavily since this is the position of the eyes in reading. Diplopia away from fixations in other quadrants is considered much less important.

Visual Efficiency (VE) of One Eye

The percentages of efficiency for the 3 measurements are multiplied to give the total visual efficiency.

Example: Visual acuity = 73%
Visual field = 57%
Motility   = 90%

$0.73 \times 0.57 \times 0.90 = 37\%$ VE or 63% loss.

Visual Efficiency (VE) of 2 Eyes

The 2 eyes are calculated separately and the better eye is weighted 3 times and the poorer eye once. Thus one blind eye and one normal eye gives 75% visual efficiency.

VISUAL STANDARDS FOR THE ARMED FORCES*

The visual acuity requirements outlined below apply for all branches of the services. For aircraft pilots and service academy candidates, the requirements are much more rigid.

Standards for Disqualification

Any strabismus of over 20° deviation is disqualifying, as is the presence of diplopia. Any active or progressive disease of the eyes is disqualifying even though the minimal visual standards can be met.

Minimal Standards for Officer Personnel

Officer candidates must have uncorrected visual acuity of 20/200 each eye, correctable to 20/20 in the better eye and 20/40 in the poorer eye. The maximal allowable hyperopia is +5.00 sphere. The maximal allowable myopia is −3.00 sphere.

In special branches of service such as the Adjutant General's Office, the Nurse, Medical, and Dental Corps, and in transportation, these standards are more liberal (20/400 in each eye correctable to 20/20 in the better eye and 20/40 in the poorer eye).

Minimal Standards for Enlisted Personnel

Enlisted personnel must have at least 20/400 visual acuity in each eye, correctable to 20/40 in the better eye and 20/70 in the poorer eye, 20/30 in the better eye and 20/100 in the poorer eye, or one blind eye and at least 20/100 in the other eye, correctable to 20/20.

VISUAL STANDARDS FOR DRIVERS' LICENSES IN THE USA

Most states have different visual standards for persons applying for drivers' licenses, and some have none. In general, no fixed limits are placed upon applicants although the failure to meet certain minimum standards may result in suspension of driving privileges until a cer-

*Subject to change. Local recruiting offices are supplied with the latest data.

$$\frac{3 \times (\% \text{ VE better eye}) + \% \text{ VE in worse eye}}{4} = \text{binocular VE (\%)}$$

Example: RE = 90%; LE = 30%.

$$\frac{3 \times 90 + 30}{4} = 75\% \text{ binocular VE.}$$

tification is obtained from an ophthalmologist or optometrist.

The 1967 Survey of State Requirements for Motor Vehicle Operators is a convenient summary of the requirements. It is published and distributed by the American Optical Co.

EDUCATIONAL VISUAL STANDARDS IN THE USA

Twelve percent of the pupils in elementary schools have significant eye difficulty. One in 100 to one in 1000 (statistics vary) requires special educational facilities because of severe visual deficiencies. Although a medical examination is mandatory for school children in 21 states, ophthalmologic examinations are seldom included. It has therefore been found necessary to devise procedures by which it will be possible, without a highly specialized staff, to give preliminary screening tests.

The Snellen test is the single most important test. Visual acuity tests may be given by nurses, parents, or trained volunteer teachers. Visual acuity testing of preschool children is far more important than visual acuity testing of school age children.

Even if a child has a significant visual handicap, it is best if he tries regular school. If he cannot keep up with regular school work, special "sight-saving" classes are necessary.

Education of Visually Handicapped Children

Education must be provided for partially seeing pupils at all school levels. (For educational purposes, a partially seeing child is one who has a corrected visual acuity of 20/70 or less in the better eye.) Experience indicates that it is best to establish the first class on an elementary school level, since the earlier help is given the better will be the prospect of success. In communities in which the school population is too small to warrant the establishment of more than one class, it may be advisable to give the advantages of the special class to children above the second grade, since much less close eye work is required in the first and second grades and a great deal of material in large, clear print is available for younger children. In general, well motivated partially sighted children have good learning potential.

Education of Blind Children

Children with visual acuity correctable to 20/200 or less are ineligible for ordinary visual educational methods and must be entered either in special schools for the blind, where emphasis is placed upon learning by touch (Braille), or (preferably) in integrated schools where facilities are available for special training but where the child is not deprived of all contact with normal persons in his age group.

PRACTICAL FACTORS IN ILLUMINATION

The physical aspects of illumination discussed below are of practical interest to the physician who may be called upon to evaluate the adequacy of light sources in factories, shops, schoolrooms, and homes. Of principal interest is light intensity, which is conveniently measured in foot-candles. One foot-candle is the intensity of light falling upon 1 square foot of a surface located 1 foot from a point source of one international candle. Foot-candles can be measured directly with special light meters.

Proper illumination minimizes eyestrain and increases the speed and efficiency of reading. Poor lighting does not cause eye disease but increases eye fatigue. The most common error students make in adjusting their lighting arrangement is to place a desk lamp opposite to them on the desk. From this position the light is reflected into the reader's eyes, causing glare. For reading, the best light source is an incandescent or fluorescent lamp coming from above which produces a diffuse light with a minimum of glare and shadows. For writing, the light source should be so adjusted that the shadow of the arm and hand on the page is eliminated.

The most common sources of light are daylight, incandescent light, and fluorescent light. Daylight is an excellent light source but quite variable, and it is difficult to control its intensity. Incandescent lamps simulate daylight and provide a steady, diffuse flow of light. Ordinary fluorescent tubes operate on an alternating current which causes flickering, but it is possible to link 2 fluorescent tubes in a couple so adjusted that when one is on the up-phase the other is on the down-phase, thus eliminating the flicker.

Illumination Factors Affecting Visibility

A. Intensity: The amount of illumination is directly related to reading efficiency. A reader employing 5 foot-candles reads much slower and less efficiently than if he were to utilize a 30 foot-candle source. In practice the following minimum intensities are recommended (assuming that all undue reflections resulting in glare have been eliminated): Reading black print on white paper, 30-40 foot-candles; schoolrooms, 30-40 foot-candles at the desk and 40-50 foot-candles at the black-board; passageways, halls, and closets, 5 foot-candles; eye charts, 80-100 foot-candles; operating room illumination at the point of surgery, 100 foot-candles.

There is a close relationship between a person's age and the magnification and illumination he will require. For example, because they have great powers of accommodation, children can read small print in semidarkness by holding the page close to their eyes. (This does not hurt the child's eyes although it may bother the parents.) On the other hand, a 48-year-old, slightly far-sighted presbyope cannot read under ordinary illumination without magnifying glasses because he has lost his power of accommodation. He can read by putting in a stronger light bulb or by taking the printed material into sunlight. The presbyope also can improve his visual performance by holding printed matter farther away. ("I need longer arms.")

The basic requirement in illumination is to have enough light to see by. Once this is accomplished, the intensity of illumination and the magnification (eye glasses) can be adjusted to increase the efficiency of visual performance.

The intensity of light on an object is inversely proportionate to the square of the distance from the light source. Therefore, if a reading lamp 2 feet from the page is moved to a distance of 4 feet, there will be 4 times less light on the page.

B. Contrast: It is much easier to read black letters on a white page than black letters on a blue page. Eye fatigue is minimized when the surroundings are about 30-40% darker than the object being observed. Thus in watching a television screen it is best not to have a completely darkened room.

C. Diffuseness: Shadows and spotlight phenomena should be avoided. However, diffuseness is overdone by manufacturers of indirect lighting fixtures. Indirect "reading lamps" are usually inadequate because of the vastly decreased amount of illumination on the printed page. This can be demonstrated by observing the unwarranted amount of light cast on the ceiling by the average indirect reading lamp.

D. Age of Subject: Illumination requirements and age are closely related, as evidenced by the increased illumination required by the 45-year-old presbyope compared with his teen-age daughter. Although it is not recommended, children in the 7-16 age group can read adequately in semi-darkness, whereas the same person 30 years later may be able to read the telephone book only by "taking it to

the window." Conversely, many people in the 50-65 year range who require full correction for their presbyopia can still read fine print without glasses in sunlight.

In general, illumination should be sufficient to perform the task at hand efficiently and comfortably.

REHABILITATION OF THE VISUALLY HANDICAPPED AND SPECIAL SERVICES AVAILABLE TO THE BLIND

Although no completely reliable statistics are available, the most widely used estimates place the legally blind population of the USA at 2.14 per thousand (ie, approximately 500,000). Approximately 50,000 become legally blind annually, and many others have enough visual loss to constitute a serious employment problem.

Blindness does not necessarily imply helplessness. Individual adjustment to marked visual impairment or total blindness varies with age at onset, temperament, education, economic resources, and many other factors. The older patient, for example, may accept blindness quite stoically, whereas for the younger patient the vocational or social impact of blindness is often catastrophic. Blindness is accepted more easily by persons who are born blind and by persons of any age who lose their vision gradually rather than suddenly.

The responsibility of the physician clearly does not end with the diagnosis, prevention, and treatment of ocular disorders which might result in blindness. The physician caring for the patient who is suddenly faced with actual or imminent blindness is in a position to be of great assistance. When blindness is a possibility but is not inevitable (eg, during acute ocular inflammation), optimism and reassurance are warranted. However, it is unwise to offer false hopes or to delay "breaking the news" when blindness is inevitable. If it is certain that blindness will occur, it is important to extend to the distraught patient and to his family the warmth, understanding, encouragement, and assistance so desperately needed. The physician should be alert to the severe depressive reactions which may occur.

It is especially important to assist the patient in making the adjustment to blindness while some vision is still present. Early referral to rehabilitation agencies is essential for recently blinded adults and those with irreversible progressive visual loss. Training programs or reeducation for the many changes involved in daily living and employment are greatly simplified if the patient has the partial support which is provided by even limited vision.

It may be valuable to have the patient talk with a blind person who has made a satisfactory adjustment to blindness.

Many special services are available for blind persons. The aim of the rehabilitation program is to enable the patient to lead as nearly normal a life as possible. More than 25,000 blind persons in the USA are regularly employed. An additional larger number of blind home-makers are able to perform their household duties without assistance or are able to live independently of others.

The physician should work actively with the patient and his family and with other professional people concerned with rendering services to the blind.

Rehabilitation must be individualized for each patient. Guide dogs, for example, may be extremely valuable for certain persons but totally unsatisfactory for others. The methods of sightless reading and writing must be adapted to the capabilities, needs, and preferences of each patient. Mobility training is most important; 2 universities* have postgraduate programs in mobility training for the blind.

State Services

The physician should be familiar with the many special services available to the blind. Services vary from state to state but may be illustrated by the diversified programs for the blind conducted by the State of California.†

A. Educational Services for the Blind:
1. California School for the Blind - A residential school for general education from kindergarten through the secondary grades; also provides field service, guidance, and assistance to preschool children and students in advanced courses.
2. California State Library - A repository for magazines and books in raised type (Moon and Braille), talking books and machines for use with the books, games adapted for use by the blind, and writing appliances. These materials may be secured directly from the library or by mail (postage-free).
3. Bureau for Physically Exceptional Children - Coordinates the establishment and operation of special public school programs

---

*Boston University and Western Michigan State University.
†The services referred to are those provided by public-sponsored agencies for the blind and do not include the many religious organizations, private or voluntary health and welfare agencies, sheltered workshops, and community and recreational facilities.

for visually handicapped children in selected school districts and counties throughout the state. This program enables blind and partially seeing students to live at home and attend school with normal children.

B. Reader Services for Blind Students: Provides reader services for blind students in high schools, junior colleges, vocational training schools, colleges, and universities.

C. Rehabilitation Services for the Blind:
1. Field Rehabilitation Services - Counselor-teachers provide services to the blind within their homes or in hospitals and other institutions so that individuals may learn the skills necessary to meet the demands of daily living. Counseling in adjustment to blindness is given to the visually disabled person and his family.
2. Orientation Center for the Blind (State of California Department of Rehabilitation) - Provides intensive orientation and pre-vocational training, including training in technics of daily living and travel, physical conditioning, sensory training, instruction in Braille, typing, and business methods and training in hand and machine work, homemaking, and other vocationally useful skills. Limited residence facilities are available.
3. Vocational Rehabilitation Service - Provides, for the adult blind, vocational counseling to help work out suitable employment objectives, supervised vocational training, and job placement. The following services may also be provided if needed for employment and if the applicant is unable to pay for them: medical and surgical treatment, including hospitalization; prosthetic appliances and glasses; maintenance and transportation while undergoing treatment or training; and tools or equipment needed in training, job placement, or self-employment.
4. Business Enterprise Program - Assists blind persons to establish and operate vending stands, snack bars, and cafeteria or other businesses they may be qualified to operate.
5. Industrial Rehabilitation for the Blind - California Industries for the Blind consists of 3 manufacturing plants offering work adjustment, job training, work experience, and employment to blind workers. There are also 3 Opportunity Work Centers which provide work adjustment, job training, and sheltered employment, largely in assembly and packaging jobs. These programs are for those blind patients who are unable to secure private employment.

D. Social Welfare Programs for the Blind:
1. Aid to Needy Blind - Financial assistance paid by the county, state, and federal governments to the adult blind who, because of

loss or impairment of sight, are unable to provide themselves with the necessities of life.

2. Aid to Partially Self-Supporting Blind Residents - Financial assistance by the county and state to the adult blind who, because of loss or impairment of sight, are unable fully to provide themselves with the necessities of life but who are working on a plan for self-support.

3. Prevention of Blindness - A program designed to prevent blindness or restore vision by providing necessary medical or surgical treatment.

E. Provisions for Prevention of Blindness, Division of Preventive Medical Services:

1. Prevention of Blindness in Newborn Infants - Enforces legal requirement of (1) silver nitrate or penicillin prophylaxis for the eyes as a preventive measure against ophthalmia neonatorum; (2) prenatal serologic test of parents for syphilis; and (3) control of excessive use of oxygen in the care of premature infants as a preventive against retrolental fibroplasia.

2. Control of Communicable Diseases Which Are Apt to Cause Loss of Vision - Requires reporting, isolation, treatment, and control of ophthalmia neonatorum, trachoma, and syphilis.

3. Aid to Physically Handicapped Children - Provides for the necessary medical care of children suffering from eye conditions leading to loss of vision if the parents or legal guardians are unable to meet these costs in whole or in part.

4. Vision Conservation in Industry - Studies and makes recommendations for the elimination or control of eye hazards in industry.

F. Guide Dogs for the Blind: The State Board of Guide Dogs for the Blind was established for the purpose of ensuring that guide dogs are trained and that their owners also are trained to use the dogs as guides. Minimum requirements, licensing, and supervision of Guide Dog Schools are functions of the Board.

National Services

The following organizations will provide information and send literature and catalogues upon request:

(1) American Foundation for the Blind, 15 West 16th Street, New York, New York 10011. Provides information on almost all phases of problems of the blind; sells special watches, home appliances, etc for the blind.

(2) American Printing House for the Blind, 1839 Frankfort Avenue, Louisville, Kentucky 40206. Prints and sells Braille publications.

(3) Guide Dogs for the Blind, Inc., San Rafael, California 94901. Training of guide dogs and training of blind persons to use dogs as guides.

(4) Hadley Correspondence School, 620 Lincoln Avenue, Winnetka, Illinois 60093. Provides home study vocational and avocational courses from 6th grade through college.

(5) Howe Memorial Press, 549 East Fourth Street, South Boston, Mass. 02127. Manufactures script writing boards, books, alphabets, and games for the blind.

(6) Howe Press of Perkins Institute, Watertown, Mass. 02172. Distributes Perkins Brailler (portable Braille machine) and Braille paper of all types.

(7) Library of Congress. Extensive repository of magazines and books in raised type, talking books and machines for use with books, games adapted for use by the blind, and writing appliances. These materials are usually supplied through the state libraries.

(8) Office of Vocational Rehabilitation, US Dept of Health, Education, and Welfare, Washington, D.C. 20014. Conducts a nationwide program for the vocational rehabilitation of the blind; provides pamphlets and other information regarding rehabilitation services available to the blind.

(9) Readers Digest. Publishes Readers Digest in Braille and on records for the Talking Book; may be secured from the American Printing House for the Blind.

(10) Recording for the Blind, Inc., 121 East 58th Street, New York, New York 10022. Records textbooks and educational materials free of charge for blind persons for educational, vocational, or professional use.

(11) Seeing Eye, Inc., Trenton, New Jersey. Provides a program similar to that of Guide Dogs for the Blind (see above).

(12) Veterans Administration Hospital, Blind Section, Hines, Illinois 60141. Center for blind veterans.

(13) Xavier Society for the Blind, 154 East 23rd Street, New York, New York 10010. Provides free monthly publication ("Catholic Review") to any interested Braille reader. Also will lend or sell hand-transcribed Braille books on religious and other subjects.

•   •   •

Bibliography

American Foundation for the Blind. 1970 Catalog of Publications.

Carroll, Rev. T.J.: Blindness. Little, Brown, 1961.

Cholden, Louis: Psychiatric Aspects of Informing the Patient of Blindness. American Academy of Ophthalmology and Otolaryngology, Instruction Section, Course No. 221, 1953.

Cholden, Louis: Some Psychiatric Problems in the Rehabilitation of the Blind. Bulletin of the Menninger Clinic, Vol. 18, No. 3, May 1954.

Connor, G.B. (editor): Blindness 1964. American Association of Workers for the Blind, Inc., 1964.

Coordinating Council for State Programs for the Blind: State Services for the Blind in California, Revised. California State Printing Office, 1968.

If Blindness Occurs: The Seeing Eye, Inc.

US Department of Health, Education, and Welfare, Office of Vocational Rehabilitation: Opportunities for Blind Persons and the Visually Impaired Through Vocational Rehabilitation, Revised. US Government Printing Office, 1958.

VOCABULARY OF TERMS RELATING TO THE EYE*

Accommodation: The adjustment of the eye for seeing at different distances, accomplished by changing the shape of the crystalline lens through action of the ciliary muscle, thus focusing a clear image on the retina.

Agnosia: Inability of a person to recognize common objects despite an intact visual apparatus.

Albinism: A hereditary deficiency of pigment in the retinal pigmented epithelium, iris, and choroid.

Amaurosis fugax: Transient recurrent unilateral loss of vision.

Amblyopia: Uncorrectable blurred vision due to any cause.

Amblyopia ex anopsia: Uncorrectable blurred vision due to disuse of the eye with no organic defect.

Aniridia: Congenital absence of the iris.

Aniseikonia: A condition in which the image seen by one eye differs in size or shape from that seen by the other.

Anisometropia: Difference in refractive error of the eyes, eg, one eye hyperopic and the other myopic.

Anophthalmos: Absence of a true eyeball.

---

*Modified and reproduced, with permission, from Publication 172 of the National Society for the Prevention of Blindness, Inc.

Anterior chamber: Space filled with aqueous bounded anteriorly by the cornea and posteriorly by the iris.

Aphakia: Absence of the lens.

Aqueous: Clear, watery fluid that fills the anterior and posterior chambers.

Asthenopia: Eye fatigue caused by tiring.

Astigmatism: Refractive error which prevents the light rays from coming to a single focus on the retina because of different degrees of refraction in the various meridians of the cornea.

Binocular vision: The ability of a person's 2 eyes to focus on one object and to fuse the 2 images into one.

Blepharitis: Inflammation of the eyelids.

Blindness: In the USA, the usual definition of blindness is corrected visual acuity of 20/200 or less in the better eye, or a visual field of no more than 20° in the better eye.

Blind spot: "Blank" area in the visual field, corresponding to the light rays that come to focus on the optic nerve.

Buphthalmos: Large eyeball in infantile glaucoma.

Canaliculus: Small tear drainage tube in inner aspect of upper and lower lids leading from the puncta to the common canaliculus and then to the tear sac.

Canal of Schlemm: A circular modified venous structure in the anterior chamber angle.

Canthus: The angle at either end of the eyelid aperture; specified as outer and inner.

Cataract: A lens opacity.

Chalazion: Granulomatous inflammation of a meibomian gland.

Choroid: The vascular middle coat between the retina and sclera.

Ciliary body: Portion of the uveal tract between the iris and the choroid. It consists of ciliary processes and the ciliary muscle.

Coloboma: Congenital cleft due to the failure of some portion of the eye or ocular adnexa to complete growth.

Color blindness: Diminished ability to perceive differences in color.

Concave lens: Lens having the power to diverge rays of light; also known as diverging, reducing, negative, myopic, or minus lens, denoted by the sign (−).

Cones and rods: Two kinds of retinal receptor cells. Cones are concerned with visual acuity and color discrimination; rods, with peripheral vision and vision under decreased illumination.

Conjunctiva: Mucous membrane which lines the posterior aspect of the eyelids and the anterior sclera.

Convergence: The process of directing the visual axes of the eyes to a near point.

Convex lens: Lens having power to converge rays of light and to bring them to a focus; also known as converging, magnifying, hyperopic, or plus lens, denoted by the sign (+).

Cornea: Transparent portion of the outer coat of the eyeball forming the anterior wall of the aqueous chamber.

Corneal contact lenses: Thin plastic lenses which fit directly on the cornea under the eyelids.

Corneal graft (keratoplasty): Operation to restore vision by replacing a section of opaque cornea with transparent cornea.

Cover test: A method of determining the presence and degree of phoria or tropia by covering one eye with an opaque object, thus eliminating fusion.

Crystalline lens: A semi-transparent biconvex structure suspended in the eyeball between the aqueous and the vitreous. Its function is to bring rays of light to a focus on the retina.

Cycloplegic: A drug that temporarily puts the ciliary muscle at rest, paralyzes accommodation, and dilates the pupil.

Cylindrical lens: A segment of a cylinder, the refractive power of which varies in different meridians.

Dacryocystitis: Infection of the lacrimal sac.

Dark adaptation: The ability of the retina and pupil to adjust to decreased illumination.

Diopter: Unit of measurement of strength of refractive power of lenses.

Diplopia: Seeing one object as 2.

Ectropion: Turning out of the eyelid.

Emmetropia: Absence of refractive error.

Endophthalmitis: Extensive intraocular infection.

Enophthalmos: Abnormal retrodisplacement of the eyeball.

Entropion: A turning inward of the eyelid.

Enucleation: Complete surgical removal of the eyeball.

Epiphora: Tearing.

Esophoria: A tendency of the eyes to turn inward. .

Esotropia: A manifest inward deviation of the eyes.

"E" test: A system of testing visual acuity in illiterates, particularly pre-school children.

Exenteration: Removal of the entire contents of the orbit, including the eyeball and lids.

Exophoria: A tendency of the eyes to turn outward.

Exophthalmos: Abnormal protrusion of the eyeball.

Exotropia: A manifest outward deviation of one or both eyes.

Farsightedness: See Hyperopia.

Field of vision: The entire area which can be seen without shifting the gaze.

Floaters: Small dark particles in the vitreous.

Focus: The point to which rays are converged after passing through a lens; focal distance is the distance between the lens and the focal point.

Fornix: The junction of the palpebral and bulbar conjunctivas.

Fovea: Small depression in the macula adapted for most acute vision.

Fundus: The posterior portion of the eye visible through an ophthalmoscope.

Fusion: Coordinating the images received by the 2 eyes into one image.

Glaucoma: Abnormally increased intraocular pressure.

Gonioscopy: A technic of examining the anterior chamber angle, utilizing a corneal contact lens, magnifying device, and light source.

Hemianopsia: Blindness of one-half the field of vision of one or both eyes.

Heterophoria (phoria): A tendency of the eyes to deviate.

Heterotropia: See Strabismus.

Hippus: Spontaneous rhythmic movements of the iris; iridokinesia.

Hordeolum, external (sty): Infection of the glands of Moll or Zeis.

Hordeolum, internal: Meibomian gland infection.

Hyperopia, hypermetropia (farsightedness): A refractive error in which the focal point of light rays from a distant object is behind the retina.

Hyperphoria: A tendency of the eyes to deviate upward.

Hypertropia: A manifest upward deviation of the eyes.

Injection: Congestion of conjunctival blood vessels.

Iris: Colored, circular membrane, suspended behind the cornea and immdiately in front of the lens.

Ishihara color plates: A test for color vision based on the ability to trace patterns in a series of multicolored charts.

Jaeger test: A test for near vision using lines of various sizes of type.

Keratoconus: Cone-shaped deformity of the cornea.

Lacrimal sac: The dilated area at the junction of the nasolacrimal duct and the canaliculi.

Lens: A refractive medium having one or both surfaces curved. (See also Crystalline lens.)

Limbus: Junction of the cornea and sclera.

Macula lutea: The small avascular area of the retina surrounding the fovea.

Microphthalmos: Abnormal smallness of the eyeball.

Miotic: A drug causing pupillary constriction.

Mydriatic: A drug causing pupillary dilatation without affecting accommodation.

Myopia: A refractive error in which the focal point for light rays from a distant object is anterior to the retina.

Nearsightedness: See Myopia.

Nystagmus: An involuntary, rapid movement of the eyeball.

Oculist or ophthalmologist: Terms used interchangeably; a physician who is a specialist in diseases of the eye.

Ophthalmia neonatorum: Conjunctivitis in the newborn.

Ophthalmoscope: An instrument with a special illumination system for viewing the inner eye, particularly the retina and associated structures.

Optic atrophy: Optic nerve degeneration.

Optic disk: Ophthalmoscopically visible portion of the optic nerve.

Optician: One who makes or deals in eyeglasses or other optical instruments, and who fills prescriptions for glasses.

Optic nerve: The nerve which carries visual impulses from the retina to the brain.

Optometrist: A nonmedical person trained in the measurement of refraction of the eye.

Orthoptist: One who gives training to those with ocular muscle imbalances.

Oscillopsia: The subjective illusion of movement of objects that occurs with some types of nystagmus.

Palpebral: Pertaining to the eyelid.

Pannus: Infiltration of the cornea with blood vessels.

Partially seeing child: For educational purposes, a partially seeing child is one who has a corrected visual acuity of 20/70 or less in the better eye.

Perimeter: An instrument for measuring the field of vision.

Peripheral vision: Ability to perceive the presence, motion, or color of objects outside of the direct line of vision.

Photocoagulation: A method of causing artificial inflammation of the retina and choroid for treatment of certain types of retinal disorders, particularly retinal detachment.

Photophobia: Abnormal sensitivity to and discomfort from light.

Posterior chamber: Space filled with aqueous anterior to the lens and posterior to the iris.

Presbyopia ("old sight"): Physiologically blurred near vision, commonly evident soon after age 40.

Pseudoisochromatic charts: Charts with colored dots of various hues and shades forming numbers, letters, or patterns, used for testing color discrimination.

Pterygium: A triangular fold of tissue which extends from the conjunctiva over the cornea.

Ptosis: Drooping of the eyelid.

Pupil: The round hole in the center of the iris which corresponds to the lens aperture in a camera.

Refraction: (1) Deviation in the course of rays of light in passing from one transparent medium into another of different density. (2) Determination of refractive errors of the eye and correction by glasses.

Refractive error (ametropia): A defect in the eye that prevents light rays from being brought to a single focus on the retina.

Refractive media: The transparent parts of the eye having refractive power.

Retina: Innermost coat of the eye, formed of light-sensitive nerve elements.

Retinal detachment: A separation of the retina from the choroid.

Retinitis pigmentosa: A hereditary degeneration and atrophy of the retina.

Retinoscope: An instrument especially designed for the objective aspect of refraction.

Rods: See Cones and rods.

Sclera: The white part of the eye, a tough covering which, with the cornea, forms the external protective coat of the eye.

Scotoma: A blind or partially blind area in the visual field.

Slit lamp: A combination light and microscope for examination of the eye, principally the anterior segment.

Snellen chart: Used for testing central visual acuity. It consists of lines of letters or numbers, in graded sizes drawn to Snellen measurements.

Strabismus (tropia): A manifest deviation of the eyes.

Sty: External hordeolum.

Sympathetic ophthalmia: Inflammation in one eye following traumatic inflammation in the fellow eye.

Synechia: Adhesion of the iris to cornea (anterior synechia) or lens (posterior synechia).

Tonometer: An instrument for measuring intraocular pressure.

Trachoma: Serious infectious keratoconjunctivitis.

Uvea (uveal tract): The iris, ciliary body, and choroid.

Uveitis: Inflammation of one or all portions of the uveal tract.

Visual acuity: Detailed central vision, as in reading.

Visual purple: Photosensitive pigment in retinal cones.

Vitreous: Transparent, colorless mass of soft, gelatinous material filling the eyeball behind the lens.

Zonule: The numerous fine tissue strands which stretch from the ciliary processes to the lens equator (360°) and hold the lens in place.

Zonulolysis: Lysis of the zonule, as with chymotrypsin, to facilitate removal of the lens in cataract surgery.

SELECTED REFERENCE BOOKS

Abrahamson, I. A.: Color Atlas of Anterior Segment Eye Diseases. Blakiston, 1964.

Adriani, J., & others: Symposium on Ocular Pharmacology and Therapeutics. Transactions of the New Orleans Academy of Ophthalmology. Mosby, 1970.

Allen, J. H.: May's Manual of Diseases of the Eye, 24th ed. Williams & Wilkins, 1968.

Apt, L. (editor): Diagnostic Procedures in Pediatric Ophthalmology. Little, Brown, 1964.

Armaly, M. F., & others: Symposium on Glaucoma. Transactions of the New Orleans Academy of Ophthalmology. Mosby, 1967.

Arruga, H. M.: Ocular Surgery, 3rd ed. Blakiston-McGraw, 1963. Translated from the Spanish by Hogan and Chapparo.

Ballantyne, H. J., & I. C. Michaelson: The Fundus of the Eye. Williams & Wilkins, 1963.

Beard, C., & M. H. Quickert: Anatomy of the Orbit: A Dissection Manual. Aesculapius, 1969.

Becker, B., & R. C. Drews: Current Concepts in Ophthalmology. Mosby, 1967.

Berens, C., & J. H. King, Jr.: An Atlas of Ophthalmic Surgery. Lippincott, 1961.

Berens, C., & J. Zuckerman: Diagnostic Examination of the Eye, 2nd ed. Lippincott, 1964.

Blodi, F. C., & L. Allen: Stereoscopic Manual of the Ocular Fundus in Local and Systemic Disease. Mosby, 1964.

Burian, H. M., & others: Symposium on Strabismus. Mosby, 1971.

Caird, F. I., Piri, A., & T. G. Ramsell: Diabetes and the Eye. Blackwell, 1969.

Callahan, A.: Surgery of the Eye: Diseases. Thomas, 1956.

Callahan, A.: Surgery of the Eye: Injuries. Thomas, 1950.

Cogan, D. G.: Neurology of the Visual System. Thomas, 1965.

Duke-Elder, S. (editor): The Eye. Vol. 2 of Clinical Surgery (Rob & Smith). Butterworth, 1964.

Duke-Elder, S.: Parsons' Diseases of the Eye, 14th ed. Little, Brown, 1965.

Duke-Elder, S.: System of Ophthalmology. Mosby. Vol. I, The Eye in Evolution, 1958. Vol. II, The Anatomy of the Visual System, 1961. Vol. III, Normal and Abnormal Development, 1963. Vol. IV, The Physiology of the Eye and of Vision, 1968. Vol. V, Ophthalmic Optics and Refraction, 1970. Vol. VII, The Foundations of Ophthalmology: Heredity, Pathology, Diagnosis and Therapeutics, 1962. Vol. VIII, Diseases of the

Outer Eye—Conjunctiva, Cornea and Sclera, 1965. Vol. IX, Diseases of the Uveal Tract, 1966. Vol. X, Diseases of the Retina, 1967. Vol. XI, Diseases of the Lens and Vitreous—Glaucoma and Hypotony, 1969. Vol. XII, Neuro-ophthalmology and Motility, 1971.

Duke-Elder, S.: Textbook of Ophthalmology, 7 Vols. Mosby, 1938-1954.

Ellis, P.P., & D.L. Smith: Handbook of Ocular Therapeutics and Pharmacology, 3rd ed. Mosby, 1969.

Fasanella, R.M. (editor): The Management of Complications in Eye Surgery, 2nd ed. Saunders, 1964.

Fedukowicz, H.B.: External Infections of the Eye, Bacterial, Viral and Mycotic. Appleton-Century-Crofts, 1963.

Fonda, G.: Management of the Patient with Subnormal Vision, 2nd ed. Mosby, 1970.

Fox, S.A.: Ophthalmic Plastic Surgery, 3rd ed. Grune & Stratton, 1963.

Ganong, W.F.: Review of Medical Physiology, 5th ed. Lange, 1971.

Girard, L.J.: Corneal and Scleral Contact Lenses. Mosby, 1967.

Harrington, D.O.: The Visual Fields. A Textbook and Atlas of Clinical Perimetry, 3rd ed. Mosby, 1971.

Havener, W.H.: Ocular Pharmacology, 2nd ed. Mosby, 1970.

Hogan, M.J., & L.E. Zimmermann: Ophthalmic Pathology: An Atlas and Textbook, 2nd ed. Saunders, 1962.

Hughes, W.F.: Year Book of Ophthalmology, 1970. Year Book, 1970.

Jawetz, E., Melnick, J.L., & E.A. Adelberg: Review of Medical Microbiology, 9th ed. Lange, 1970.

Kaufman, H.E., & B. Rycroft (editors): Viral Diseases. Corneo-Plastic Surgery. Little, Brown, 1964.

Keeney, A.H.: Ocular Examination: Basis and Technique. Mosby, 1970.

Kempe, C.H., & others: Current Pediatric Diagnosis & Treatment. Lange, 1970.

Kestenbaum, A.: Methods of Neuro-ophthalmic Examination, 2nd ed. Grune & Stratton, 1960.

Kimura, S.J., & E.K. Goodner (editors): Ocular Pharmacology and Therapeutics and Problems of Medical Management. Davis, 1963.

King, J.H., & J.A.C. Wadsworth: An Atlas of Ophthalmic Surgery, 2nd ed. Lippincott, 1970.

Kolker, A.E., & J. Hetherington: Becker-Schaffer's Diagnosis and Therapy of the Glaucomas, 3rd ed. Mosby, 1970.

Langham, M.E. (editor): The Cornea, Macromolecular Organization of a Connective Tissue. Johns Hopkins Press, 1969.

Leopold, I.H. (editor): Symposium on Ocular Therapy, Vol. 4. Mosby, 1969.

Linksz, A., & D. Guerry III (editors): Pleoptics. Light Coagulation. Little, Brown, 1961.

Lyle, T.K. (editor): May and Worth's Manual of Diseases of the Eye, 13th ed. Davis, 1968.

Mann, I.: Culture, Race, Climate, and Eye Disease. Thomas, 1966.

Moses, R.A.: Adler's Physiology of the Eye. Clinical Application, 5th ed. Mosby, 1970.

Newell, F.W.: Ophthalmology: Principles and Concepts, 2nd ed. Mosby, 1969.

Paton, R.T., & H.M. Katzin: Atlas of Eye Surgery, 2nd ed. Blakiston-McGraw, 1962.

Philps, S., & J. Foster: Ophthalmic Operations, 2nd ed. Williams & Wilkins, 1961.

Reed, H.: The Essentials of Perimetry. Oxford, 1960.

Salzmann, M.: Anatomy and Histology of the Human Eyeball in the Normal State. Chicago Medical, 1912.

Scheie, H.G., & D.M. Albert: Adler's Textbook of Ophthalmology, 8th ed. Saunders, 1969.

Shaffer, R.N., & D.I. Weiss: Congenital and Pediatric Glaucomas. Mosby, 1970.

Somerset, E.J.: Ophthalmology in the Tropics. Williams & Wilkins, 1963.

Sorsby, A. (editor): Modern Trends in Ophthalmology, Vol. 4. Appleton-Century-Crofts, 1967.

Troutman, R.C., Converse, J.M., & B. Smith: Plastic and Reconstructive Surgery of the Eye and Adnexa. Butterworth, 1962.

Walsh, F.B., & W.F. Hoyt: Clinical Neuro-ophthalmology, 3rd ed. Williams & Wilkins, 1969.

Wilmer, W.H.: Atlas Fundus Oculi. Macmillan, 1935.

Wolff, E.: The Anatomy of the Eye and Orbit, 5th ed. Blakiston-McGraw, 1961.

Index